Dr Craig Hassed is a general pract
Monash University Department o
teaching, research and clinical int
stress management, mind–body m
otion, holistic healthcare, compl
ethics. He is regularly invited to speak around Australia
on these topics. He is published widely in peer-reviewed journals, and
has written three previous books.

Also by Craig Hassed

*New Frontiers in Medicine: the body as the
shadow of the soul* (Volumes One and Two)
Know Thyself

the essence of health

The Seven Pillars of Wellbeing

DR CRAIG HASSED

EBURY
PRESS

The information in this book is not intended as a substitute for consulting with your physician or other health care provider. While much care has been taken to provide the most recent research and accurate information, the author, copyright holder and publisher do not accept responsibility for any problems arising out of the contents of this book.

An Ebury Press book
Published by Random House Australia Pty Ltd
Level 3, 100 Pacific Highway, North Sydney, NSW 2060
www.randomhouse.com.au

First published by Ebury Press in 2008

Addresses for companies within the Random House Group can be found at www.randomhouse.com.au/offices

National Library of Australia
Cataloguing-in-Publication Entry

Hassed, Craig.
The essence of health.

ISBN 978 1 74166 704 2 (pbk.)

Holistic medicine.
Health.
Lifestyles.

613

Cover illustration and design by Sarah Maxey Design
Internal design by Midland Typesetters, Australia
Typeset in 11.5/15pt Garamond Classico by Midland Typesetters, Australia
Printed and bound by Griffin Press, South Australia

Random House Australia uses papers that are natural, renewable and recyclable products and made from wood grown in sustainable forests. The logging and manufacturing processes are expected to conform to the environmental regulations of the country of origin.

On a regular basis I remember an ancient invocation which helps to give my work purpose and direction. It was also sounded when Nelson Mandela was inaugurated as the president of South Africa, and goes as follows:

May all be happy;
May all be without disease;
May all creatures have wellbeing;
And none be in misery of any sort.
Peace, peace, peace.

Contents

Acknowledgements

I would like to thank the following for their valued contributions towards this book: my friends and colleagues at the Monash University Medical Faculty, and particularly the Department of General Practice, for the space and support for innovation within the medical curriculum and for the encouragement and opportunity to make this material available to a wider audience; the medical students and tutors whose enthusiastic and committed participation in the Monash Health Enhancement Program is not only a source of joy but also encouragement for a better future for healthcare; 'Dooky', a Monash medical student, for the part he played in the birth of the ESSENCE mnemonic; and Margie Seale, Meredith Curnow and Random House Australia for their sincere interest and support in publishing this work.

I would also like to thank and acknowledge the following people for permission to adapt content for sections of this book: George Jelineck (multiple sclerosis), Rob Moodie (promoting health), Rick Kausman (healthy eating), Bernie Crimmins (exercise), David Morawetz (sleep), and Michelle Allen and Nicola Graham (nutrition). Thank you, as ever, to my wife, Deirdre, without whose support my work would be difficult, if not impossible. Lastly, I would like to thank the teachers, too many to name, who have inspired and instructed me over the years, either directly or by the example they set.

Introduction

The Essence of Health is a comprehensive and holistic approach to health-care. It is the foundation of maintaining wellness, preventing illness and treating any condition, particularly the chronic illnesses which modern healthcare finds so difficult to deal with. Essence stands for:

- E   Education
- S   Stress Management
- S   Spirituality
- E   Exercise
- N   Nutrition
- C   Connectedness
- E   Environment

The Essence program has been used in the core Monash University medical curriculum since 2002.

Why the Essence of health?

The Essence of Health fills important gaps which currently exist in healthcare. It is a useful and informative resource for people dealing with serious illnesses, people who want to prevent illness and increase their wellbeing, and healthcare students and practitioners. It provides a practical and systematic approach that empowers us to take a more active role in our own healthcare and that fosters a collaborative partnership with our health practitioners. The greatest advances in future healthcare will not be scientific ones as in past centuries, but for us to learn to change our own attitudes and healthcare practices.

It may be that the greatest challenge we face is to understand ourselves and to govern our own health behaviours so that most of modern medicine is made redundant. Perhaps the highest aim of a healthcare system is to educate and empower the community to such an extent that they are rarely in need of medical help. In other words, the highest aim of healthcare is to prevent illness. The next highest aim is to intervene in the simplest and safest way at the earliest stages of illness, addressing its causes not just its symptoms. The last aim – and there will always be a need for this – is to provide treatment for serious, advanced illnesses and in the case of accidents and emergencies. Even then, the best option will always be the simplest and safest.

The iceberg

Examining modern healthcare may be likened to looking at an iceberg, not because hospitals are sometimes described as being cold and clinical, but because most of it is hidden. The 10% that we see above the surface is the healthcare system which we know and experience on a daily basis. It largely consists of the GP consultations, referrals to specialists, tests, drug prescriptions, hospitals and medical procedures which are done to us. The 90% which we don't see is made up of what we can *do for ourselves*. This 90% comprises what we eat, how active we are, our state of mind, how we relate to the world and those around us, the environment we live in. This 90% is what keeps the 10% afloat and it is all too easy to ignore.

This is not to say that the 10% is not useful or important. Science has made some wonderful technological advances over recent centuries, particularly in the field of emergency care. This is what Western medicine does best, but it would be easy to believe that this is all healthcare is. The 'essence' of something is the essential, indispensable part of it – and that is what we are seeking in *The Essence of Health*: the essential, indispensable elements of health and wellbeing. For example, nutritious food is essential to good health, but cholesterol-lowering drugs aren't. Physical activity is essential to health, but liposuction isn't. Good mental health, social support and finding meaning in life are essential to health, but antidepressants aren't. These drugs and procedures may have a place but their place is secondary, not primary.

The healthcare stories which seem to attract the most frenzied media attention tend to be the high-cost, technologically sophisticated discoveries. A supposed medical breakthrough in the management of lung cancer is a lot more exciting than a story about the benefits of quitting cigarettes. Of course, what escapes the headlines is that the reality of medical breakthroughs aimed at managing chronic diseases rarely measure up to the media hype.

The Australian state of Victoria is a world leader in the field of health promotion, principally through the wonderful work of VicHealth and the Victorian Health Promotion Foundation. Anti-smoking campaigns remain a major priority for them and have led to enormous savings in terms of human suffering, lives and money. The prevalence of smoking in Victoria fell from 34% in 1983 to 17% by 2006. Interestingly, VicHealth is funded by tobacco taxes and has bipartisan political support. It has also been the main driver in providing education and guidance on anti-smoking legislation over that time. Even as a world leader, Victoria still only spends just over 1% of its health budget on health promotion and the rest largely on treating diseases which should have been preventable in the first place. Even a small shift in resources towards promoting health would save huge amounts of suffering, energy, time and money. For each year of life saved, smoking prevention programs cost approximately one five-hundredth of what it costs to treat lung cancer.[1]

Projections about global health in the year 2030 provide sobering reading.[2] By 2030, depression is expected to rank easily as the greatest non-fatal burden of disease in affluent countries. It is expected to be followed by heart disease, dementia, alcohol abuse, diabetes, stroke, hearing loss and lung cancer, in that order. These are chronic diseases which are largely caused by lifestyle factors. They are, therefore, largely preventable with simple lifestyle measures.

The foundations

Our body can be likened to a house. Over time cracks may appear in the walls, doors may jam up and gaps may appear between the floorboards. It would be all too easy to believe that a cosmetic repair has fixed the problem, such as a bit of putty and paint, sanding the door, or putting a rug on the floor. 'Out of sight, out of mind,' as the saying goes. The problem, however, keeps recurring ever worse than before because we have not given attention to the foundations – unseen, underneath – that support the house. In terms of heart disease, the cracks in the wall are things like high blood pressure, high cholesterol and diabetes. They are signs that a disease process is underway and it needs to be rectified before major 'structural damage' – a heart attack – occurs. If we wait until that stage the solution will be a lot harder and more expensive.

Much of the time healthcare resources are spent on the cosmetic solutions but the deeper problem remains. The problem, of course, lies in the foundations. If they are not strong and well aligned then everything above is in an unstable state. The foundations of good health are laid out in *The Essence of Health*. We will call them the seven pillars of health.

Becoming educated about health

As any of us who have tried to change to a healthier lifestyle will note, it is not so easy. It requires education, quality information, skills in behaviour change, a supportive environment and, importantly, supportive healthcare practitioners.

The word 'doctor' literally means 'teacher' but the doctor's educative role in healthcare is often pushed to the side by the pressures of time or faith in pharmaceuticals. 'Education' is a word derived from a word meaning 'to draw out'. True education draws out the strengths, insights, common sense and capacities that we have within us. Drawing them out takes a little time, effort and art, and the healthcare system does not always make it easy for a doctor to play this role. The volume of work confronting doctors and the fact that the system tends to financially penalise them the longer they spend with the patient make it difficult to practise medicine with a holistic perspective. This is despite research suggesting that longer consultations often lead to better outcomes, save money and allow room for broader health issues to be dealt with.[3]

Many people are becoming increasingly dissatisfied with conventional healthcare and are actively looking for a more holistic model.[4] Prime reasons why increasing numbers of people go to complementary medicine practitioners are that they spend extra time with their clients and are generally perceived to take a more holistic approach. Why is it that many people feel they have to look outside conventional healthcare to get support and information that is central to their health? Going outside the conventional healthcare system and using complementary therapies can be valuable, and complementary medicine practitioners are often well informed, balanced in their approach and skilled in lifestyle management. But going outside conventional healthcare can also be a concern. Many patients don't speak to their doctors about what other therapies they are employing. Some people, particularly vulnerable, sick ones, access expensive 'cures' for their conditions that are of questionable value. A small number of people reject conventional healthcare entirely even when their life may depend upon it. At the end of the day, what is needed is an integrated and holistic approach, not two competing systems of medicine.

The most important thing that a doctor can teach us as patients is how to care for ourselves so that we are as independent in our health-care as possible. If we become ill, we need to be active participants in our own healthcare, combining self-help strategies with the most effective and safe medical and complementary therapies available.

Unfortunately, trainee health practitioners are rarely taught at university to look after their own mental, social and physical health. This may go some way to explaining why these issues tend to be ignored in the GP's or specialist's clinic.

There are promising signs that attitudes to healthcare are changing. Indeed, the healthcare system is quite a sick patient at the moment and many patients cannot wait too much longer for it to recover. Our experience of applying the Essence model with our medical students has shown us that they can learn valuable information and skills they will need in their practice one day while at the same time deriving significant personal benefits.[5]

A more holistic model of health

Hippocrates said, 'The human being can only be understood as a whole.' In many quarters around the world the importance of adopting wellness, holistic and lifestyle approaches to the prevention and management of chronic diseases is being increasingly recognised. The term 'Integrative Medicine' refers to a philosophy and method of medical practice which is by nature holistic. It blends lifestyle changes with the judicious use of evidence-baesd conventional and complementary therapies. Although a holistic approach can solely be delivered by practitioners, it heavily encourages the involvement of the patient in their own healthcare. As such, Integrative Medicine extends conventional medical practice and is more appropriately seen as 'best practice' rather than 'alternative practice'. Importantly, it is not a rejection of conventional healthcare, nor is it in competition with it.

'The doctor of the future will give no medicine, but will interest his patients in the care of the human frame, in diet, and in the cause and prevention of disease.' This quote is attributed to Thomas Edison. In many ways, this concept is not new, but what is new is the gathering momentum for implementing it. *This* momentum for change is being driven by changing community attitudes. Many people desire safe, non-invasive but effective treatment, and they want to be empowered and involved in their own healthcare. Increasing numbers of people have become dissatisfied with the management of their chronic health conditions, because they haven't been informed of effective self-care and lifestyle changes they can make. Evidence is gathering that involving patients in managing their health delivers far better outcomes than conventional medicine alone. This will be important in the future as the costs of conventional healthcare spiral and become unsustainable.

Despite its potential, the lifestyle management of chronic conditions is often less effective than it could be for a number of reasons. The most important is that lifestyle advice is often delivered without supportive or enabling strategies like behaviour change skills, stress management, goal setting, and follow-up. *The Essence of Health* therefore provides information together with supportive strategies.

The drug culture

There is much talk about the drug culture which revolves around illicit drugs, but there is a bigger and far more lucrative drug culture which revolves around prescribed medications. Undeniably there is a place for some prescribed medications but our faith that drugs are able to solve just about any health concern is misplaced.

'You need to keep an open mind, but not so open that your brain falls out.' A professor of obstetrics and gynaecology said this in relation to considering the use of complementary medicine. But keeping an open mind while not letting our brains fall out is just as important when we are considering using conventional medical treatments. Research on pharmaceuticals, for example, is very selectively published in order to create an inflated perception of the benefits and downplay potential harms. Drug-company-sponsored research in the US is nearly three times more likely to report positive findings and 20 times less likely to report negative findings – such as that the drug didn't work or had major side effects – than independent research.[6] Conflict of interest – when a researcher is funded by a pharmaceutical company while being paid by them to promote their drugs – is very common. Many health stories in the media are based on press releases from drug companies and the experts giving their opinions in such stories commonly have such conflicts of interest.

To illustrate further, in the US, the Food and Drug Administration (FDA) monitors all drug trials, whether the trials' results are published and therefore known to the public, or not. A recent review[7] found that 31% of trials on the 12 most widely prescribed antidepressants were not published – and nearly all of these were the trials showing that a drug was not effective. Of the studies that were published, in some cases researchers had clearly put a positive spin on the data to make a drug seem more effective than it was. From the published studies it appeared that 94% of drug trials were positive but an FDA analysis of the data showed that only 51% were positive – that is, half of the trials of antidepressants really suggested that they were not effective. They work largely through the placebo effect.

Obviously market forces have a significant effect on the independence and credibility of research. Potentially this makes a mockery of the 'evidence-based medicine' doctors use to make informed decisions for the benefit of their patients. A balanced approach would not reject the use of pharmaceuticals out of hand but we would be well advised to take greater note of independent rather than industry funded research. It is undeniable that drugs have a place in preventing and treating some illnesses but there is far too much promotion and use of drugs with questionable evidence, marginal benefits, exorbitant costs and major side effects.

Expert opinion

It is a hard thing for doctors and patients alike to sort out what holds true and what does not in our knowledge of health. We tend to believe what we have been told, believe what most of our peers believe and ignore what most of our peers ignore. It is human nature. Many widely held attitudes and beliefs among doctors have little foundation, while other commonsense and evidence-based ideas are either ignored or even vigorously resisted. A study in a leading journal called *Medical Education* found that in the medical lectures delivered in hospitals by senior medical staff, called 'grand rounds', most of the medical opinions given, though expressed with great confidence, were contrary to scientific evidence.[8] Much of the time fixed or long-held opinion masquerades as fact. Attitudes shift slowly and it often takes a new generation to move beyond the limitations of previous generations.

It may seem like a strange thing to do at the start of a book: to potentially undermine the whole basis of expert opinion. That is not the intention. All of us – doctors, experts, patients and the general public – are trying to sift what is true from what isn't so that we can discover what we need to do to advance the wellbeing of ourselves and others. Evidence and expert opinion are certainly important in helping us to sift information, but so are intuition, common sense and experience. In proceeding through the Essence program, try to keep all these actively engaged.

How to use this book

Part 1 of this book introduces and explains the seven core concepts – or the seven pillars – of the Essence program: education, stress management, spirituality, exercise, nutrition, connectedness and environment. The chapters in this part discuss why each of the seven pillars is so important, and the science and evidence behind them; it also explores general principles for introducing them into your daily life.

In Part 2, we see how to transform the principles in Part 1 into real change in our lifestyle and wellbeing. This part focuses on how to change our daily habits and behaviours, to introduce Essence into our life. We learn about how to change our behaviour, along with goal setting and motivation. And there is detailed guidance on how to apply the Essence program to a range of situations, from personal use to running courses for groups, to educating healthcare practitioners.

For information concerning specific illnesses and health issues, turn to Part 3, which shows how the Essence principles can be applied to the prevention and management of individual chronic diseases, from cardiovascular disease and cancer through to arthritis and dementia. They are, if you like, the Essence of managing heart disease, or the Essence of managing cancer, and so on.

In the appendices at the end there is a helpful questionnaire to assess stress levels and healthy lifestyle, useful health websites and an outline for an eight-week Essence course, of interest for anyone who wishes to run a course for a group, or use it in health education or schools.

This book is based on valid scientific evidence and is referenced throughout, making it a valuable resource for those who wish to read further. There is a vast amount of information we can read but it is worth keeping in mind that underlying all this often complex information there are simple principles. We should aim to understand the principles before we get too concerned about the details.

It is important to also remember that we should not make changes to our lifestyle at the expense of having necessary medical care and monitoring. It is easy to think that if we are applying self-help strategies we won't need the help of doctors or other healthcare practitioners. This is a potentially dangerous assumption.

It may be difficult to change many aspects of our lifestyle at the same time. If we are able to make wholesale changes then that is well and good, but for many of us it might make more sense to change one aspect at a time, like improving our nutrition and then moving on to exercise, and so on. We can set one goal at a time and get that firmly established before moving on to the next. For example, we might wish to reduce our risk of heart disease and choose exercise as the first goal. After a few weeks, when we have established a graded exercise program, we might choose to start working on stress management. By this time it is likely we will have gathered momentum and can make changes to other aspects of our lives.

Part 1
The Seven Pillars of Wellbeing

The first part of this book looks in detail at each of the seven pillars of the Essence model. The following chapters lay out why each element is important and some of the science and evidence behind each one, and also explore some general principles for introducing them into your daily existence. For information concerning specific illnesses and health issues, Part 3 shows how the Essence model can be applied to the prevention and management of individual chronic diseases, from cardiovascular disease and cancer through to arthritis and dementia.

1

Education

In many ways, this whole book, and the Essence program, is all about education. It underpins how the other six pillars of wellbeing can be introduced practically into our lives by:

- Providing information;
- Giving instruction in applying skills;
- Teaching us how to think and find answers to questions;
- Drawing out wisdom.

In terms of personal health, education is crucial as far as learning about illnesses and understanding prevention and treatments. If we are more educated about our health, the cause of illness and the reasons for treatment and prognosis, then we're far more likely to take preventive steps, seek treatment when necessary, use those treatments effectively and have more positive results.

Socrates, the great Greek philosopher, continually encouraged his fellow Greeks to 'Know Thyself', so another really important aspect of education is understanding ourselves, what motivates us, and the physical and psychological barriers within us which impede our progress. Knowing these things gives us a great advantage; without this kind of awareness we have little chance of being able to take steps to change our patterns of behaviour and improve our lives. It would be like trying to fix a car without understanding how it is put together. As psychologist Daniel Goleman revealed in his groundbreaking theory, self-awareness is also one of the five domains of emotional intelligence but it influences a lot more than just our emotions.

Education has a fundamental role in improving our health for a number of other reasons. Independent of other factors, simply having an adequate level of education is associated with better health from the outset. People who are more educated tend to come from higher socio-economic backgrounds and are more likely to have healthier lifestyles and better health outcomes. Poor health behaviours are consistently linked to lower educational status, and this is one of the great challenges in providing better health outcomes for the disadvantaged in society.

Because those with more education are more likely to have a higher socio-economic background, they are also more likely to have better access to healthcare services. Across the board, education provides people with a greater ability to deal with problems, make decisions and assimilate health-related information. Importantly, education is also associated with a greater level of autonomy, self-empowerment and self-determination, meaning that people who have had an adequate level of education are more likely to make informed choices and feel more in control of their direction in life. Put another way, an inadequate education is associated with social disadvantage, a lack of choice, a sense of disempowerment and greater difficulty in being able to understand information.

Of course, this doesn't mean that people need a university education in order to be healthy, but it does mean that if people feel they have the resources to work through issues in a systematic and logical way, if they are able to appreciate basic concepts and if they are able to take on information and appreciate its relevance, then they will be far better able to navigate their way through life and the health challenges that come their way. The support of a health practitioner who is interested and able to take the time to assist in this process also cannot be overestimated.

The concept of education is dealt with in a number of ways throughout this book. Attention is given to understanding our behavioural patterns, habits and motivations, how to set achievable goals, and basic health information about various illnesses. Of course, in the great spirit of education, there is always more that we can learn, so if you finish reading this book and feel more confident to make your own decisions, to access further information and to put questions you have to your doctor, then you will be well on the way to greater self-confidence and a healthier life overall.

2
Stress management

In the Essence model, 'stress management' covers the broad area of mental health, as well as the important mind–body link. It includes 'stress', in the conventional sense of the word; our emotional state and level of happiness; whether we experience anxiety, depression or other mental health problems; the impact of our mental and emotional state on physical wellbeing; and how at peace we feel with ourselves and the world.

As this chapter demonstrates, fostering good mental health is a vital part of the prevention and management of any health condition. If our mental health is suffering, not only does it have direct effects on the development of illness, but it also accelerates ageing and has an impact upon our ability to cope with the symptoms of an illness if we do fall ill. As this is such an important issue, this is a significant chapter in this book and is split into two parts. The first part lays bare essential background details and research about stress and how it impacts on our lives; the second part introduces important stress reduction techniques that can be woven into daily life.

Background about stress

WHAT IS STRESS?

'Stress' is a much-used, abused and, many would say, overused word in the world today, and can mean different things to different people. When a person says they are 'stressed' it could mean any number of things. One person could mean that they feel under pressure, anxious, fearful or irritable. Another might mean that they are suffering physical symptoms like palpitations, tremulousness or lethargy. Another might mean that they find themselves burnt out or that their performance is dropping. For some it means being unable to cope or motivate themselves; for others, stress will be used synonymously with depression. And although many of the physical consequences of stress will be the same as for say, depression, quite different approaches may need to be taken in order to manage them.

'Stress' is sometimes described as a 'perceived inability to cope'. If we are confronted by certain challenges but don't believe we have the ability to deal with them, we will experience stress. If this is going on continuously then it might be said that we have 'chronic' stress. Stress is also sometimes described as when 'demands exceed means', like our resources being stretched beyond their capacity. Stress can also be used interchangeably with anxiety. Regardless of all these uses, however, research has consistently proven that stress has tangible impacts upon both mind and body.

In conventional usage, the word 'stressor' refers to the event, person or situation which has stimulated the stress response with all its physical and psychological effects. If, for example, we are in a hurry and we get caught at a traffic light then it could be referred to as a stressor. If someone loses their job then that might be considered as a more major stressor (provided they were not relieved to have lost it). But as will be discussed later, events like these are not inherently stressful in themselves; it is how we see or experience the event which determines whether it is a stressor or not. To think that our stress is entirely dependent on the events around us is very disempowering and makes it seem we are helpless in a world full of unpredictable threats. To realise that our stress responses are actually in our own hands means we can begin to take responsibility and control over our own lives. This requires awareness, practice, discernment and courage, but the benefits for our overall health are worth it.

Our mental and emotional states can produce a wide variety of symptoms but it is also worth bearing in mind that before we attribute particular symptoms to stress it's important to first make sure that the symptoms are not due to a medical condition. For example, an overactive thyroid can masquerade as anxiety, anaemia can masquerade as lethargy and, although uncommon, brain tumours can masquerade as headaches. If you are in any doubt about where your symptoms are coming from then it's important to have a health check and any relevant tests to help exclude other things.

MENTAL HEALTH TODAY

By any indicators, mental health in most developed countries has not been heading in a positive direction over recent decades. In 1996 the World Health Organisation (WHO) issued figures suggesting that depression was expected to be a leading burden of disease and that prophecy has progressively moved closer to being fulfilled.[1] According to Australian research, over 20% of adults are expected to have a major depressive episode at some time in their lives and among one in six elderly people have persistent symptoms.[2] In European societies, a syndrome related to mental ill health, which includes depression, suicide, abuse, risk-taking and violent behaviour, as well as 'vascular morbidity and mortality', has been observed, despite recent clinical and research advances in health sciences in general.'[3] To give an indication of how significant these increases have been, one study estimated that there was a 45% increase in daily stress over the last 30 years.[4] The rise in mental illness seems paradoxical considering that developed countries are meant to be enjoying unprecedented levels of physical health, relative affluence, technological advancement and social freedoms. Also paradoxical is that suicide rates generally go down during times of adversity such as during a major war[5]; so although we don't generally look forward to adversity, it certainly can teach us something about ourselves if we pay attention to the lesson it is trying to teach us.

This decline in mental health is due to many factors, which could include an increased awareness of stress – we might be seeing more of it because we're looking for it more. The increase can also be explained by the more stressful, insecure and busy lives we tend to lead these days. Factors like the rapid increase in the amount of social change, job insecurity, the speed of life, competitiveness, substance abuse and many other factors probably all contribute. In addition, as a people living in modern times, we now want more than ever before; but to want more, no matter how much we may already have, will always leave us in want.

Measuring which illnesses have the greatest impact upon the community is not an easy thing to do. Statisticians use the so-called 'DALY' (Disability-Adjusted Life Year) to try and measure the impact or 'burden of disease' caused by various illnesses on the community's health. The DALY measures both the level of impact which a condition has on a person's life as well as the duration or number of years that that condition impacts upon the person's life. For example, Ischaemic Heart Disease (IHD), contributes a significant number of DALYs as it causes a significant impact and is very common, but it tends to affect people in later life. Dementia also has a very major impact upon a person's life and is relatively common but also generally affects people very late in life. Mental health problems in general, however, especially depression, have a very major impact on wellbeing, are increasingly common, but affect people of all ages, and therefore contribute a significant numbers of DALYs.

Currently depression 'causes the largest amount of non-fatal burden, accounting for almost 12% of all total years lived with disability worldwide.'[6] Predictions estimate that, in Australia, mental illnesses, principally depression and anxiety, will soon be the major burden of disease[7] and this is independent of the secondary effects that mental health has on physical health. Depression, for example, is a major independent risk factor for heart disease and poor immunity and is also associated with other 'co-morbidities' such as unhealthy lifestyle and substance abuse.

Stress and depression often present as a mixed picture and evidence suggests that stress hormones may play a role in the development of various psychiatric disorders, including depression.[8] From a superficial and purely biochemical perspective, depression is due to low serotonin levels in the brain – but what lowers the serotonin production in the brain? Stress, among other things, has effects on our brain's production of serotonin.[9] Antidepressant medications largely aim to work by increasing the brain's production of serotonin – but too much serotonin can also be associated with anxiety and even mania. Drugs like amphetamines, for example, seek to give the brain a surge of serotonin and so make a person feel euphoric for a time, but psychosis is a well-known side effect of these substances and the person who takes them will also experience a post-drug low as the brain is depleted of serotonin for some days afterwards.

One aspect of the modern social landscape is the fact that we are seeing higher rates of depression occurring at younger ages. One marker of this is suicide, and suicide rates in the under-25 age group have gone up fourfold within the last 50 years. Thinking about suicide – this is called 'suicidal ideation' – is alarmingly common in adolescents. One study estimated that one in two young people were experiencing high levels of psychological stress[10] and also found that as many as one in four 15–24-year-olds presenting to GPs for any reason had recently experienced suicidal thoughts. Despite the fact that evidence shows the use of antidepressant medications in children and adolescents provides no benefit, they are still widely used in this age group. Depression is being diagnosed in younger age groups but serious concerns about the use of antidepressant medications in this age group have been raised in recent major reviews.[11][12]

A large part of the reliance on antidepressants, which is understandably encouraged by concerned families and practitioners, is market-driven. The pharmaceutical industry makes a lot of money out of these medications despite the evidence but thankfully, increasing attention is starting to be directed to the social causes of poor mental health and non-drug treatments, through education and community programs. These programs encourage the development of resilience and 'protective' factors, like feeling connected at home or school, having supportive relationships including with respected elders, having a spiritual or religious dimension to life[13] as well as various lifestyle factors like regular exercise. Young people are far less likely to run into problems with mental illness, drugs or violence, even in the presence of risk factors, with these kinds of protective factors.

HAPPINESS AND PLEASURE ARE NOT THE SAME THING

The causes of declining mental health in the general community no doubt depends upon a wide range of factors including physical inactivity, poor nutrition, substance abuse and social influences. Popular culture and pleasure-seeking behaviour may also be factors. It has been a widespread opinion that adolescents 'self-medicate' for depression with high-risk behaviours like substance use and promiscuity, but one population study tested whether substance use and promiscuity precede and predict depression or vice versa.[14] Interestingly, what they found was that sex and drug behaviours were more likely to cause depression, particularly among young girls, rather than the other way around. It is therefore not surprising that building up community, supportive relationships, positive role models and a sense of belonging all protect against risk-taking behaviour among adolescents.

It's natural that human beings pursue happiness, and there are countless ideas about what happiness is and how to attain it. The monk who meditates in the cave and learns to master his desires and impulses is pursuing happiness every bit as much as the extreme sportsman, or the stockbroker, or the drug-addicted adolescent. There are those of us, like the monk, who wish to transcend attachment to worldliness, pleasure and pain; there are those of us who pursue happiness by completely immersing ourselves in the pursuit of worldliness and pleasure and the retreat from pain; and there are those of us who seek it by trying to find moderation or a balance between these extremes. Each of us, according to our understanding, pursues happiness. But how do we know if we are on the 'right' track? A good way of measuring this is whether we grow in happiness over time.

Differing pathways in the brain correspond with these differing approaches to pleasure. Dopamine, a brain neurotransmitter closely linked with our brain's reward pathways, is associated with the ability to experience pleasure and motivation,[15] and these pathways ensure that we do the necessary things associated with survival, like eat, reproduce and protect the body from harm. Most people experience pleasure and pain in daily life without being overly moved by the one or repelled by the other, but when they are pursued in excess, our reward pathways trigger addictions. If the addiction can't be fed then we experience withdrawal – anxiety and pain. This withdrawal response has enormous ramifications in the community – many social ills, like smoking, drinking and gambling, revolve around feeding people's addictions and then taking advantage of them. It is a vicious cycle and this is probably why many traditions have thought of pleasure as leading to a false and fragile form of happiness. When pursued as an end in itself it seems to bring as much pain as it does pleasure and leaves the person with little self-determination. Pursuing it without restraint is a false form of freedom which eventually resembles living under a form of tyranny.

Even though unhealthy behaviours are more likely to cause depression, mood, neurochemistry and behaviour in general are all intertwined. As we can all understand, mood affects behaviour – for example, depression and anxiety increase susceptibility to peer influence to take up risk-taking behaviour – so building resilience and emotional intelligence may therefore have a number of benefits, including an ability to avoid unhealthy behaviours. Stopping smoking is associated with high levels of depression and depression is often associated with relapse.[16] This may help to explain why cognitive behavioural therapy reduces relapse rates for smokers.[17]

Part of the modern mental health problem may well be linked with the common assumption that pleasure and happiness are the same thing. They are not. Pleasure-seeking behaviour tends to require increasingly intense and more frequent stimulation to produce the same response. This seems to 'tire' the reward system over time, and what begins as a 'lunge into pleasure' soon becomes a 'retreat from pain', i.e. the discomfort and anxiety associated with withdrawal. This leads to problems such as an inability to experience pleasure (anhedonia), apathy and disturbed mood (dysphoria).

Another way our reward pathways can be affected is if we experience stress early in childhood or adolescence, which has implications for the way these reward pathways operate throughout life.[18] This in turn has implications later on for how easy or hard we find it to deal with impulsivity and emotional reactivity. Interestingly, just like the pleasure response, the relaxation response is associated with an increase in dopamine release in the brain's reward centres[19] but is also associated with reduced impulsivity, greater self-control and better mood. This may go some of the way toward explaining why practising things like meditation is associated with better emotional health, impulse regulation and healthy lifestyle change.

THE 'FIGHT OR FLIGHT' RESPONSE

The fact that our body has a stress response is a good indication that it fulfils an important function. Our nervous system has many different aspects to it, some of which are under more conscious control than others. Moving our limbs, for example, is obviously under our control. Regulating our heart rate or digestion, on the other hand, is not easily controlled. These involuntary bodily functions are being constantly monitored and adjusted according to moment-by-moment needs by what is called the 'autonomic nervous system' (ANS). The ANS has two parts – the 'sympathetic nervous system' (SNS) which is all about activation, and the 'parasympathetic nervous system' (PNS) which is all about rest and maintenance. If we had to consciously think about regulating all these bodily functions ourselves we wouldn't have time to do anything else, so it is a great blessing to have nature do this for us automatically.

Many of the symptoms we associate with stress, anxiety or fear – such as muscle tension, tremulousness, clamminess, or rapid heart beat – are a result of SNS activity, and are known as the 'fight or flight response'. They can lead on to tiredness, headache and many other symptoms associated with chronic stress. Chronic stress can be precipitated by one major stressor which extends over time, but more often it is the result of an accumulation of a large number of minor daily stresses and hassles.

When needed, the fight or flight response is a natural, necessary and appropriate physiological response to an exceptional situation. For example, if we are about to be bitten by a snake, chased by a tiger, or run over by a truck, then we need to respond quickly in order to fight off the threat, or to fly away from it. 'Fight or flight', if based on a clearly perceived threat, is encoded into our physiology to *preserve life* by activating changes in the body through chemicals like adrenaline. These are outlined in the following table.

The stress response

Physiological change	Reason
Elevation of blood pressure and heart rate	To increase the blood flow and fuel distribution around the body
Diversion of blood flow to muscles and away from the gut and skin	The muscles are being prepared for a high level of exertion: digestion is not an important priority in the face of a short-term threat
Platelet adhesiveness (platelets becoming 'stickier' and thereby the blood being more ready to clot)	In anticipation of tissue injury and blood loss
Short-term mobilisation of white blood cells and a surge in white blood cell numbers	To help protect the body from infection if it becomes injured
Activation of inflammatory chemicals such as cytokines and interleukins	These chemicals assist the body in repairing damaged tissues and mobilising immunity if injury occurs
Mobilisation of energy stores (glucose and fats) into the blood stream	This is fuel to assist the body in being able to produce a short-term burst of energy
The body becomes sweaty and clammy although it feels cool	The perspiration is in order to keep the body cool under high exertion and the cold clamminess is because the blood has been diverted away from the skin to the muscles
Respiration increases	The body needs oxygen in order to burn the fuel and to breathe off carbon dioxide to maintain chemical balance
Pupils dilate	To facilitate distance vision

All of these changes take place for good reason. If we didn't have this ability to adapt to threats in this way our species wouldn't have survived for very long. Fundamentally, though, these changes are about mobilising energy, increasing performance, defending the body against damage and assisting healing. They help the body cope with demands and potential injury.

MEN AND WOMEN UNDER STRESS

Most of the early research on the stress response was done on men and so the fight or flight response was the predominant model. There is, however, more to it than that. Men and women both have the capacity to activate fight or flight, but men are especially built for maintaining the activation response, largely due to the presence of testosterone.[20] There is now growing evidence to suggest that women do not respond to stressful situations in entirely the same way as men, emotionally, socially, behaviourally or physiologically. When stressed, women initially experience the fight or flight response but then activate what is now called the 'tend and befriend' response, where they 'tend to' or look after children, as well as 'befriending' a social group or network which can offer her and her children resources and protection.'[21]

Thus, when stressed, women are more likely to communicate, express emotion, and nurture. Also, as the female of most species is involved in tending the young they have the biological or behavioural *disposition* to 'tend and befriend'. Men, on the other hand, are more likely to take physical action or assert control over the situation. If one of those tigers comes to the mouth of the cave the woman is more likely to say to the man, 'You get the tiger please, dear, while I look after the kids.' In any case, the SNS activation response in women is down-regulated by various female hormones, most importantly oxytocin and oestrogen.[22] Levels of oxytocin are highest while nurturing, as in breast-feeding, social interaction and caring physical contact like massage or intimacy, and it has a calming or settling effect on SNS activation.[23] Of course none of this suggests that men can't tend and befriend or that women can't activate the fight or flight response when required, but it does mean that each gender is more 'specialised' for one or other response which, taken together, helps the species to adapt more completely to threats.

There are harmful ways in which these male and female responses are expressed. For example, excessive testosterone levels in men are associated with excessive physical aggression and crime. Female aggression, on the other hand, is more 'cerebral' or emotional.[24] Many men and women know what it feels like to be subject to such aggression and how difficult it can be to cope with a pattern of behaviour about which we have little understanding or control.

FREEZING UNDER STRESS

There is another possible response to a threat, and that is to freeze. There are two 'ways to freeze' when under stress; one not adaptive and the other adaptive. When we need to respond and find ourselves confused, tense and not knowing what to do, we 'freeze under pressure'; this is the non-adaptive way. We all know what it feels like and it is anything but enjoyable or useful. The other sort of freezing, the adaptive way, is seen in some animals, although humans can do it, too, and is one response that can protect us from danger when fight or flight are not possible. When an animal is under imminent threat it 'plays dead', and in this state there is a sense of deep stillness and such a profound down-regulation of bodily responses and breathing that it's hard to tell if the animal is alive. This can sometimes lead to a predator leaving the animal alone as it won't attack something it thinks is dead.

IS STRESS GOOD OR BAD?

Is stress of any use? All things have their place and in their proper place all things can be useful, and this goes for unhappiness and stress also, but only if they are used intelligently. The appropriate activation of the fight or flight or tend and befriend response can help us to adapt to threatening situations. Stress can also be a very useful motivator to overcome inertia and procrastination and improve performance.

We can also look at emotional and psychological pain in a similar way to physical pain – it's there for a reason. If we break a leg, we know that the physical pain is trying to give us some very useful information, albeit unpleasant, about a part of the body which is hurt and in need of healing. If we attend to it then the required healing takes place, and function and strength are eventually restored. However, if we numb pain with a strong painkiller, we might feel more comfortable but we may not give due care to the injured part and then do more damage in turn. Often, dealing with stress and unhappiness is like this. For example, we can try to block out or numb the stress with aggression, denial or drugs but these will give only the appearance of temporary relief. Meanwhile the problem, which has to do with ways of seeing and thinking or coping, gets more deeply entrenched. If we pay attention to emotional distress with an interested and compassionate curiosity then we have the opportunity to recognise its source, learn from it, and to do something constructive about it, so although stress or depression may not be pleasant or desirable they can be used constructively.

If the stress response is about preserving life, then why are stress and poor mental health often said to be bad for our health? The answer lies in the fact that the stress response can be activated appropriately or inappropriately. In other words, stress is activated by whatever we *perceive* to be a threat, whether it really is a threat or not. Seeing our GP coming towards us in order to measure our blood pressure is enough to put our blood pressure up, enough, in fact, for one-quarter of patients to be diagnosed inappropriately with hypertension (high blood pressure).[25] This is called 'white-coat hypertension'.

The activation of the stress response is not bad for our health so long as it is activated when it needs to be, is deactivated when it is no longer required, is not over-activated, and is not prolonged. Unfortunately, the vast majority of occasions in which the response is activated are unnecessary – we activate it over something which is not really there, or activate it far in excess of what the situation demands. Much of this has to do with stress related to an anticipation of future events and replaying of past events. The word 'anxiety' even comes from the Latin word 'anxius' meaning 'to anticipate some future event'. If we imagine being chased by a tiger, and if we take the imagination to be real, then the body activates the response as if the tiger was really there. Unfortunately, about 99% of the tigers we find ourselves running from are only in our imagination! This is where approaches such as mindfulness can be so invaluable.

The replaying of an event in the mind can reproduce the stress response even though the event is long over, particularly if that event is replayed with a significant level of emotional response. Emotions are powerful in 'burning' events, for better or for worse, into our memories. It is for this reason that learning to be less emotionally reactive to memories has such a significant effect on helping us to be free of the burden of past events. In the most extreme cases this 'replaying' can lead to what is called 'post-traumatic stress disorder' where the memory, emotion and physiological response have become strongly wired into the circuitry of the brain. As soon as the memory is recalled, the emotional response arises and the physiology reacts. But if such a response can be wired in it also means that it can be unwired again.

WEAR AND TEAR

Extended activation of the stress response leads to what is called high 'allostatic load'[26] or prolonged wear and tear on the body, much like a car being driven hard and having heavy demands placed upon it. Any mechanic knows that the parts of that car will wear out a lot faster under such circumstances, and it is no different with our bodies. High allostatic load is found in chronic stress and anxiety and also depression. It is associated with poor immunity and acceleration of atherosclerosis, otherwise known as 'hardening of the arteries'. It also increases the incidence of 'metabolic syndrome', the cluster of common symptoms in developed countries, which is made up of Type-2 diabetes, central obesity, hyperlipidaemia (high blood fats, lipids or cholesterol) and hypertension. Allostatic load is also associated with osteoporosis because of the chronically high cortisol levels, which leaches calcium out of the bones. Importantly, high allostatic load is associated with a loss of nerve cells in certain parts of the brain (atrophy) – in particular, the frontal lobes of the brain, associated with higher reasoning, and the hippocampus, associated with memory. Even more interesting is the recent finding that the long-term practice of mindfulness meditation not only reduces allostatic load but also can preserve and possibly even regenerate nerve cells in these important regions of the brain.[27] We are finding that the brain is a far more malleable organ than was previously appreciated.

Stress chemicals, like cytokines, whether released appropriately or inappropriately, have important effects on mood, behaviour and emotion.[28] They activate many of the symptoms associated with depression and produce similar effects on the immune system as those seen in depressed patients. This may be part of the reason why depression occurs more frequently in those with chronic medical disorders associated with immune dysfunction. The symptoms associated with an illness, like a significant infection, are in part due to the activation of the immune system. It induces 'sickness behaviour' – apathy, lethargy, lack of motivation and appetite – which is a good way for nature to keep us in bed while the body is trying to recover.

Activating these chemicals when we don't need to, such as when we ruminate on problems, is not so helpful and may explain in part why depression is associated with the symptoms that it is. The important thing to remember is that we can learn to reverse these effects over time by learning better coping strategies.

THE MIND–BODY CONNECTION

The father of Western medicine, Hippocrates, said 'the human being can only be understood as a whole'. So what is the 'whole person'? To the ancient Greeks – as with other ancient Eastern, Western and indigenous healing systems – the whole person includes the physical body, mind, and spirit or consciousness. These are also said to be interdependent with the body, mind and spirit or consciousness inherent in the universe. The physical body, being the most superficial aspect of ourselves, is governed by the mind and enlivened by consciousness. Consciousness is primary and is synonymous with 'being' or 'self'. Thus, 'the body is the shadow of the soul', according to the great Renaissance philosopher Marsilio Ficino.

This holistic idea as a basis of healthcare is not dissimilar to the WHO definition of health. They define it as 'a state of dynamic harmony between the body, mind and spirit of a person and the social and cultural influences which make up his or her environment'. Medical science has increasingly validated this intimate link between mind and body and has gone a long way to explaining why we become ill or recover.[29]

Much of what has dominated modern science and healthcare has been 'reductionist' and 'materialistic' in its approach. Reductionism is when something is broken down or reduced into so many parts that we forget that those parts have meaning and purpose only within the whole. Materialism relates to the view that the physical world is the only world and everything can therefore be reduced to chemical reactions and physical forces. This reductionist and materialist philosophy is superficial and, when applied to healthcare, has often proved expensive, invasive and dehumanising, and has shown only very limited success in preventing and treating many common and chronic conditions. Although, for example, depression does involve chemical changes in the brain, a reductionist and materialist approach would say that is *all* depression is. Such an approach deals with the symptoms or manifestations of diseases but not with their causes.

As a result, many people are returning to more holistic and/or integrative approaches to healthcare.[30]

The materialistic view of the mind, psyche or soul has a long history. Attempts to find the seat of the soul somewhere in the brain date back to ancient Egypt and can be traced through ancient Greece right up to the modern day. Today, with the rise of the neurosciences, brain-scanning techniques and genetics, we are discovering connections between mental and emotional states and the corresponding biochemical states. This is sometimes called 'mind-mapping' or, perhaps more accurately, 'brain-mapping'. Even spiritual experiences are being reduced to the mere activation of neurons in a particular part of the brain called the temporal lobe. For some, this is as a direct challenge to metaphysical explanations of the human condition, but for others it is a fascinating elucidation of the physical details underpinning the metaphysical view.

From the early twentieth century, specific functions were being mapped to particular parts of the brain. This early work led to a rather primitive understanding of the brain and some naïve and simplistic approaches to treating mental illness and behavioural problems, such as the relatively widespread use of frontal lobotomy in the 1940s.[31] Psychosurgical techniques like these have understandably been relegated to history and the mainstay of the modern approach to mental illness since the 1960s has increasingly been the use of pharmaceuticals. Now the pendulum seems to be swinging back to psychological therapies. We are increasingly realising that to manage psychological and emotional problems requires more than just altering the level of a particular chemical in the brain.

The intimate mind–body connection means that the mind and con-sciousness are profoundly important in determining health and ill-health, whether it's through direct physiological effects or effects on behaviour. Acknowledging the importance of the mind doesn't deny the also important role of physical risk factors and treatments. Recognising, for example, that emotion plays a role in exacerbating asthma symptoms doesn't ignore the importance of taking asthma medications, monitoring, and seeking emergency care if needed.

In the mind–body view, such as the wisdom traditions might have understood it, the mind is non-physical. It is made up of thought and emotion which have flow-on chemical effects in the brain. The brain, on the other hand, is the physical organ which translates thought and emotion into biological, electrical or chemical activity. Through hormones and neurotransmitters it regulates all the other functions throughout the body. If someone says, for example, that an illness, pain, or stress is 'in the mind' they are correct, but this does not mean that it is not also 'in the body'.

THE EFFECT OF THOUGHT ON THE BRAIN

Thought and emotion drive brain activity. Depression, for example, is a symptom which is experienced emotionally but has a number of effects on the body. Through brain scans we can see that the placebo response in the brain – where someone is given a 'sugar pill' thinking it is an active drug – is biologically similar to that in people who receive the active drug.[32] This placebo effect is estimated to account for at least 80% of the clinical effect of antidepressants. In fact, more recent reviews of unpublished data suggests that antidepressants may be no better than placebo for mild to moderate depression.[33] This tells us that the major part of what is happening in the brain is based on belief rather than chemicals. Such scientific observations are difficult to understand if we think that the cause of the recovery from depression is purely a chemical one. Recovering from depression through psychotherapy or cognitive therapies uses different pathways to the ones used by antidepressants.[34] Changing thought has a far more widespread effect.

In a similar way, brain scans indicate that giving a placebo to people who believe that it is a painkiller leads to a different cascade of chemical changes specific to pain pathways.[35] Interestingly, empathy, or experiencing another's pain, has been shown with brain scans to be associated with similar changes in the loved one and the one actually experiencing the pain.[36]

In drug trials the placebo effect has long been the bane of the researcher's life. It is hard to explain and confounds the ability to determine the effectiveness of medications. It can also produce unwanted 'side effects', a phenomenon sometimes called the 'nocebo' effect. Harnessing its clinical potential raises ethical issues and drawing a patient's attention to it has the potential to remove perhaps the major part of the clinical response for many treatments.

Conditions which seem to be most responsive to the placebo effect also seem to be the ones most susceptible to emotion, perception and interpretation. These include things such as mood, sleep and pain perception. Placebos are clearly more effective in people who have higher hopes of beneficial outcomes, have had positive experiences with therapies in the past and have higher trust in the therapist giving them the treatment.

Rarely are surgical techniques subjected to placebo-controlled trials but when they are the results are interesting. For example, a trial on arthroscopic surgery of the knee found that arthroscopic lavage (washing out the joint) or debridement (removing fragments from the joint) were no better than those of a placebo procedure (a small incision while under anaesthetic).[37]

The effect of thought on the brain can be illustrated in other ways. When a person has a stroke, a part of the brain has died which results in a loss of function and the person having to relearn skills. 'Mental practice' of a motor skill activates the same neural pathways as physically practising the same skill. A study on stroke patients demonstrated that rehabilitation was more effective when mental practice was included for 30 minutes twice a week for six weeks. These patients with moderate motor deficits showed clinically significant reductions in impairment, increases in arm function and new ability to perform important activities of daily living.[38] The thought was stimulating the brain to repair the damaged pathways to some extent.

It seems that for many people with chronic pain there are changes in how the brain registers pain. If people become very reactive to pain then it sensitises the brain to increasingly experience pain with relatively low-level stimuli. The brain is literally becoming sensitised and maintained by 'sustained attention and arousal'.[39] In other words, the person has become highly vigilant and reactive to pain messages. This is a possible reason why chronic pain is such a prominent part of conditions which involve social isolation, psychological stress or lowered mood and may also be part of the reason why strategies such as social interaction, mindfulness and relaxation techniques help in chronic pain syndromes. They help us not to be so reactive to pain and may help to rewire the brain's pain circuits.

There are undoubted physical effects of depression, stress and other emotional states. To change the chemistry and activity of the brain, for better or for worse, one must change thought and emotion, or at least the thoughts and emotions we give our consciousness to. These skills will be explored in the section on mindfulness-based stress management.

To explain how our thoughts can affect our brains, we need to look at what is known as brain remodelling. A neuron, or brain cell, has many, many connections with other brain cells through its axon (main connecting cable), dendrites (branches) and synapses (points of connection). Through the dendrites and synapses, the brain is remodelling itself all the time depending on how it is being used.

With the rapid advances in neuroscience many of the long-held myths about the brain are being challenged. Daniel Siegel's book *The Mindful Brain* gives a fascinating and comprehensive coverage of this emerging field.[40] For example, it had long been believed that there was very little modification in the brain after its initial development during childhood and adolescence. In early childhood many new cells are still being born and in childhood and adolescence the connections are largely being laid down. Some connections are 'pruned' and others are reinforced. Now we know that the process doesn't end there. Extensive and ongoing modification of the brain takes place throughout the whole of one's life, although this remodelling is easiest when we are young. This remodelling, for better or for worse, is in response to experience, memory, attention and emotion. This is called 'neural plasticity': like plastic, the brain can be moulded.

The adaptability of the Central Nervous System (CNS) is exemplified by recent experiments examining the effects of stress on the animal brain.[41] If you stress an animal, it secretes certain chemicals that are crucial in the remodelling of the brain's anatomy, particularly the part of the brain called the amygdala, which is associated with fear-based emotions and anxiety. This 'rewiring' is reversed if the animal is allowed to return to a stress-free environment.

Modern brain scanning and imaging techniques are giving scientists the opportunity to examine the human brain under a range of psychological states. We can have a genetic predisposition to anxiety and depression, and many of us may be unconsciously conditioning ourselves for these conditions by the way we learn to respond to events from an early age. Memory of emotionally traumatic events with a high level of reactivity reinforces this wiring and plays a significant part in post-traumatic-stress-disorder. The region called the hippocampus, which is important for consolidating new learning and memory, is negatively affected by stress through cell loss (atrophy). The prefrontal cortex – which is located behind the forehead and plays a role in working memory and higher functions like reasoning, decision-making, emotional regulation and our sense of self – is also subject to atrophy in chronic stress and depression. The amygdala, on the other hand, thrives and grows with stress because it is stimulated so often.[42] It is an important role of the frontal lobes to exercise a mediating and moderating effect upon the emotional and fear centres of the brain and they will do this if these patterns of behaviour are reinforced.

Brain scans show that anticipation as well as physical events have significant effects upon brain activity. The thought of eating chocolate, for example, will most definitely 'light up' parts of the brain associated with rewards and pleasure.[43] A cheaper wine labelled as expensive produces more drinker satisfaction and stimulation of the brain's pleasure centre than the same wine bearing its correct price tag. Likewise, an expensive wine labelled as a cheap one produces less satisfaction and brain stimulation.[44]

The brain responds to what we believe and will be remodelled based upon what we think, how we feel and what we do. The reward centres are located in what is called the mesolimbic system, lying just under the limbic system of the brain which is intimately involved with emotions. The reward system drives us to pursue behaviours associated with survival, like eating, sex and other pleasant sensations. If it is natural for the brain to respond to pleasant 'rewards' it is also natural for it to have a tendency towards addiction if those rewards are over-stimulated, particularly in those who have a genetic predisposition to addictive behaviours.

More peaceful states of mind, such as those induced by meditation, are associated with altered levels of activity in the brain, specifically an increase in activity in the left frontal lobe, which is associated with better mood, optimism and also improved immunity.[45] This was demonstrated in a trial in which one group undertook an 8-week program in mindfulness-based stress reduction and a second group did not. At the end of the 8-week period, both groups were vaccinated with influenza vaccine. Among the mindfulness group there were significant increases in left-sided anterior (prefrontal) activation, which is associated with positive mood, and this also correlated with a significant increase in antibody response to the influenza vaccination. This demonstrates the interconnectedness of psychology, brain and immunity and shows that there is much a person can do to enhance their own health and resilience to stress and illness. Other studies have shown that when positive emotions are stimulated, such as when watching a film of a loved one, then not only do these areas of the brain activate but the immune system is more responsive.[46]

Studies link the practice of meditation to specific changes in brain activity, particularly those areas associated with the regulation of attention, sensory perceptiveness, mood, memory and control of the autonomic nervous system.[47] Even more interesting are the studies showing that long-term meditation practice slows age-related degeneration of the brain.[48] It had long been assumed that the brain did not have the ability to generate new cells but, like many other medical myths, we now know this not to be true.[49] We do not know the full potential of the brain's ability to regenerate, but we do know that it can be stimulated by education and training, exercise and by mindfulness throughout the whole life span.[50] This is called 'neurogenesis'. These effects are probably a combination of activating neuron growth through healthy lifestyle, mental stimulation and reduction of stress hormones.

Other behaviours, like lying, also have effects on the brain.[51] Those who have grown up being conditioned to pathologically lie, cheat and deceive show structural abnormalities suggesting that it gets hard wired into the brain, making it less and less easy for the person to recognise or change. Initially the thinking patterns and behaviour govern the wiring of the brain and then the wiring tends to perpetuate the thinking and behaviour.

THE MIND AND THE IMMUNE SYSTEM (PSYCHONEUROIMMUNOLOGY)

Jonas Salk, the discoverer of the polio vaccine, is quoted as saying, 'The mind in addition to medicine has powers to turn the immune system around.' How true this seems to be. This section will discuss basic elements of the immune system and why some strategies protect us from becoming ill or help us to manage illnesses. This section also provides relevant background for the chapter in Part 3 called 'Healthy immunity'.

Although many people have an intuitive sense of the close link between our mental state and resistance to disease, it has only been formally studied in recent years. This field is called psychoneuroimmunology, or PNI for short. It had previously been thought that the brain and immune systems had their own memories and worked independently. Nothing could be further from the truth. Put simply, PNI has shown that the mind is connected through the nervous and hormone (endocrine) systems to the immune system. The findings of PNI have major implications for our susceptibility to infections and cancer, response to allergens, and the progression of autoimmune and inflammatory conditions.[52] In fact, it would be hard to find a disease process not profoundly influenced by immune function. Even heart disease is now known to have an immunological basis.

Every part of our body communicates with every other part. This communication takes place via 'hard-wiring' through nerves – like a cable network – and also via a blood-borne 'postal system' which uses hormones and neurotransmitters. Hormones are chemicals which are released by one cell and tell other cells in a distant part of the body to perform or cease some function. Neurotransmitters are chemicals which are secreted by nerves to communicate with other cells – usually other nerves – to activate them in some way. By these two means the nervous system communicates with every system in the body including our immune defences. Both the nervous and immune systems are two-directional, meaning that the immune system also sends messages back to the CNS.[53 54] Especially important in the feedback loop are the areas of the brain called the limbic system, which is involved with emotions, and the frontal lobes, involved with emotional regulation and higher functions like decision-making and appraisal.

The immune system protects the body through the direct action of white blood cells (WBCs), its 'combat troops' which identify and destroy viruses, bacteria and cells which are infected or cancerous. Some WBCs also produce another specialised part of the immune system – immunoglobulins. These compounds are specifically formed to latch on to foreign antigens like bacteria and viruses and immobilise them or make them easier for the WBCs to recognise. Low WBC counts, underactive WBCs or low levels of immunoglobulins leave us open to infections.

Over 100 neurotransmitter and hormonal receptors have been found on the surface of WBCs. The chemistry of thought is not localised to the brain, which goes some way to explaining why emotional states like stress, anxiety and depression can cause distant physiological effects and susceptibility to disease. Sayings such as having 'butterflies in the stomach' start to take on a different meaning when we consider the intimate mind–body link. Furthermore, drugs which have psychoactive properties also affect the functioning of immune cells because they have the same receptors as our brain cells.

The way our mental state affects immunity is not just a matter of stress suppressing immunity. If that was the case, stress would be useful for reducing inflammation, which is an effect of immune over-activation. In fact, negative emotional states suppress the beneficial immune function that is meant to be protecting us from infection but increases inflammation at the same time. This is called immune dysregulation. Immune regulation is where the immune system is more balanced and is therefore better able to do what it should do – protect the body from infections and cancer – and do less of what it shouldn't be doing – causing inflammation and tissue damage.

The most commonly used test of immune status is to simply measure the number and types of WBCs in our blood. This tells us how large the army is but tells us little about how well the army is functioning. On the other hand, tests of immune function, which are more specialised and expensive, are designed to tell us how well the cells are performing their designated roles.[55] Such tests include measuring how quickly the WBCs multiply in response to an infection. Another test is to measure how quickly and well Natural Killer (NK) cells – a specialised form of WBC – kill infected or tumour cells. Other tests measure the body's ability to stimulate antibodies in the allergic response. They are not the sorts of test a doctor would normally be able to order.

Negative emotional states have a negative effect on immunity largely by affecting how well immune cells carry out their core functions[56][57] rather than by affecting cell numbers. For this reason, compromised immune function due to stress or depression is harder to pick up on standard blood tests, which give only WBC counts. Of course, if immune cell numbers diminish markedly, such as during chemotherapy, then that can be a major threat to health. Therefore, much like a defence force, our immune system can function poorly either because the 'soldiers' are too few, too under-active or over-reactive.

Immune cells are meant to discriminate 'self' from 'non-self'. An antigen is like a label on a cell which helps the body to distinguish the difference. It is as if our cells have got our names written all over them. This way, our body recognises germs as being non-self if they are in a place where they shouldn't be. This is an important defence against certain cancer cells that carry antigens on their surface. Cancer cells, mutating as they do, will often start to 'misspell' their surface labels so that they start to look like foreign tissue. In such a case the body will recognise and reject the cancer because it is no longer acting as a part of the self. (However, there are other cancers that don't wear their antigens on the surface which makes them difficult for the immune system to recognise and attack.)

Immune dysfunction takes place when the immune cells lose

their ability to discriminate between self and non-self. They might attack healthy tissue inappropriately, leading to inflammation and autoimmune disease; or they might not attack things they should such as viruses or cancer cells, which can predispose to infection and cancer. Autoimmune diseases, such as inflammatory bowel disease, rheumatoid arthritis and MS, are becoming increasingly common and nobody is sure why, although factors like stress, infections, genetics, and possibly vaccinations for some individuals, may play a role.

Immune cells mirror emotional states. Negative emotional states have been associated with a variety of diseases, whether due to an accumulation of small stressors or the impact of one or two large ones. An accumulation of small daily stressors can be as detrimental if not more detrimental to health than major stressors.[58] Changes in immune cell numbers and function start to occur within five minutes of an event a person perceives to be stressful.[59] Depending upon the reaction to the stressor, measurable changes in immunity can remain for up to 72 hours afterwards.[60] Those who perceive that they have some control over their situation are buffered from stress and the resulting immuno-suppression, whereas those who perceive that they have no control, especially if they are anxious to be in control, experience prolonged effects. 'Control' denotes being in control of the situation and, more importantly, being in control of one's response to the situation. Being able to choose an attitude of acceptance of an unavoidable but challenging situation buffers one enormously from the health effects of adverse life events. States of ongoing stress and depression are associated with immuno-suppression.

Acute stress alters the number and function of immune cells, with individuals varying markedly in the magnitude of their response. Those who are most psychologically and physiologically reactive to stress – for instance, having the greatest increases in blood pressure, heart rate, cortisol, adrenaline, etc. – are the ones most likely to have the biggest disruption to immunity. Therefore they have the greatest susceptibility to infection during stressful periods in life.[61] For example, in one study, healthy subjects listed stressful events in their life and were then tested to assess how reactive they were to stress, by measuring their response to an assumed stressor (making a speech). Participants were then followed weekly for 12 weeks. Those who tended to produce a high level of the hormone cortisol when under stress – or 'high cortisol reactors' – with high levels of stressful life events had a far greater incidence of coughs and colds than did high cortisol reactors with low levels of stressful life events. 'Low reactors' – people who did not tend to overreact to stressful events – had fewer coughs and colds, irrespective of their life-event scores.[62] Similar findings were found among hospital doctors.[63] Those who coped better with the stress of being on call had the least disruption to their WBC count. Conversely, if there is an inflammatory process taking place somewhere in the body, such as in rheumatoid arthritis, then stress and anger will aggravate the inflammation.

The mechanisms are infinitely complex but the principle is infinitely simple: a healthy and happy mind is fundamental for a healthy body. Being inflamed emotionally – that is, having a stressed and angry mind – is associated with physical inflammation. It is interesting to note that the Sanskrit word for attachment, 'raga', from which we derive our English word 'rage', also means anger, red, passion and inflammation.

Stress in all its forms can impair the body's ability to heal itself. Anger, for example, and the inability to feel in control of it, also means that our wounds heal more slowly.[64] This confirms previous studies showing that stresses like marital disharmony not only lead to significantly higher secretion of inflammatory hormones including cytokines but also disrupt wound healing.[65] Similar effects are seen in depression.[66]

What are the implications? One is that stress increases our susceptibility to infection.[67] We are roughly twice as likely to come down with a cold if we are stressed and then exposed to a cold virus. Not surprisingly, if one gets a viral illness, like influenza, higher stress levels are associated with more severe symptoms.[68] There is also a strong link between stress and relapse for chronic infections such as herpes viruses.[69] In chronic and latent infections there is a balance between the ability of the infecting agent – say, a virus – to spread and the body's defences, which are trying to keep it in check. These viruses lie waiting until times when the immune system is suppressed and they can re-emerge.

Relaxation can elevate resistance to infection.[70] Data shows that those with HIV infection who are above average for stress and have below-average levels of social support are two to three times more likely to progress to AIDS over a five-year period.[71][72] Another study on HIV-positive patients,[73] in the *American Journal of Psychiatry*, showed that for every one severe stressor per six-month period, the risk of early disease progression from HIV to AIDS was doubled.

Such observations need to be turned into interventions. In one such intervention, which gave Cognitive Behaviour Therapy (CBT) to HIV-positive men, the reductions in depression and anxiety were paralleled by reductions in stress hormones, improvements in WBC counts[74] and elevation of DHEA (dehydroepiandrosterone),[75] all important markers of a good prognosis. DHEA is also thought to be an important hormone in patients with chronic fatigue syndrome.

Another study, on medical students,[76] looked at immune function over the exam period and revealed profound immune suppression before and during exams compared to low-stress periods. This corresponds with the general observation that students frequently succumb to illness during or just after exams. When students were randomised into two groups, one being taught relaxation techniques and the others not, it was found that those who were not taught relaxation had the predicted poor immune function, but those who were taught and practised relaxation had far more effective immunity and fewer infections. Those who learned relaxation and did not practise it might as well not have learned in the first place. Even keeping a journal about significant events is associated with improved immune function and fewer doctor visits for infectious disease.[77]

One of the easiest markers of immunity to measure is Salivary Immunoglobulin A (S-IgA), one of our first-line defences against infection in the respiratory, gastrointestinal and urinary systems. Low levels of S-IgA are associated with an increased risk of infection.[78 79] S-IgA levels have been found to be reduced by stressful life events such as sporting competitions, stress, exam pressure, social isolation, grief and anxiety and was also low in those with the 'need to have power and to influence others'.[80 81 82 83 84] The relaxation response and positive emotional states, on the other hand, are associated with enhanced immunity, although some studies have shown variable results depending on how the emotional state was induced.[85 86 87] One group of researchers measured the levels of S-IgA in people before and after they had induced positive (care and compassion) or negative (anger and frustration) emotions for only five minutes. On the day that the positive emotions were induced the group had increased S-IgA levels for approximately four hours afterwards whereas on the day the negative emotions were induced the group had a short burst of increased S-IgA followed by five hours of immuno-suppression.[88]

Early PNI research was hampered by apparently inconsistent

findings. For example, in response to stressors some people have immuno-enhancement and others immuno-suppression. On this basis one could easily conclude that there is no reliable and predictable effect of stress on immune function. If some have enhancement and some have suppression then when the results are averaged out over the whole group there would be little overall change. Some studies looking at life stress and its impact on cancer incidence have made similar findings. The factor these studies did not measure was that it was the individual's *reaction* to the stressor which really mattered. It is another example illustrating what the philosopher Epictetus said: 'Man is not disturbed by events but by the view he takes of them.'

When researchers take into account individuals' perceptions and coping styles it is found that those with positive ones consistently have immuno-enhancement, making them more resistant to disease. Those with negative perceptions and coping styles consistently have immuno-suppression, putting them at greater risk of disease.[89][90][91] So if one person's football team loses they may get angry or depressed – and therefore experience significant immuno-suppression – whereas another person will be philosophical about it and might experience enhanced immunity.

Carers of those with chronic illnesses are prime candidates for poor immunity. For example, those caring for loved ones with Alzheimer's disease have been found to exhibit immune suppression proportional to the level of distress they feel.[92] Similarly, the immuno-suppression observed in those going through marital separation is proportional to the amount of negative emotion and difficulty the person experiences in letting go. Such studies illustrate the fact that the person's perception of a situation and their coping abilities are central in determining the physiological response.

THE EXPERIENCE OF PAIN

The experience of pain is 'holistic' in the sense that every part of our mental, emotional and physical makeup can be affected by it. Pain is not localisable to any one centre of the brain but is dependent on the interaction of many centres which register and modify pain signals. They include the ones involved with attention, mood, emotion, fear and thought. This means that the causes of chronic pain are many and varied and therefore the management of it needs to address a range of issues.

Stress, fear and depression not only affect pain perception but also the chemistry of the nerve endings and pain pathways, so chronic pain syndromes are understandably very common in those who are finding it difficult to cope or feel helpless and hopeless. Conditions often associated with chronic pain and psychosomatic illnesses include burnout, multiple chemical sensitivity, chronic musculoskeletal and low back pain, chronic fatigue syndrome and fibromyalgia. It is not that the pain is imaginary but that the brain can be receiving pain messages disproportionate to the level of tissue damage. Evidence suggests that, in these cases, neural loops in the brain are sensitised and maintained by 'sustained attention and arousal'.[93][94] This means that the person is hyper-vigilant and preoccupied with the pain. They become over-reactive to it, emotionally and psychologically, when they notice a sensation of pain. Over time the same pain stimulus produces greater suffering, and a vicious cycle begins. Practices like mindfulness that reduce arousal and reactivity help to gently shift the focus of attention. They have excellent long-term effects in the management of chronic pain and other symptoms.[95][96] Neural plasticity may be part of the reason why. Chronic pain conditions such as irritable bowel syndrome seem to be responsive to a range of mind–body interventions such as hypnosis. For example, a study found that 71% of patients initially responded to hypnotherapy and of these, over time 81% maintained improvements in quality of life, anxiety or depression scores, visits to health professionals and medication use.[97] These benefits were still demonstrable after five years.

Relaxation is associated with greater pain tolerance because it seems to enhance the brain's responsiveness to endorphins.[98][99] These are the body's own painkillers, which are about 100 times stronger than morphine. The relaxation response also has an anti-inflammatory effect which is important in conditions where chronic inflammation is a part of the problem. It is associated with muscle relaxation and a reduction in muscle spasm. It also desensitises the pain pathways in the brain, enhances mood and helps us not to over-react to pain when it is experienced.

In managing pain, if emotional issues are amplifying the problem then simply increasing doses of painkillers is not likely to improve the outcome and it increases the risk of addiction. A combined approach where emotional and social issues are dealt with as well as physical problems is far more likely to produce long-term benefits.

STRESS AND PERFORMANCE

We often use stress to motivate and drive performance. As stress becomes habitual, tension can begin to drive even the most mundane daily activities. It often takes the pressure of impending lateness to get us to eventually fling off the bedclothes and get moving in the morning. Hence, many of us are reluctant to reduce stress, fearing that this will undermine our productivity.

The classic Yerkes-Dodson 'stress peformance curve' is often used to illustrate the effect of arousal on performance. As it illustrates, inertia and procrastination are, initially at least, low-stress states: no stress means no performance. As stress increases, perhaps before an exam or at the approach of a deadline, performance tends to improve. If the stress is not too high or prolonged then all is well and we tolerate the temporary increase in pressure and are able to maintain performance. If, however, we are performing somewhere near the peak of this curve but the demands escalate further or something goes wrong, having conditioned ourselves to driving performance with stress, we push harder. Now we really begin to run into problems as the stress escalates but performance drops off rather than improves. This is what we might call a lose–lose situation, in which despite higher stress and energy consumption our performance starts to drop off rather than go to a higher level. We have, as it were, gone over the top.

Stress performance curves

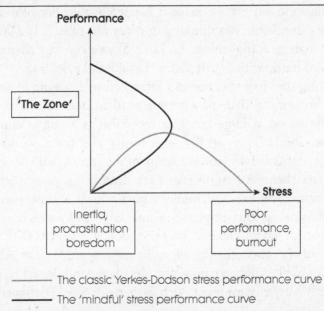

———— The classic Yerkes-Dodson stress performance curve

———— The 'mindful' stress performance curve

If this is prolonged then we burn out and are much more likely to make mistakes. An Australian study found that eight months into their intern year 75% of interns qualified as having burnout.[100] Burnout is associated with things like depersonalisation, emotional exhaustion, and lack of motivation and personal accomplishment. It is not an uncommon occurrence nor is it a sign of being 'weak', but it may be a sign of inattention, inefficiency, lack of self-awareness and self-care. Burnout is associated with poor performance but also puts us at risk of depression. A study of US hospital paediatric residents found that depressed doctors were six times more likely to make drug prescribing errors than their non-depressed colleagues.[101]

But it is possible to function at our peak when demands are high, as illustrated by the 'mindful' stress–performance curve. Athletes talk about being in 'the zone'. In this state there is no stress; in fact, quite the opposite. We feel calm, in the flow, in touch, responsive, efficient and energised. This is the most enjoyable and sustainable level of performance.

It is achieved through increasing our focus so that we are in a state of effortless concentration, or restful alertness. It has two significant effects. Firstly, because our attention is less on anxieties, fears, ruminations and concerns, there is a reduction in stress. This is associated with a feeling of inward calmness. Secondly, we are alert and responsive to the situation we are in because the mind is less agitated and distracted.

As attractive and desirable as this state is, we cannot think our way into the zone nor can we make it happen at the click of our fingers, but we can practise not thinking our way out of it. It is a 'letting go' rather than a 'doing' thing. As Luke Skywalker was advised in his *Star Wars* battle with Darth Vader, 'Let go, Luke, let go.'

Taking the time to settle and focus before engaging in an activity is not something that most people tend to do nor is it something that the world at large tends to recognise as being a valuable use of time. Increasingly we live in a busier and faster world and are being bombarded by stimuli from more fronts, with less time to assimilate them. Attention spans are decreasing, particularly in the younger generations and modern media have a large part to play in conditioning this response. Some have even suggested a new neurological phenomenon: attention deficit trait (ADT),[102] a close cousin of the phenomenon of multi-tasking. ADT (not ADHD or attention deficit hyperactivity disorder) is a conditioned response to an overly busy environment, such as many people experience at work and home. Those who coined the term ADT suggest that in trying to deal with too much input we tend to become increasingly agitated, adopt black-and-white thinking, and find it difficult to stay organised, set priorities and manage time. In ADT there exists a constant low level of panic and guilt. This can be managed by learning to regulate or direct attention, lifestyle maintenance, changing the environment to be less frenetic and learning how to switch off. These issues will be taken up in the section on mindfulness-based stress management.

MODERATION IN ALL THINGS

An ancient principle of health and happiness exhorted by the Greek philosophers was 'moderation in all things'. This is a good adage for life. For instance, too little exercise is associated with poor health and so is too much: very intense or prolonged exercise can reduce immunity and increase allostatic load.[103] Sleep deprivation and poor-quality sleep are strongly associated with depression and, not surprisingly, many depressed people can largely cure their depression by improving the quality of their sleep. Being employed is good for health but too little or too much work is associated with poor health.[104] Unemployment is as detrimental to health as over-employment, and this is quite independent of the financial disadvantage associated with lack of income. Those who abstain from alcohol do not seem to have an advantage over healthy individuals who drink moderately – but high alcohol intake leads to a host of problems, including poor immune function.

A healthy and balanced lifestyle helps the immune system to function at the level it is supposed to, as we can see from the table below showing the increase in activity of the immune system's NK cells, which play a crucial role in fighting infections and cancer.

THE EFFECT OF LIFESTYLE ON NK CELL ACTIVITY[105]

Behaviour	Increase in NK activity
Moderate exercise	47%
Managing stress	45%
Enough sleep	44%
Balanced meals	37%
Not smoking	27%
Eating breakfast	21%
Working moderate hours	17%
Avoiding alcohol	0%

It has been well documented that an unbalanced lifestyle is promoted by stress and depression, and is reversed by effective stress management.[106] [107] [108] Meditation, psychological techniques, a positive attitude and humour all help to reverse the immuno-suppressive effect of stress.[109] [110] [111]

WORKPLACE STRESS

This is an issue of particular relevance to an increasing number of people including health practitioners themselves. For many people today there are ever greater demands at work with fewer resources and personnel to meet them. Workplaces are often far less stable, employment more tenuous and workplace restructuring a more frequent occurrence. Time pressures seem greater than before, with deadlines appearing more urgent.

For many, long hours are an issue, but for many people the most troubling issue is the emotional aspects of the work environment. Where workplace stress is common, anger and interpersonal conflicts with colleagues, customers (and families, when we get home) are also common. These conflicts tend to leave us with far more baggage at the end of the day than if we had high work demands but worked in an emotionally supportive environment. Much of the interpersonal problems in workplaces are caused by an atmosphere of competitiveness where employees believe that their success must come at the expense of the success of others. Building a supportive and collegial atmosphere in the workplace is a vital aspect of improving wellbeing and performance. The investments that many workplaces are now making in this direction, as well as providing healthy lifestyle programs for employees, are signs of a far more progressive attitude. In the long run, these will prove to be resources well spent.

Workplace stress is associated with substance abuse, depression, sleep problems, an increased error rate and marital disharmony. These issues are interrelated. For example, a combination of high demands and low control in the workplace account for a large proportion of workplace stress and account for 13% of depression among men and 17% among women.[112] Sleep problems are common among hospital-employed doctors like interns, with 66% getting less than six hours of sleep per night.[113] The 20% of doctors who consistently had less than five hours' sleep a night had a significantly greater risk of drug and alcohol abuse, conflict and weight change, and made more medical errors.[114] Despite this being such a common scenario, denial is common among senior doctors, as it is in other workplaces. This has a significant influence on the culture and attitudes into which new employees are immersed.[115] Some professions, such as the airline industry, have taken a far more sensible approach to worker fatigue and wellbeing because the risks of not doing so could be catastrophic for employees and passengers alike.

Among the working population it has been consistently observed that Monday morning is the peak period for heart attacks[116] and strokes.[117] (Strangely, peak period for headaches is Tuesday.[118]) The increased risk for cardiovascular events is largely for those who already have risk factors, including significant atherosclerosis, or 'hardening of the arteries'. Weekends, on the other hand, are associated with a reduced risk of cardiac events.[119] [120] Regular vacations can reduce the risk of heart attacks by nearly 30%, according to a nine-year study.[121]

The mechanisms behind the high incidence of heart attacks associated with stress will be described in more detail in the later section on heart disease but suffice to say here, waking up on a Monday morning with a sense of dread or impending doom leads to a surge in SNS activity and creates a 'biochemical soup' which is just right for triggering a cardiac event. This, of course, is independent of the fact that at that stage of the morning the stressors are in our imaginations as the day hasn't even begun yet. Imagining our workload, things going wrong at work, arguments with our boss, or the replaying of past stressful events, will needlessly activate the system.

Other stress factors also increase the cardiovascular risk of workers. In a study on job stress and heart disease in over 10,000 men and women who were followed for over five years, it was found that an imbalance between personal efforts and rewards was associated with a more than double risk for heart disease.[122] Having a low level of control in the workplace was an even higher risk.[123]

The Western lifestyle, which has been adopted by an large number of countries around the world, seems to value activity and productivity so highly that it has become addicted to it. Many people have forgotten that it is the time we spend in quiet that allows us the energy, clarity and creativity to be productive during our active hours. Little wonder that so many people are searching for 'sea changes', 'tree changes' or any change from the daily grind. A failure to recognise the need for balance between activity and rest leads to burnout. On a long-term basis, between seven and nine hours of work a day seems optimal. [124]

Work is not all bad, though. Despite the fact that chronic stress can be a risk factor for dementia, having complex work where we are exercising our brain is protective against dementia.[125] It is not only the act of working, but the attitude with which we work, which determines whether work is beneficial to our health or stress-laden. People can work harder and for longer periods when they have commitment and a positive attitude to their work; when it is a 'labour of love' as we say.

Research on workplace stress and health by Karasek and Theorell[126] suggested that the three main dimensions of workplace stress are control, support and demands. To achieve sustainable performance and enjoyment of our work, we need to understand them.

Control

There are two aspects to control, the so-called external locus and internal locus. External refers to having control over the people and events around us, whereas internal means having control over ourselves, in particular our responses and attitudes. Managing workplace stress can therefore involve modifying the external environment. This could include things like involving people in decision-making processes, developing systems that work on cooperation not competition, varying workers' activities and offering workers choice over things like work conditions and roster.

It is often the case that we have little control over what is happening around us and so in such situations the ultimate and more important form of control is over our responses to the events and people around us. The aim is to increase the level of control we have over our thoughts, feelings and attitudes so that we are not controlled by unhelpful or destructive thoughts and feelings which might understandably arise at work. When we are confronted by a challenge, for example, changing our attitude from unwillingness to willingness can have an enormous impact on how we experience the situation and on the level of mental and physiological stress we subsequently have to bear. This ability to respond in a way which we feel happy about is the very essence of autonomy, responsibility and empowerment. Self-control means we are able to be more expressive of emotions in a socially acceptable manner and to cope with interpersonal and other stresses.

Support

For many people workplace support is a rare commodity, especially in very competitive environments where it is far more common to experience a sense of being undermined by colleagues rather than supported. The illusion of separateness allows this pattern to flourish. Cooperation and support flourish when we collectively appreciate that we are all part of the one organisation, one community, one nation and, indeed, one humanity.

Time and resources spent on building adequate support into workplaces seems to be an expense, but in the long run it's really an investment, not only in staff's wellbeing but also efficiency. Support can be built in as a formal process of adequate training, briefing, debriefing, professional development and fostering of effective communication strategies. Equally, if not more, importantly the workplace culture needs to sustain and support people.

Demands

There are three main issues related to dealing with workplace demands: clarifying perception, reducing demands or improving capacity. As demands escalate in our working life, the first step is to clarify actual versus imagined demands. We often anticipate that things will be far more demanding than they actually are. We might have found ourselves feeling overwhelmed before we have even attempted a task and as a result will have already expended significant amounts of time, energy and mental activity in anticipation and resistance. However, if the actual demands are high then we have to either reduce them or improve our ability to perform, in a sustainable way.

Just like when we go to a smorgasbord, in working life it is easy to put too much on our plate. We can moderate demands by reducing the busyness of our lives, cutting out certain demands and activities.

Sometimes demands are beyond our control and we can't cut push them off our plate, so how we meet them becomes the important issue. Rather than praying for more time, resources and energy, we might need to learn to improve our capacity by making better, more focused and efficient use of the time, resources and energy we have. Thus, skills like focusing, mindfulness, relaxation, time management and problem solving can be very helpful. Many postgraduate and professional development courses are beginning to address these issues.

Stress reduction

THE RELAXATION RESPONSE

The 'relaxation response' was a term originally coined by Herbert Benson of Harvard Medical School. The relaxation response helps to undo the harmful effects of inappropriate stress that can lead to cardiac risk factors, high blood pressure and blood sugars, immune dysfunction, alterations in genetic function and negative lifestyle choices such as smoking, lack of exercise and poor diet. It incorporates a deeply relaxed physical condition and a focused, clear and alert mental state. This combined state of body and mind is sometimes also called 'restful alertness' or 'active calmness' because it enables us to take effective action while feeling inwardly calm. It is associated with a reduction in allostatic load as indicated by the following changes.

Relaxation response: benefits for the body

- Better digestion through increased blood flow and gut motility
- Reduction in blood pressure and heart rate due to reduction in adrenaline
- Metabolism: signs of physiological rest
  - Reduced metabolic rate and respiration
  - Positive impact upon Metabolic Syndrome
  - Demobilisation of energy stores, which reduces blood glucose and cholesterol
  - Reduced thyroid hormones
- Reduced platelet adhesiveness and 'thinner' blood
- Improved immune regulation and function
- Reduced inflammatory and stress hormones (e.g. cortisol, cytokines, interleukins, etc.)
- Improved wound healing
- Changes in brain activity
  - Greater EEG (electroencephalogram) coherence, more alpha and theta waves associated with rest and focus
  - Increased serotonin, which improves mood
  - Increased cerebral blood flow
  - Quicker reflexes and improved sensory perception
  - Reduced reactivity to pain and increased effect of endorphins
  - Neural plasticity and neurogenesis – the ability of the brain to make new cells
  - Increased (left) prefrontal lobe activity associated with optimism and better mood

Relaxation response: benefits for the mind

- Decreased anxiety
- More optimism, decreased depression and rumination
- Greater self-awareness and self-actualisation
- Improved coping capabilities and resilience to stress and challenges
- Happiness tends to be less conditional on circumstances
- Improved feeling of wellbeing
- Reduced reliance upon drugs (prescribed and non-prescribed) or alcohol
- More restful sleep, less insomnia, less sleep needed
- Reduced aggression and greater empathy
- Improved I.Q., memory and learning capabilities
- Greater efficiency and output and reduced stress at work
- Better time management
- Enhanced emotional intelligence
- Improved impulse control
- Improved pain control
- Reduction in personality disorders and increased ability to change undesired personality traits
- Adjunct to psychotherapy

How to achieve the relaxation response

- Relaxation or meditation techniques
- Some forms of music
- Hobbies or interests performed with attention
- Physical activities, e.g., yoga, tai chi or walking in nature
- Humour
- Problem solving
- Cognitive therapy
- Shifts in perception and attitude, e.g. greater acceptance
- Prayer
- Sport

Overall, in the relaxation response there is a move towards restoring a natural balance, called homeostasis. This move of the body towards balance, harmony, efficiency and health is natural and will take place automatically if it is allowed. The mind too will return to happiness and contentment if it is allowed. This state is achieved by the removal of impediments such as anxiety and depression-producing rumination which have become entrenched in our thinking. Such thought patterns are toxic for the mind every bit as much as something can be toxic for the body. Relaxation is what lies beneath the cover of thought and emotion.

THE POWER OF MEDITATION

The potential for benefit is there even in old age. A review looked at the outcomes over nearly eight years of two studies on the elderly that included the Transcendental Meditation (TM) program and other stress-reduction techniques.[127] The TM group showed a 23% decrease in death from any cause, a 30% decrease in the rate of death from heart disease and a 49% decrease in the rate of mortality due to cancer.

An audit found that 2,000 meditators had significant reductions in illness rates in every disease category compared to 600,000 non-meditators.[128] For example, there was an 87% reduction in heart disease and a 55% reduction in tumours. Follow-up over an 11-year period showed an overall 63% reduction in healthcare costs (i.e. 63 cents in the health dollar saved). This included 11.4 times fewer hospital admissions for heart disease, 3.3 times fewer for cancer, and 6.7 times for mental disorders and substance abuse, when compared to the general public who do not meditate.[129] There are undoubtedly direct physiological benefits from the long-term practice of meditation but there could be other reasons for the benefits. For example, it could be argued that those who choose to meditate are not average people; they might be more health conscious or less stress prone in the first place. More conscious and healthy lifestyle choices are natural side effects of meditation, so some of the benefits may not have been from meditation but from people eating better or exercising more. The real answer is probably a combination of all of the above but in any case, on the strength of this and other evidence, a number of insurance companies are starting to offer reductions of up to 30% on life-insurance premiums for those who regularly practise an approved form of meditation.

VARIETIES OF MEDITATION AND RELAXATION EXERCISES

In their simplest form, meditation exercises are basically mental disciplines aimed at developing our skills to regulate where our attention is focused. There are many different varieties of meditation (although some activities called meditation require a rather loose interpretation of the word). In essence, they rely on a combination of cultivating an attitude of non-judgment and directing attention, for example to the senses – such as focusing on the breath, hearing or a visual object – or a mantra, which is an inwardly repeated word or phrase.

The following list gives a little background to some meditative practices which are widely in use. There are many more variations on these and many organisations offering their own styles of meditation. Mindfulness and mantra forms of meditation both have a long tradition of use, dating back thousands of years. In the modern scientific context, mantra meditation – largely through the work of the TM movement since the 70s – mindfulness, and Progressive Muscle Relaxation have the greatest amount of evidence to prove the beneficial effects.

Progressive muscle relaxation (PMR)

The aim in PMR is relaxation of the body. This is achieved by practising a sequence of letting go of muscle tension. Some variations practise tensing the muscles first before relaxing them. Many would not call PMR a form of true meditation but rather a preparation for learning meditation. There are other variations on PMR including autogenic training and yoga nidra.

Mindfulness

This involves using a focus to bring the mind into the present moment. As the body is always present it is a useful focus. There are a number of variations of mindfulness including:

- Sequentially placing attention on the parts of the body (body scan). The main aim is to cultivate impartial awareness. Relaxation of the body is seen as a side effect of the process rather than the prime intention.
- Focusing attention on the breath – also found in yoga.
- Focusing on one or more of the five senses.
- A global awareness of all sensory and mental experiences: open or undifferentiated awareness.
- Insight or reflective practices where the attention is placed on a specific thought, question or issue, with the aim of finding resolution or illumination.
- Walking meditation – walking slowly with focused awareness on the act of walking.

Stillness meditation

Although this includes elements of PMR the main focus here is on the feeling of stillness behind the thoughts, feelings and sensations. Many would say that this is also implied in mindfulness practice.

Mantra meditation

The mantra is a word or phrase silently repeated in the mind. If the mind wanders, the focus is gently brought back to the mantra. There is a significant overlap of mantra meditation and some forms of repetitive prayer and chant. It has been practised in various cultures throughout history. Transcendental Meditation (TM) and the Christian Meditation Network are among many groups who teach mantra meditation.

Visualisation and imagery

In these practices the mind forms an image, scene or sequence of scenes as a focus for the attention. The meditators are often guided by another person or recording. Imagery can be used as a pleasant focus to redirect attention from anxiety-provoking thoughts, as a way of reinforcing a desired pattern of thought or behaviour, or as a way of tapping into unconscious thoughts and memories.

Affirmation

In this form of meditation a positive thought or attitude is frequently repeated mentally or verbally, as a way of reinforcing it and as a way of helping to minimise the impact of negative or anxiety-provoking thoughts and attitudes. It is like a 'reconditioning' of the mind rather than assisting a person to cultivate non-attachment to the mind as in mindfulness and mantra meditation. There is significant overlap with other 'positive thinking' practices.

Different forms of meditation suit different people but all need practice and perseverance in order to be effective. There is little use in thinking in terms of success or failure, but just practice. With experience comes learning how to meditate more deeply. Anxiety about results or progress impedes the process because it takes the attention away from the focus and onto mental activity about the process. Meditation should be simple and easy and if it becomes difficult or complicated then one should seek guidance.

The mindfulness-based approach, which will be explored in detail in this book, is largely aimed at remedying the problems associated with the unconscious and habitual activity of the mind. It is aimed at finding a peacefulness and stillness beneath the mental activity. It aims to transcend thought by resting in a simple awareness of our thoughts and non-attachment to them. One might consider the mind to be like the ocean; mindfulness practices are aimed at diving deep under the oftentimes turbulent surface.

When the mind is very turbulent, those who think that they have to make the mind placid will find that they struggle with the thoughts and feelings and feel swamped by them. Even if the mind is blowing with cyclonic-force winds, there is always the centre of our being – that which is watching. This might be likened to the 'eye of the cyclone' where there is peace even amidst the storm.

Imagery, visualisation and affirmation practices, rather than going beyond the thinking mind, are more directly aimed at changing the content of the mind itself. This can be helpful but a problem is that it is the mind's ability to visualise and imagine which is at the root of many of our anxieties, stresses and maladaptive coping strategies. 'Visualisation' takes many forms including 'catastrophising', 'awfulising', ruminating and prejudging events. It tends to go on habitually and unconsciously and most of us have unknowingly lost the ability to distinguish between reality and imagination. Unless we cultivate the ability to see this mental activity for what it is, and are able to engage or disengage from it as we choose, we will be dominated by it. The unconscious and habitual mental activity described above is of a different nature to the conscious use of creative imagination as used by many artists, composers and inventors. Here it is purposeful, conscious, and the mind is being used like an instrument rather than acting as a master.

MINDFULNESS-BASED STRESS MANAGEMENT

The following pages provide an overview of mindfulness-based therapies which are used for a range of clinical conditions as well as health maintenance. The two most widely known variations of mindfulness-based therapies are Jon Kabat-Zinn's Mindfulness-Based Stress Reduction (MBSR) and Mindfulness-Based Cognitive Therapy (MBCT) which is based on Kabat-Zinn's program but integrates it with some aspects of cognitive therapy. This chapter outlines an abridged form of the Stress Release Program (SRP)[130] which has been used at Monash University in our undergraduate training of medical students as well as for postgraduate training in Australia and elsewhere since 1991. Outcomes of this program have been extremely positive with siginificant improvements for mental health and quality of life.[131]

What is mindfulness?

Put simply, mindfulness is simply about awareness. Living without awareness is a little like living in a dark room. We can't see or understand what is in front of us, we can't move purposefully and our imagination gets carried away. Apart from this, the room is not functional, nor can we put the room in order. Mindfulness helps us to develop the ability to 'turn on the light'. Learning to direct attention where we want it to be also goes by the name of 'attention regulation'. It simply means that we are able to pay attention to what we choose and not be distracted.

> *The faculty of voluntarily bringing back a wandering attention over and over again, is the very root of judgment, character, and will. No one is compos sui if he have it not. An education which should improve this faculty would be the education par excellence. But it is easier to define this ideal than to give practical instructions for bringing it about.*
>
> William James, *Principles of Psychology*, 1890

Consistent evidence is accumulating that mindfulness, although gentle, is possibly the most powerful way of dealing with a whole range of problems. It is extremely effective in eliciting the relaxation response and can help to curb heart disease, ageing of the brain and poor immunity.

It is important to note that although meditation is often called a relaxation exercise it relates more to what is happening in the mind than the body. Relaxation is a common by-product of mindfulness practices but mindfulness is a distinctly different state from simple physical relaxation.[132]

Mindfulness is more than just time out. It is a method of teaching us to pay attention, not just while we are practising the exercise, but for the whole day. It is a training ground for the mind to learn to 'wake up' and to work more consciously and effectively during daily life. Hence day-to-day mindfulness is more important than trying to have a peak experience in the chair while meditating.

Over time, the practice of mindfulness meditation teaches us not to struggle against unnecessary and distracting sensations, thoughts, reactions and feelings, which are often full of anxiety, fear, negativity, criticism, etc. Reacting to them simply feeds and strengthens them and gives them greater impact. One therefore cultivates the ability to be aware of them with an attitude of acceptance, non-criticism and non-judgment. Bit by bit, they come and go more easily, causing less disturbance as they pass. When these thoughts and feelings are strong and have been reinforced for some time it takes a significant deal of patience as they are not likely to subside quickly. Importantly, one is not trying to 'get rid' of them but rather one is learning to let them come and go by themselves.

Practising mindfulness is a little like being at a train station. We can stand on the platform and watch a train of thought come and go – or we can get on board. Normally we unconsciously and habitually get straight on the train whether we want to go to the destination or not. Being more mindful means learning to watch the trains come and go, without getting on board – without becoming attached. The trick is in not fighting against the train, because then it can have considerable impact. If a train of thought comes along that is going somewhere useful then by all means get on board. Thoughts tend to come whether we want them or not, but if we consistently don't get on board unhelpful trains of thought, because of falling passenger numbers, fewer come along that line and they may eventually stop altogether. The freedom comes with non-attachment.

One may find that, like turning on a light, the greater awareness generated through mindfulness makes certain thoughts, memories, fears or anxieties more obvious and therefore initially more disturbing. This is not a negative thing or a sign that we are doing something wrong. The very fact that these things surface while we are practising mindfulness means that we are being offered the opportunity to learn to deal with them in a way other than by suppression. This is the invitation to learn to become free of them. Some of these thoughts and feelings can be quite strong and so one needs some courage and patience in learning to deal with them. It is best to proceed gently and never to force oneself (or another) to proceed unwillingly. It is important to remind oneself to see the thoughts as they are: images and feelings rising and falling on the surface of one's awareness. By being aware but not reacting to these thoughts we learn self-control. The sense of control comes not through struggling with unpleasant states of mind and body but rather in learning not to be controlled by them. It is much like watching a movie but remembering that it is 'just a movie'.

With an attitude of non-judgment and acceptance, thoughts are seen as mental events rather than facts. This ability to stand back from our thoughts and look at them objectively, rather than be consumed by them, is called meta-cognitive awareness (meta – beside; cognitive – thoughts). The state of non-attachment is quite different to 'depersonalisation'. In depersonalisation a person feels removed, cut off, detached, cold and surreal. Studies now suggest what mindfulness practitioners have known for a long time: the non-attachment associated with mindfulness is quite different to depersonalisation.[133] In mindfulness there is a sense of not being caught up in events but at the same time one feels connected to the present moment. The present is warmly and compassionately embraced by our awareness and so we can be more responsive to it.

What we give our attention to is, in a sense, what we meditate upon, for better or for worse. In due course this is what influences us. As the saying goes, 'As a man [or woman] thinketh, so he [or she] becomes.' If we feed a lot of angry thoughts with attention then we are practising anger and we soon become expert at it. It is like meditating on anger and it literally gets wired into our brain. Unfortunately, this process is unconsciously going on most of the time, unless we become more mindful in our daily lives.

Unlike many conventional medical treatments, the side effects of mindfulness-based therapies are beneficial, as they are for all the Essence elements. Studies on undergraduate students[134] found that those who practised mindfulness were at a lower risk for depression, anxiety and neuroticism, and saw increases in their Emotional Intelligence (EI). EI encompasses capacities like self-awareness, an ability to regulate one's emotions and behaviour, empathy, deeper motivation and social skills like the ability to cooperate. Some of the advantages of mindfulness are listed in the table below.

Benefits of mindfulness therapy

- Improved immunity
- Reduced anxiety, distress and depression
- Increase in empathy and spiritual experiences
- Improved knowledge about stress
- Treatment of obsessive-compulsive disorder (OCD) and personality disorder
- Improved sensitivity towards oneself, one's peers and – for health practitioners – patients
- reduced sense of isolation
- Greater use of positive coping skills such as engagement and prioritising, and less use of negative coping skills such as avoidance

- Greater ability to resolve workplace conflicts
- Enhanced ability to cope with cancer and related symptoms
- Improved sleep
- Treatment of fibromyalgia
- Reduction of chronic pain
- As an adjunct to the management of eating disorders, particularly binge-eating
- Preservation and possible regeneration of nerve cells in some parts of the brain
- Enhanced knowledge of alternative therapies

Sources[135 136 137 138 139 140 141 142 143 144 145 146 147 148 149 150 151 152]

Self-awareness relates to being aware of not only what is happening in the body, but also of what is taking place in the mind. It is surprising and more than a little disconcerting to find that we are often oblivious to what is going on in our own minds or where our attention is. Mindfulness soon reveals this to us and so if after starting mindfulness practice one becomes aware of how distractible the mind is then one should see that as progress. Self-regulation, another key component of EI that is boosted by mindfulness, is our ability to exercise self-control. It is closely related to self-discipline, IQ and performance. For students, self-discipline predicts many things, including their school marks, school attendance and selection into competitive educational programs. A study has suggested that a major reason for students falling short of their intellectual potential is their failure to exercise self-discipline, which only reinforces the importance of mindfulness practice.[153]

Some very interesting studies are showing that long-term mindfulness practice is associated with thickening of brain regions associated with attention, self-awareness and sensory processing. Meditation might offset age-related thinning of the brain's grey matter (cortex). According to a study reported in the journal *Neurobiology of Ageing*, 'The regular practice of meditation may have neuroprotective effects and reduce the cognitive decline associated with normal aging.'[154] What an interesting prospect: to be able to renovate your brain.

Mindfulness can be used by itself; as an adjunct to other forms of psychotherapy, where it has been found to result in more rapid alleviation of symptoms, increased achievement of therapeutic goals and a decrease in the number of therapy sessions required[155]; or as part of a cognitive therapy–based program such as Mindfulness-based Cognitive Therapy (MBCT). MBCT cultivates a moment-by-moment awareness of negative thoughts – such as rumination of suicidal thoughts in depression – without getting entangled in them and reacting to them.

Mindfulness practice must be tailored to the individual's agenda. For one person the agenda might be learning to relieve anxiety; for another to help prevent relapse in depression; for another to cope with cancer, fibromyalgia or chronic pain. For a student, mindfulness might be relevant in terms of being able to study better. It could be used as an adjunct to the management of eating disorders, hypertension or asthma, etc. So although the principles are universal the application must be made to fit an individual's needs.

In most cultures and meditative traditions the ultimate aim of contemplative practices is spiritual and philosophical insight. Although this may not be the initial goal when people take up mindfulness for health reasons, it may open up as time goes on. This should come from the person themselves, if it comes at all. It is not helpful for someone learning meditation to have someone else's agenda imposed upon them. We all need to proceed at our own pace and in our own way, according to our own culture and beliefs. One may, of course, find over time that what was originally of central importance, such as the prevention of a relapse of depression, leads into a far deeper philosophical inquiry into the nature of suffering.

When not to use mindfulness practice

There are a few possible contraindications to meditation such as some psychiatric conditions. For example, people with acute psychosis – such as is found in schizophrenia, bipolar disorder or severe acute depression – may have insufficient insight and objectivity to be able to practise effectively and remain objective about the state of mind or emotion. Perhaps a more appropriate practice in such circumstances would be a mindful physical activity that engages the attention such as hobbies, music, crafts, tai chi or yoga.

There is little evidence about the effect of mindfulness meditation when a person is in remission from psychosis and one should proceed carefully and with adequate supervision in such a circumstance. If mindfulness-based therapies are being used as part of the management for a person with a past history of psychosis then it might be advisable to avoid intensive practice or retreats as there is some evidence to suggest that, although uncommon, they can cause vulnerable individuals to relapse. Furthermore, mindfulness or other forms of meditation should not be seen as replacing the appropriate use of necessary medication for people with a history of mental illness.

How to practise mindfulness meditation

For people with already full lives it is recommended that the meditation be practised initially for 5 minutes twice daily. Before breakfast and dinner are good times because our metabolism is at a low point after we eat and we get sleepy more easily then. The duration of practice can be built up to 10, then 15, 20 and even up to 30 minutes or longer, depending on time availability, motivation, needs and commitment. Many people find that starting with longer sessions is too onerous and it is difficult to get the practice established. Well-respected and widely used programs like MBSR and MBCT do start with longer periods of practice – say 40 minutes a day – but this is generally for people dealing with major illness or pain, whose motivation is already very high.

Sessions of 5 to 30 minutes of meditation might be compared to full stops punctuating our day. Regular short mindful pauses of 30 seconds to 2 minutes might be compared to commas. Inserting commas during the day can help to reinforce our ability to be mindful at all times. Even pausing only for long enough to take a couple of deep breaths can help break the build-up of tension and mental activity throughout the day. Any activity done mindfully is really a form of meditation and so the mindfulness practice should be seen as a reminder to live mindfully.

It is helpful, wherever possible, to have a quiet place to practise without interruption. This is not to say that mindfulness cannot be practised anywhere, any time – indeed, it is important for the practice to be as portable as possible, whether the environment is active and noisy or not. We can, for example, pause while waiting at red lights (eyes open preferably), or before a meal.

If interruptions to our meditation do occur then it helps not to be concerned, but rather just deal with them mindfully and then, if possible, go back to the practice. When sitting down to practise it helps to have an idea of how long you will be practising for. Having a clock within easy view can help to reduce anxiety about time. Simply open the eyes to check the time if need be.

Position

It is preferable to sit, as one is less likely to go to sleep in an upright position. In sitting for meditation it is best if the back and neck are straight and balanced, requiring a minimum of effort or tension to maintain the position. Lying down can also be useful, particularly if deep physical relaxation is the main aim of the practice, or if the body is extremely tired, in pain or ill. It is much easier to go to sleep while lying down, which may not be desirable unless it is late at night. Having settled into the preferred position, it would be usual to let the eyes gently close. Meditation can also be practised with open eyes, in which case they would generally be cast gently down, resting on a point a metre or two in front of the body.

From here one can begin practising mindfulness using the sense of touch focused on the body (body scan) or the breathing, or one can use another sense such as hearing. One can also practise using a combination of these. The important thing about the body and the senses is that they are always in the present moment so they help to bring the mind into the present moment. Contact with any of the senses will automatically draw the attention away from the mental distractions which otherwise monopolise our attention.

The body scan

Initially, be conscious of the whole body and let it settle. Now, progressively become aware of each individual part of the body, starting with the feet and then moving to the legs, stomach, back, hands, arms, shoulders, neck and face. Take your time with each part. The object of this practice is to let the attention *rest* with each part, simply noticing what is happening there, what sensations are taking place, moment-by-moment.

Practise cultivating an attitude of impartial awareness, that is, not having to judge experiences as good or bad, right or wrong. Simply accept them as they are. There is no need to change your experience from one state to another or to 'make something happen'. The harder we try to make something happen the more we get in our own way. When the mind judges, criticises or becomes distracted, for example, these are simply mental experiences to observe non-judgmentally as they come and go. As often as the attention wanders from an awareness of the body simply notice where the attention has gone and *gently* bring it back to an awareness of the body. It is not a problem that thoughts come in or the mind becomes distracted. They become a problem only if we view them as a problem.

Breathing

The attention can be rested on the breath as it passes in and out of the body. The point of focus could be right where the air enters and leaves through the nose, or it could be where the stomach rises and falls with the breath. Again, no force is required and in mindfulness there is no need to try and regulate the breath; let the body do that for you. Again, if distracting thoughts and feelings carry the attention away with them, just be aware of them but let them come and go by themselves, letting go of any notion that one needs to battle with them. There is no need to try and stop these thoughts coming into the mind, nor to try and force them out. Notice that trying to force thoughts and feelings out just feeds them with attention, makes them stronger and increases their impact. We are simply practising being less reactive to them, even if the thoughts are about the meditation practice and how well or poorly we think it might be going.

Listening

Here we are simply practising being conscious of the sounds in the environment both near and far. As we listen we let the sounds come and go and in the process also let any thoughts about the sounds – or anything else for that matter – come and go. Keep gently bringing the attention back to the present when it wanders. The value of listening is that the attention is not being used to feed the usual mental commentary running so much of the time in our minds. It is this commentary which is so full of habitual and unconscious rumination, and is almost constantly reinforcing ideas about ourselves and the world.

Finishing

After practising for the allotted time gently come back to an awareness of the whole body and then slowly allow the eyes to open. After remaining settled for a few moments, move into the activities of the day which need your attention. The mindfulness practice is not finished when you get out of the chair: it has just begun! Move back into your day-to-day life with the intention of doing it mindfully.

Variations of mindfulness

There are a number of variations of mindfulness practice but it is useful to be well established in the practices described above before moving on to these variations.

Open awareness

Here one practises simply sitting with an open awareness focused on no particular object or sense. In the process one is simply observing thoughts, feelings and sensations as they come and go. Many people find that because the mind does not have a particular focus of attention in this form of meditation, it is far easier to become distracted.

Reflection or insight meditation

Here one is letting the mind intentionally rest upon a particular thought, decision or issue. There is no particular attempt to solve the problem but rather, with an attitude of quiet interest, to observe with non-attachment what the mind presents in relation to it. As the surface activity of mind settles, a solution may come from a deeper or more intuitive level of the mind. If at some stage an insight does arise out of the blue then it will have a different quality to the surface mental activity which is usually busy covering those insights. Such insights generally arise from quietness and stillness. They have a clarity about them and seem strangely impersonal or impartial compared to all the deeply personal preoccupations that usually take up our mind. When we have made mistakes in life, we may find that we have ignored such intuitive insights.

Managing stress mindfully: The Eight-week Stress Release Program

To practise mindfulness meditation is profoundly useful and will slowly retrain the mind to be more attentive, objective and less reactive. This will be extremely helpful in dealing with stress. But in order to be more aware of the thought patterns which generate or reinforce stress, it is also useful to explore the following series of eight tasks. It is helpful to practise one of these tasks per week. Keeping a journal and recording our insights, observations and questions will help to deepen our learning over the eight-week program.

As we proceed, we should try not to criticise what we might perceive to be failures, nor get carried away with what we perceive to be successes. The really useful thing about so-called 'failure' is that we can learn so much from it, and if we learn from it then we are better off than we were before. If we put the emphasis on learning as being the only true objective, rather than trying to 'get it right' or berating ourselves when we think we 'get it wrong', then we will learn much more quickly and happily.

Week 1: Perception

A stressor is a situation, event, circumstance or person which triggers the stress response. As we have seen, misperception will inappropriately activate the fight or flight response. For instance, the actual physical discomfort that we experience in the dentist's chair is generally minor compared to the level of suffering we produce for ourselves. If that pain were not amplified through the lens of fear and anticipation, or if it were experienced as a part of something we willingly participated in like a sporting activity, then it would barely raise an eyebrow let alone the pulse. The remedy is to pay attention to what is *actually* being experienced rather than just blindly reacting to what we *think* is happening.

Our state of mind and habitual thoughts unconsciously colour the way we see the world and interpret events in it. For example, to a person with a more stable sense of self, a criticism may be seen as an opportunity to learn or perhaps as a reflection of the fact that the person criticising them is under a lot of stress. To someone with very low self-esteem the same criticism may be seen as a major threat, triggering an unthinking and overly defensive or aggressive response. This can lead to conflict and a downward spiral of thought and mood. The most unfortunate thing is that, being on automatic pilot as we often are, we may be totally unaware that this whole process is taking place.

To reduce stress mindfully is not a matter of replacing a stress-laden perception with a falsely positive one, like looking at life through rose-coloured glasses. It is important to remember that from the perspective of mindfulness, pleasant misperceptions, expectations and mental projections are just as distracting and problematic as unpleasant ones. It does not matter whether we are having an anxious daydream or a pleasant one when we take our attention off the road; it is just as dangerous either way. It doesn't matter that we enjoy the flattery of someone with dishonest motives; it is just as deceptive. It does not matter that drugs feel like a legitimate path to happiness; they still produce addiction and misery. It does not matter that a person dying of thirst thinks a mirage to be made of water; it won't quench their thirst.

In mindfulness, all one asks is to see things as they are.

Practice for the week: In your day-to-day life, when you feel the effects of stress – anxiety, fear, anger, depression or any other negative emotional state – ask yourself if the stressor you are reacting to is real. How often do you imagine stressors that don't actually exist? How often do you get things out of perspective by making mountains out of molehills? How often do you fail to see things which do need your attention? What is the effect of these examples of misperception? What is the effect of standing back from the so-called stressor and having a fresh and unbiased look at it?

Week 2: Letting go and acceptance

To relax, mentally or physically, we do not have to *do* anything. We merely have to *stop doing* something: holding on. In this sense, mindfulness is about non-doing. The non-attachment of mindfulness is not about cutting-off or denial, it is about not being bound to sensations, thoughts and feelings. Much of the time we make the understandable mistake of thinking that they have a hold of us. We feel bound by them, imprisoned by them, influenced by them and even dominated by them. Through lack of awareness and investigation, we have lost the ability to choose how we respond to things. With mindfulness we soon discover that it is the other way around: we have a hold of our sensations, thoughts and feelings, and we experienced tension because we didn't know that we could let them come and let them go.

Being bound by our experiences is an unconscious habit, not a necessity. It feels like a great relief to let go, not because it is foreign to us but because it is natural. We are so habituated to tension that we have come to believe that tension is our natural state, but we were not born anxious, preoccupied and distracted; we have managed to think our way into that state over a long period of time.

Practical examples may help to illustrate what is meant by 'holding on' and 'letting go'. We each have an image of ourselves. It could be that we are smart or stupid, kind or selfish, of one nationality or another. When that image is challenged we soon realise how attached to it we are and how much tension it causes. If we think that we are smart then being confronted by our own lack of knowledge will be a painful experience. We may desire to win the argument whether we are right or wrong, or we may find ourselves defending or denying the obvious rather than being thankful for being corrected. If we were able to let go of our preconceptions about ourselves perhaps in that situation we would act more like Socrates, who was always happy to be corrected; he never felt attacked nor did he have a need to attack others.

We hold on to opinions rather than consider them. We hold on to desires whether they are useful or not. For example, we might maintain a larger mortgage than we can comfortably afford and thus find our life is dominated by it. We can cling to a relationship long after it has passed and so cause ourselves enormous grief. We might cling to a fixed plan for how an event should go even when circumstances are telling us that's not possible.

There are common misconceptions about letting go, such as that it is about failing to respond to life even when a response is called for, or that it is about giving everything away. Letting go merely means viewing the flow of sensations, thoughts, feelings and events with non-attachment. Letting go doesn't mean becoming inert; on the contrary, in letting go we tend to become more able to respond freely and without the limiting effects of anxiety, worry or preconceived ideas. This is the very heart of responsibility – the ability to respond.

An important principle in mindfulness which is related to letting go is acceptance. Whatever is happening is happening. There is no denying that. If there is comfort, peace and happiness then so be it; but equally, according to mindfulness, if there is pain, anxiety and depression then so be it. Life is constantly trying to teach us that experiences – both pleasurable and painful – are coming and going whether we like it or not. The crucial factor in how much impact those experiences have is the attitude and relationship we cultivate towards them. If our body has chronic pain then learning to be at peace with the pain will help to reduce our suffering significantly. If a depressing thought or feeling comes to our awareness, fighting against it may merely bind us to it all the more. But with acceptance comes a growing ability to be less moved by negative thoughts and feelings, to let them flow through so that we can be less preoccupied by them and then bring our attention gently back to the present moment.

Accepting, or being at peace with, the things we find very painful is not easy and takes time, patience and courage. True acceptance is not about trying to make something go away, thinking to ourselves, 'If I accept this then it will go away.' That is not true acceptance but is non-acceptance masquerading as acceptance in order to get rid of something about which we have a negative attitude. It there is a problem that needs a response then first accept that it is happening but then get on and deal with it with attention.

Practice for the week: What attitude of mind is predominant when you notice stress or conflict, whether in yourself or with others? What are we holding on to in stressful or conflict-filled situations? What effect do letting go and acceptance have on stress? How do holding on and letting go, or acceptance and non-acceptance, change your experience of day-to-day events?

Week 3: Presence of mind

The present moment is the only moment that can rightly claim any relationship to reality; the past and future cannot.

When we say that someone has 'presence of mind' we are often describing a state of being calm, focused, responsible and capable. 'Absent-mindedness' is the opposite of presence of mind. If the mind is absent it means that it is not in the here and now. It has probably slipped off to some other time and place, generally without us even noticing. This is not a mental state conducive to effective action or understanding.

Without knowing it, we spend much of our lives in an imaginary world which we are taking to be real while the reality of moment-by-moment life is not getting the attention it deserves. If we take a little time to investigate what is going on in the mind when we experience anxiety, fear, depression or worry we will notice that the mind has slipped into a future that hasn't happened or a past that has already come and gone. On the other hand, when the attention is on the here and now, thoughts of the past or future don't have the ability to cause the emotional upset that they often do.

Mindfulness teaches us how often the mind is distracted with thoughts about the past and future. In the recreated past we tend to replay old events – oftentimes embellishing them – ruminate on regrets, re-experience old hurts and criticise ourselves for old mistakes. In the imaginary future we tend to imagine problems which will never happen, a process sometimes called 'catastrophising'. As Mark Twain is quoted as saying, 'I've had a lot of catastrophes in my life, and some of them actually happened.' We also concoct anxiety and fear, dwell on rigid ideas about how things must turn out, and prejudice situations and conversations long before they happen, if they ever happen. We often become anxious about how to get things to go the way we assume they must, and feel frustration or grief because they don't go according to those pre-conceived ideas. We prejudice events, prejudging them.

'What about planning and preparation?' one might say. Planning and preparation can be as much a present-moment activity as anything else can be. It needs our attention, but not worry or rumination. Living for the here and now does not mean not caring about the future, or having no plans or goals, but it does mean that we let the future come to us moment-by-moment, as we practise dealing with each moment on its merits and directing our attention to what the moment requires.

For example, we can be so preoccupied about a future exam that we can't focus on the study required to prepare for it. We can be so anxious about the outcome of an interview that we present as tense and unfocused. An athlete can be so concerned with the outcome of a game that they lose concentration on the game or behave in a way that they might later be ashamed of. We can be so preoccupied about all the jobs we have to do that day that we feel exhausted before we have even done anything. We can keep replaying a past unpleasant experience to the extent that we totally distort current events and relationships. This can reinforce a pattern of stress and avoidance.

When not present in the here and now, we are much less able to see and understand the thoughts and feelings which are actually driving and motivating our actions. The question is, are we going to keep living under the tyranny of the past and our imagination about the future, or are we going to live the life we are meant to be living now?

> **Practice for the week:** How much of the time do you find yourself living in the past or future? What is the effect of this? Where is the mind when you experience stress? What is the effect of living in the here and now? What is the effect of using the mindfulness practice – particularly connecting with your senses – to bring your attention back into the present moment? What is the effect of focusing on the one task which is relevant at any given time? If you make a mistake, what was your mind fixated on at the time?

Week 4: Limitations

It is worthwhile to ask ourselves the question, 'Have I reached my full potential?' The answer will almost surely be 'No.' In that case, it is worth asking ourselves, 'What stands in the way of me reaching my potential?' Many of the thought patterns that govern our actions are full of limiting ideas we hold about ourselves and the world around us. Because we tend not to examine or question these thought patterns, they may be needlessly limiting our sense of fulfilment as well as generating stress and avoidance.

Some limitations are not stress laden or problematic, such as setting reasonable limits on how much we eat, sleep, exercise and work. This is a natural and adaptive part of a healthy and balanced life. There are also limitations which are not problematic because we have no desire or need to overcome them. We may not need or desire to climb Mt Everest, for instance. What we are interested in here are the potentially stress-laden, unconscious, habitual and stifling limitations which dominate much of our life. What form do these problematic limitations take? They can be ideas such as 'I can't speak in public' or 'I'm not bright enough for maths' or 'I can't cope with pressure' or 'I can't draw' or 'I can't cook' or 'I'm hopeless with computers'. They can be habits such as 'I always drive fast' or 'There is only one way to do this job'. They can be likes and dislikes such as 'I never eat foreign food' or 'I hate exercise'. They can be assumptions about the way we are obliged to respond to a situation such as 'Everyone gets stressed before exams' or 'If you fail you have to be devastated' or 'If someone insults you, you have to get angry'.

The reason these types of limitations are problematic is that when we are presented with an opportunity to do something, like speak in public or learn about computers for a new job, we see it as a stressor rather than an opportunity to learn, grow or have some fun. We therefore experience stress, perform poorly, don't learn quickly or we make convoluted efforts to avoid the things we think we can't do. Children are not born with this mentality but they can take it on early in life depending upon the ideas and examples they are exposed to by adults. Young children naturally sing, draw, and wish to learn and expand their horizons. They do not live in fear of failure or what everyone will think of them. As such their lives tend to be full of enjoyment and fascination and they learn quickly.

To transcend problematic limitations first requires that we see them, then see the effects they have on our lives, and then to start to exercise a conscious choice about whether we wish to continue to live under their tyranny. The object is not to put pressure on ourselves in terms of success and failure but simply to get the attention on the activity and off the idea. For example, if we need to speak in public then the idea that we're a bad public speaker is likely to come up quickly, but we can choose not to feed the idea with attention and to instead give our attention to preparation. Part of our preparation may be to practise not feeding ideas such as 'It has to go well' or 'If I make a mistake then it is a total failure'. The only true success is that we had a go.

Practice for the week: What stress-laden or problematic limitations do you notice in your day-to-day life? What is their effect on your sense of wellbeing, on your performance, on learning, or on your actions? What is the effect of reinforcing the limitation by acting upon it again? What is the effect of seeing it but choosing to gently give the attention to the task at hand rather than the limitation? What is the effect of taking the focus off so-called 'success and failure' and putting it on just having a go?

Week 5: Listening

During day-to-day life, what do we spend our time listening to? It might be the birds singing in the trees, or the drops of rain falling on the ground, or the sound of children playing. It might be traffic noise on the way home from work. Chances are, however, that we don't listen to life. Mindfulness practice shows us that we spend most of our time listening to an endless internal dialogue going on in the mind. When stressed, worried, afraid, angry or depressed this internal dialogue has a particular tone to it and is constantly reinforcing and justifying the attitudes and feelings we hold about ourselves and the world. One of our favourite forms of internal chatter is to endlessly criticise, particularly ourselves.

One example of internal chatter we may be familiar with is anticipating an argument with a family member while we drive home. We can find ourselves indignant, insulted and even outraged at all the things they have said to us despite the fact that we are alone in the car. We are taking imagination to be reality when in reality we are merely arguing with ourselves and projecting it onto others. If they have been doing the same thing, we may find that when we arrive home we walk into a barrage of criticism and blame.

When we are unmindful we have no choice or awareness of what we listen to. Our internal chatter has a personal sound about it, as if it is 'me' talking to myself. But who is 'me'? Who is talking and who is listening? In a more mindful and objective state, when we view this mental chatter objectively, we realise that the mind is just talking away to itself, trying to convince itself of something. Mental chatter is just mental chatter. With mindfulness we can simply notice it and remain quite unaffected; we don't have to believe it or react to it. Like the radio, we can change channels by shifting our attention.

If we give our internal chatter free rein it only allows us to give partial attention to what actually is going on around us, in particular, to our conversations with others. Miscommunication is the source of much stress and fosters misunderstanding, conflict and loneliness. How often have we noticed, for example, that when we are having an argument with someone, we don't actually hear what they are saying? While the other is speaking we are generally listening to the mind formulate what we are going to say in reply, based on what we assume they are saying. In turn, we don't feel heard because the other person is probably doing the same thing. If you observe an argument objectively you may get the impression that neither person is actually hearing what the other is saying. The simple reason for this is that they're probably not. A person could be forgiven for assuming that raising the volume will get their message through, which of course it doesn't. Listening does that. Effective and attentive communication breaks down barriers between people and resolves conflict.

It doesn't have to be as dramatic as that. Being unmindful can simply mean that we don't hear what the other person is saying because we're having a little conversation with ourselves such as, 'What am I going to do when I get home?' or 'I'll never understand what the teacher is trying to tell me' or 'What impression am I making?' How often are we introduced to someone and immediately forget their name as if we had never heard it?

True listening means listening with attention and a quiet mind. It is more than just hearing words. It includes seeing under the surface to what the person is really experiencing. For instance, if we pay attention, we might notice that underneath a person's angry words, fear predominates. The anger is just a cover. If we are attentive we can often understand an enormous amount about their needs, feelings and grievances, and in the process become more helpful, compassionate or conciliatory as needed.

If we wish to be less oppressed by negative emotions and also to facilitate effective communication, then we need to recognise when we are listening to our internal chatter and then redirect our attention back to what is taking place in front of us. Next we need to remember the principle of 'letting go' and surrender our preconceived and rehearsed ideas about how conversations should go.

Practice for the week: How often do you find yourself listening to an internal dialogue? What is the tone of this chatter? What is the effect of it on your body, mind, emotions and performance? Are you attentive when listening to others or anticipating what they're saying? What is the effect of not listening to others? What is the effect of practising listening with attention, whether to a conversation or the sound of birds singing?

Week 6: Self-discipline

Have you ever found yourself not getting on with what you need to? Have you ever put things off until it is too late or the pressure is so high that you get agitated? Have you ever worked too long, not worked enough, eaten too much or slept in? If so then you, along with the rest of the human race, have demonstrated a lack of self-discipline. If you criticise yourself for your lack of self-discipline then please go back to the exercise for week five and practise not getting caught in a mental dialogue about it. The aim is not to criticise ourselves but rather to observe and understand the effect that a lack of self-discipline has on our life and wellbeing.

'Discipline' is a word which tends to carry a lot of baggage and assumptions with it. Self-discipline is not about oppression. It is about using our better judgment to govern our lives and decisions, rather than our unreasonable and oftentimes whimsical lesser judgment. The better judgment is based on reason and insight while the lesser judgment most commonly revolves around strong desires, aversions, inappropriate and outdated habits, unreasonable beliefs, whims and misguided emotions.

What does this mean in practice? Take the experience of picking up a message from the body that it has had enough to eat. A 'quiet but impartial inner knowing' tells us, 'It's time to stop now' but within about three milliseconds a somewhat noisier and more partial desire asserts itself: 'But I would just love another serve of dessert.' If we are not careful we will say yes to our generous and eager-to-please host who will place another plate of dessert before us, which we will struggle to finish and then regret for the rest of the night. We might notice that 'quiet but impartial inner knowing' prompting us the next morning that now is a good time to do some exercise but about three milliseconds later a whining and very partial voice protests: 'I'm tired. I don't want to exercise.' This is despite the fact that experience has taught us many times that we feel better for exercising. The mind always seems to be able to find something else to do in order to put off an important or pressing job we would like to avoid. The task is to start to realise the cost of being ruled by this lesser judgment. Start to experiment with making decisions based on our better judgement and see what the effect is. We feel better for getting on with the thing we have been avoiding and feel worse for being dominated by unreasonable impulses, whims and desires.

The better judgment tends to work on 'need' and the lesser works on 'want' or 'don't want'. Not all of the things we want are necessarily good for us, and many of the things that are good for us we try and avoid. At least if we can begin to see what is happening we can start to realise that underneath our impulses, we do actually have a choice. In a state of unawareness we seem to have no choice and self-deception flourishes. Choice and freedom require awareness.

Mindful self-discipline is not brought about by force. Rather it is fostered by seeing what is going on and letting go of that which is of no use. We are really learning to acknowledge and respect what we know within ourselves. Being self-disciplined does not mean that you can't enjoy things or that you must work all the time. In fact, knowing when to stop working and take time for play, rest or self-care is an important but much ignored aspect of self-discipline.

> **Practice for the week:** What governs your day-to-day decisions and actions? In what ways do you see your better and lesser judgments playing out? What are the effects on your wellbeing and functioning when you follow your lesser judgment; and what if you follow your better judgment? What is the effect of putting off something you need to get started on? What is the effect of getting started?

Task 7: Emotions

Emotions are the powerhouse or energy store behind our thoughts, actions and physiology.

Often we get caught up in negative emotions no matter how much harm, divisiveness or discontent they may be causing to us or others. Even when we do notice the effect of a negative emotion we often replace it with another, like replacing anger with self-criticism. The more we fight against or dwell on these emotions the more they seem to impact upon us. The more we react to them the more they wire themselves into the circuitry of the brain. Rather than feeling trapped by this fact we should feel empowered by it because the reverse is also true. The less we react to them, through acceptance and non-judgment, the less binding they become; they become unwired in the brain. As paradoxical as it may seem, the less we try to get rid of negative emotions or criticise ourselves for having them, the more they will recede of their own accord.

Negative emotions tend to overlay the quite natural disposition for the positive. Compassion, for example, is quite natural among those we might think of as being more enlightened. When we become less preoccupied by negative emotions we make space for the deeper, stronger and more useful emotions to surface. We can observe the emotions – negative or positive – just like we observe thoughts. We can choose whether to go with our emotions or not, remembering that those we hold on to will be the ones which control us. It is not implied that we should suppress certain feelings or try not to have them. We may not be able to stop the trains coming, but we can decide which ones to get on. If we let them go by, negative emotions begin to lose their strength and frequency until after a while they cease to come at all. Sometimes, however, negative emotions can be quite strong and persistent, as in clinical depression or panic attacks, and it is often useful to seek specialised help and support to deal with such conditions.

Having a more positive emotional state does not necessarily equate with agreeing with everyone or being at their whim. There may be times when we need to confront an issue or stand up for a principle with clarity and conviction. Here, we may need to let go of fear so that courage and resolution might surface.

Any emotion can have its time or place. Even anger can have its place and as such is not always negative. It may be appropriate in a given situation and to suppress it would be harmful. Appropriate or mindful anger is born of a clear perception of a situation, is not excessive, lasts only as long as it is needed and never has any harmful intent towards self or others. It is supported by reason, embodies an emotional strength to deal with a situation and doesn't leave baggage after the event is over. We feel in control of it, not controlled by it. Inappropriate or unmindful anger is the opposite of all these things. It is unfortunate that about 99% of the anger we express or are on the receiving end of is unmindful.

The person we punish most with negative emotions is ourselves. Others, being in the same predicament as ourselves, also take them out on us, and so the cycle keeps repeating itself, not just among individuals but on a large scale, even between nations.

Negative feelings tend to have their origins in, and are fuelled by, the past. We replay unpleasant memories and so continually reexperience and reinforce deeply entrenched hostility, negativity and the stress which inevitably goes with them. The mindful way out of this predicament is by impartially observing emotional states, being present and exercising a moment-by-moment choice of which emotional trains to get on and which to let pass. It can be useful to gently shift the attention to what we are giving rather than what we are receiving. Forgiveness and opening the heart, for example, can be something to experiment with, firstly in small situations and then bigger ones. Once we come to understand the effect that negative emotions have on us we tend to understand that others are dealing with the same challenges. Over time, mindfulness breeds self-understanding which leads to compassion and tolerance for others. Self-criticism is not a part of the process as it tends to be destructive. Useful and objective self-evaluation is constructive, but criticism is disabling and energy-sapping, slows learning and sabotages constructive change.

> **Practice for the week:** Without self-recrimination, observe the effects on the body, mind and heart of being ruled by negative emotions. How much mental activity do you dedicate to justifying and reinforcing negative emotions? What happens when you fight with a negative emotion? What is the effect of letting go of a negative emotion and taking an attitude of acceptance? When you do let it go, what arises in its place?

Week 8: Expanding self-interest

It is surprising that with so many people around us we often feel isolated and lonely. Social isolation has as much to do with our attitude to the people around us as it has to do with the physical presence of others. We can be isolated while at a party or feel completely integrated while in solitude on top of a mountain.

It is easy to miss the fact that our own wellbeing is inseparable from the wellbeing of those around us. Although separated by things such as distance, culture, class and interest, on a planetary scale we are all like passengers on one big life raft. Our interests are inextricably linked.

When we get into a stress spiral we get more and more self-centred. Our view of the world gets smaller and smaller. Indeed, it is hard to care for others when we do not feel good about ourselves. Often, after a significant breakthrough in reducing our stress, we tend to become more connected and attentive to the needs of others.

If we feel like we are constantly battling everyone else and everyone is battling us, then how can we feel anything but stressed and tired? If we ask ourselves, 'Would I survive more happily and effectively on a life raft where people look after each other or one where people look after themselves only?' the answer is obvious. Which sporting team is more successful and enjoyable to play in: the one with team spirit or the one in which individuals play for themselves only? The latter attitude sacrifices our prosperity as well as our emotional and physical wellbeing.

These considerations can sound like niceties, but they are of immense practical importance. How can the barriers and conflicts between people be broken down? The principles have all been covered in previous weeks – paying attention, letting go, listening, emotions – but now we are also going to focus on enlarging our view from the small, claustrophobic ego boundary to include the family as a whole, workplace as a whole, community as a whole, and so on.

In the process of caring for others we must be careful to leave time for self-care. Mindful self-care is not selfish but is a vital part of being able to care for others in a sustainable and enjoyable way.

> **Practice for the week:** When stressed, how much of your thought, actions and emotions centre on yourself? What is the effect when others are preoccupied with themselves? What is the effect of being responsive to the needs of others? What is the effect when others are responsive to your needs? What is the effect of taking some time for self-care when you need it?

These eight cognitive tasks from the Stress Release Program are outlined more fully in the book *Know Thyself*.[156]

THE IMPORTANCE OF SLEEP

Good quality sleep is crucial to physical and mental wellbeing but is one of the first things to suffer when we are stressed. For the most part modern medicine has come to view the management of sleep problems as simply a matter of drug therapy. In Australia 90% or more of general practice patients with insomnia receive sedatives as the sole management of it.[157][158] This is probably due to the expectations of patients, a lack of training for doctors in non-drug treatments, a lack of consultation time and the enormous influence of the pharmaceutical industry in promoting medications.

This section examines the role of sleep in maintaining health and combating stress, and a range of simple non-drug strategies for improving sleep.

How much sleep is enough?

Sleep problems are common in most 'developed' countries and they tend to be more common the older we get. A large part of this is due to the fact that many chronic diseases, especially those that cause chronic pain, are more common as we age. At any given time, probably around 10% of the general population experience chronic insomnia, and around 1 in 7 people use sedatives on a regular basis. Factors predicting the later development of insomnia included being overweight (35% more likely than average), physical inactivity (42%), alcohol dependence (75%), and having a joint or lower back disorders (195%).[159] Having a major psychiatric disorder increased the risk eightfold.

The long-held idea that eight hours sleep a night is optimal is not entirely accurate but is a useful guide. Long-term follow-up of over 1 million adults showed that an average of seven hours sleep a night is associated with the lowest mortality rates. This is independent of other lifestyle and risk factors. Sleeping an average of nine or more hours or less than six hours per night was associated with higher mortality, as was long-term sleeping pill use.[160][161] Much of this extra mortality is due to an increased risk of cardiovascular disease.[162] These findings were confirmed in another study which found that the risk of heart disease among women was nearly doubled for those who had less than five hours sleep and nearly 60% higher for those who had more than nine hours.[163]

Therefore, the assumption that more sleep is better is not necessarily true, but there is individual variation and our need for sleep differs depending on age and illness. For instance, the very young tend to need more sleep and more than one session of sleep per day.

The benefits of having a siesta have been both supported and challenged by research. Some studies have suggested that having a regular siesta can increase the risk of heart disease and cardiovascular events[164] but other studies have suggested that siestas have a protective role[165], and indeed they are common in countries with low levels of heart disease. Part of the answer as to whether a nap after lunch is protective or harmful may depend on its duration. Shorter power naps seem to be beneficial whereas longer ones – midday sleeps – may be problematic.[166] The reason may be that a true siesta is not about sleeping for two hours; it is about taking time to relax, digest the midday meal, converse with others and to refresh for the afternoon's activity. Taking time to enjoy a lunch with family or friends followed by a short rest – rather than a deep sleep – will relax and refresh us. A longer rest – greater than 20 minutes – where we go into deep sleep is quite a different thing. It upsets various hormones including melatonin which is vital for regulating the body clock. This often makes sleep poorer and broken at night. When we come out of a deep sleep during the day or early evening we often awake feeling groggy and, to use a computer analogy, it requires greater SNS activation – such as adrenaline – to get the system 'rebooted' than it does when we are just coming out of a brief 'hibernation'.[167] Awaking from a deep sleep twice a day doubles the risk of triggering a cardiac event.

Some people are able to maintain excellent health despite relatively low levels of sleep. People who meditate regularly often report that they need less sleep over time. A person's constitution undoubtedly also plays a role as does their ability to deal with stress and the depth of their sleep.

Generally speaking, the depth of sleep is as important as the amount of sleep we get. Sleep has four stages or levels of depth: two superficial levels of dreaming sleep and two of deeper sleep. Much of the time people with poor sleep quality – sleep which is relatively superficial and easily broken – will have more tiredness than those who get less, but deeper, sleep. Severe sleep apnoea – with heavy snoring and periods of stopping breathing during sleep – is another common cause of poor sleep and sleepiness during the day.

Being active during the day, including exercising, will tend to improve sleep at night. In the absence of chronic fatigue syndrome or other significant medical conditions, there are a lot of people who oversleep and yet feel chronically tired. It would be easy to believe that the solution is to get more sleep but a better solution would be to include more activity in daily life and not to sleep past what the body and mind need.

The impact of poor sleep on health and mood

Our state of mind during the day has a profound effect upon how we sleep at night. This, of course, carries over into how we wake up in the morning and our state of mind and energy levels the next day. Significant stress and a lack of adequate relaxation during the day reflects itself in poor sleep. This can be measured in high adrenaline levels during the night. One of the flow-on effects is poor immune function (marked by poor NK-cell activity)[168] which goes some way to explaining why poor sleep problems are associated with susceptibility to infections and other illnesses.

Perhaps an even more important link is that between poor sleep, lowered mood and anxiety. Depression and anxiety affect stress hormones like cortisol which have a negative impact upon sleep patterns.[169] It is easy to get into a vicious circle of stress leading to poor sleep, lowered mood, and more stress. As a result, an increasing number of people these days try to boost their energy with stimulants such as caffeine and energy drinks. Unfortunately these can exacerbate the original problem. Quality sleep is the optimal and natural way to replenish energy and is of central importance to our mental and physical health.

It has been a common assumption in medical circles that in depressed people sleep disturbance is secondary to, or caused by, the depression and this is true, but evidence also suggests that it commonly goes the other way as well. Chronic insomnia has been found to be a major factor causing mood disorders, including nearly trebling the chance of getting depression.[170] [171] [172] In one study insomnia was found to be second only to recent bereavement as a risk factor for depression. Insomnia is a more significant risk factor for depression than having had a previous episode of depression.[173] Another study put the increased risk for depression at four times greater for women and twice as great for men if they suffered long-term insomnia.[174]

A study was done to measure the impact on depression of a non-drug program for improving sleep developed by Melbourne-based psychologist David Morawetz, called 'Sleep Better . . . Without Drugs'. The study found that approximately 75 to 80% of depressed people who went through the program significantly improved their sleep over the following one to two months. Importantly, in 57% of those who improved their sleep, depression was resolved; another 13% showed improvement in their depression.[175] These sorts of findings have been replicated in other studies[176] so we may have to start to rethink our attitudes to the cause and management of depression by giving sleep strategies a high priority.

Although the events initially leading to a sleep problem may have included things such as having a new baby, work pressures or a relationship problem, even after that factor has gone the sleep problem often remains. We develop a mental habit of not sleeping. We build a worry and then an expectation that we will sleep poorly and then proceed to take this attitude to bed with us each night.

Improving sleep

Sleeping pills can play an occasional role in improving sleep if prescribed and taken appropriately, but using sleeping pills regularly for more than a few weeks is enough to create dependency and distort our sleep patterns rather than rectify them. Only a small proportion of patients regularly taking sleeping pills note long-term improvement in their insomnia. A higher proportion report that their insomnia is worsened by them. They can be associated with a worsening of depression and reduced energy. Sleeping tablets also accumulate in the body, particularly in the elderly, and are associated with problems such as falls, drowsiness and lowered life expectancy. They are not a healthy solution to a long-term sleep problem.[177]

It only takes around four weeks to develop a chemical dependency on sleeping tablets and stopping after that time will almost inevitably mean worse sleep for a number of nights. If one has been taking sleeping tablets for a considerable time it is important to withdraw from them slowly and preferably under supervision. If they are ever needed then they are best monitored closely by the doctor prescribing them and only used in short bursts. Alternative drug measures for insomnia include melatonin, an important hormone for our sleep–wake cycle (that is, our circadian rhythm or 'body clock'). It also plays a role in regulating our immune system. For people with Seasonal Affective Disorder – or SAD, in which people experience lowered mood in the winter months – melatonin has also been found to improve sleep quality and vitality.[178] The body can be stimulated to make more melatonin through exercise, healthy diet (tryptophan-rich foods and calorie restriction), meditation, regular exposure to sunlight in the day and avoiding bright lights at night.[179][180] As a general rule, it is better to exercise four to six hours before bedtime in order to derive the maximum benefit.

Maintaining a healthy lifestyle is associated with better sleep and improvements in insomnia. Exercise and improved diet are effective if maintained over time.[181][182] A range of herbal remedies can also have some benefit but whether using melatonin or herbs, it is important to consult a trained health professional for guidance. We will now focus on the more important behavioural strategies for improving sleep.

Tools for better sleep

Following are a range of tools for improving poor sleep. Some of them will apply more to one individual's situation than another's. These strategies, and many more, are outlined in far more detail in

David Morawetz's 'Sleep Better ... Without Drugs' program and other behavioural programs. If sleep problems continue despite the application of the following strategies then it is advisable to seek attention from a trained healthcare professional.

1. **Regularly apply mindfulness, relaxation or other effective stress management tools.** This will help you to not only be more relaxed during the day but also to sleep better and deeper at night. The mental and physical rest attained during meditation can be deeper than even during sleep.

2. **Avoid long naps during the day unless due to illness.** Although short naps can be useful for rejuvenating energy, naps longer than 20 minutes during the day can mean going into deep sleep which starts to alter the hormonal body clock. The body starts to think that it is day when it is night and night when it is day, making it more difficult to sleep well at night. Also avoid falling asleep in front of the television because you will often find that the sleep cycle has been disturbed by the time you go to bed. Of course, if the body is coping with a significant illness then it may well need sleep during the daytime.

3. **Deal with chronic pain and other medical problems.** A chronic health problem with symptoms such as pain or poor breathing can seriously affect sleep. One common problem affecting sleep is sleep apnoea and it needs thorough assessment and appropriate therapy.

4. **Go to bed when sleepy.** Waves of sleep come every 75 to 90 minutes and last for 10 minutes approximately. It is important to work with your body's rhythm and let the wave pick you up and take you when it arrives. Missing the wave makes it difficult and frustrating to try to sleep before the next wave has come. Often when we try to get to the end of a television show or book chapter we push through the wave and miss it.

5. **Avoid lying in bed getting frustrated about not being able to sleep.** Being frustrated and angry about not sleeping activates the stress response. If you haven't gone to sleep within 20 minutes of going to bed then either lie there enjoying being relaxed – that will give as much rest as sleep – or get out of bed and do something restful like reading until the next wave of sleep comes. If you are awoken in the middle of the night and are unable to go back to sleep within about 20 minutes then also apply this strategy.

6. **Avoid excess alcohol, coffee and other stimulants near to bedtime.** Stimulants will make sleep difficult for some hours. A regularly high alcohol intake will also have a negative bad effect on sleep patterns.

7. **Apart from sex, use bed only for sleep.** Many people use bed for things like eating, working and watching television. This can condition us not to sleep when we go to bed. The possible exception to this advice is reading which can assist with sleep for many people. Watching television or playing computer games close to bedtime, particularly for children and adolescents, is associated with poor sleep patterns whereas reading is not.

8. **Adopt a regular sleep pattern.** Going to bed when sleepy at a reasonably consistent time is an important part of sleeping well, but getting up at a regular time is even more important. Many people don't feel sleepy at night, go to sleep late and then feel tired and sleep in late the next morning. This perpetuates a poor sleep pattern and can make us frustrated for not feeling sleepy at a more reasonable hour at night. The important thing is to get up at a reasonable and consistent time in the morning. Although this may be difficult, within a few days the body clock is reset and we feel sleepy earlier in the night.

9. **Avoid being anxious about sleep.** Being angry or anxious about not sleeping has the opposite of the desired effect. We can go to bed braced not to sleep, try to force ourselves to sleep and get anxious or angry when we don't go to sleep or when sleep is broken. Sleep is something we let happen, we can't make it happen. Many people are anxious about their sleep pattern because of a belief that eight or nine hours are mandatory but as little as six hours of reasonable-quality sleep is required for good health. In any case, deep and mindful rest or listening to soothing music will give nearly as much restoration as sleep.

10. **Maintain a healthy lifestyle.** All the other things explored in the Essence model, such as a healthy diet, regular exercise and getting an appropriate amount of sun during the day will have help improve sleep quality at night. Poor sleep is often a symptom of other aspects of life being out of balance.

11. **Deal with other problems.** If poor sleep is due to chronic pain, other health conditions or unresolved problems in daily life then it is important to resolve those issues if possible. Good quality sleep will often restore itself.

3

Spirituality

Spirituality means different things to different people and there is no one way of exploring or expressing it, but it is a basic human need to search for meaning. For many people, spirituality and religion are synonymous, but others primarily pursue knowledge rather than faith, like Socrates or Einstein, and they explore and express spirituality through questioning and inquiry. In that way, philosophy and science rather than faith can be the means whereby we explore the 'big questions'. Spirituality relates to how we find meaning and purpose, how we connect with others in society, and how we understand our place on the planet and within the universe. Others find meaning through creativity, relationships, environmentalism, altruism and social justice.

Spirituality, in the broad sense described above, impacts upon stress and mental health, lifestyle choices, relationships and our coping ability. This chapter explores the relationships between spirituality, meaning and health, and how we can make spirituality an integrated element of our daily life. This exploration aims to be wide enough to be relevant to each person's personal and cultural background. Although most people who call themselves spiritual do so within a religious context, and although religion and spirituality certainly overlap, they are not the same thing. Because of its religious connotations many people would rather avoid the word 'spirituality' altogether and feel more comfortable with the term 'meaning'. For the purposes of this chapter you are encouraged to define, explore and express spirituality in a way which is relevant to your own views and background.

The search for meaning is hard to measure but being able to make meaning of life, and especially of adversity, can be enormously beneficial to mental health when we are coping with major life events. As Carl Jung said, 'The lack of meaning in life is a soul-sickness whose full extent and full import our age has not yet begun to comprehend.'

Spirituality, religion and meaning

An active search for meaning is a vital part of what makes us human. Although many deny they search for meaning, we all do it. We all look for meaning in one way or another, whether it is through:

- Meaningful relationships and how we respect others around us;
- Making a contribution to the world through our work;
- A sense of connectedness and transcending individuality, perhaps through being a member of a political cause or even supporting a football team;
- Science and nature, which give us the opportunity to experience a sense of awe over things bigger than ourselves;
- A respect for social justice, morality and rights;
- Environmentalism;
- Religion.

As individuals, the search for meaning helps to keep us healthy. Meaning is the lens through which we look at the world. Without it an individual or community is soon dispirited and many emotional and social ills follow.[1] One only has to look at the impact of a lack of meaning and purpose on indigenous communities to get a sense of how vital it is.

Most medical and psychological studies on the subject use the terms 'religious commitment' or 'religiosity'. This means taking part in or endorsing 'practices, beliefs, attitudes, or sentiments that are associated with an organised community of faith'.[2] If we adopt the trappings of religious behaviours and attitudes we are termed 'extrinsically religious'. If we hold a strong commitment to a religious ideology we are called 'intrinsically religious'. You could be both intrinsically and extrinsically religious. When it comes to protecting our mental health, intrinsic religiosity has a stronger effect than extrinsic religiosity.

'Spirituality', on the other hand, is far harder to define and measure. It could be defined as 'personal views and behaviours that express a sense of relatedness to the transcendental dimension or to something greater than the self'.[3] It is not dissimilar to intrinsic religiosity and can encompass intangible things such as belief in a higher being, meaning, purpose and connectedness. Obviously religiosity overlaps enormously with spirituality but they are not the same. You can be religious but not spiritual, or spiritual but not religious.

Spirituality and mental health

The widespread decline in mental health in developed and materially wealthy societies is probably due to a number of factors, but an important one is the lack of meaning and spiritual fulfilment which material wealth cannot replace.

In the education and practice of health practitioners issues related to religion, meaning and spirituality are often marginalised. For many years science and ethics have tended to become increasingly secular. Rather than just ignoring spiritual matters, secular science and psychology have at times been openly hostile. Admittedly, when we look at some of the ignorant, foolish or malicious things done in the name of religion it is understandable where some of the criticisms come from. Unfortunately the criticisms often go too far and become blind or aggressive rejections of the spiritual and thus 'the baby is thrown out with the bathwater'. Freud, for example, described religion as 'a universal obsessional neurosis', and the 'mystical experience of unity' as a 'regression to primary narcissism'. Jung, one of the early pioneers of a more modern and enlightened approach to human psychology, saw the search for spiritual enlightenment as the central, but often ignored, core of human experience. Their divergence of views on this subject was one of the main reasons these two pioneers of psychology parted company. The observation that long-term Freudian psychoanalysis may be associated with negative effects on people's mental and physical health throws into question the depth of Freud's understanding of human nature.[4] Despite this, many of Freud's attitudes, or at least the attitudes he gave voice to, have been deeply etched into psychiatric theory and practice. As the psychiatrist D Lukoff wrote, 'Mainstream psychiatry in its theory, research and practice, as well as its diagnostic classification system, has tended to either ignore or pathologise the religious and spiritual issues that clients bring into treatment.'[5]

The negative attitude in many quarters of contemporary medicine and psychiatry is out of keeping with the weight of evidence which clearly shows that having a healthy spiritual life is beneficial for mental and physical health.[6] The findings are consistent whether the studies follow people forward over time or look back at the past. The relationship between spirituality and mental health seems to hold whether the studies control for other lifestyle and socio-economic factors or not. It looks to hold whether or not studies examine the prevention of, coping with, or recovery from illness.

When it comes to depression, youth suicide, substance abuse and violence, we are more often concerned with risk factors than the less publicised 'protective factors'. According to studies on tens of thousands of young people, among the most important protective factors, particularly for adolescents, are 'connectedness' and the oft-neglected 'spirituality'.[7]

In the following discussion of numerous other studies, the terms 'religious commitment', 'religiosity' and 'churchgoers' are used because they are the terms used in the particular studies. However, the findings can be applied to spirituality and meaning in whatever way you personally define it.

A number of studies have linked a lack of religiosity to depression. Religious commitment is associated with a reduced incidence of depression[8] and a significantly quicker recovery from depression.[9] Furthermore, and more strikingly, 13 studies have shown that the greater our religious commitment is the smaller our suicide risk.[10] Typical of the findings is that there is a fourfold increased risk for adolescent suicide for non-churchgoers compared to those who regularly attend.[11] No study showed an increased risk of suicide for churchgoers.

Other studies suggest that religiosity protects against drug and alcohol abuse, one of the most common but maladaptive ways of dealing with mental health problems. One study showed that 89% of alcoholics lost interest in religious issues in their teenage years whereas among those without an alcohol problem only 20% lost interest.[12] Doctors are a high-risk group for substance abuse, but as one study showed, religious commitment while in medical school protects them against development of an alcohol problem in later life.[13] When doctors in the study did develop an alcohol abuse problem, religious affiliation protected them against heavy use, with all its extreme health and social consequences.

There are a number of reasons why people with an active spiritual life are protected against various problems. Such people:

- Often have a high level of social connectedness and support through their religious group;
- Are more likely to receive positive messages about healthy living;
- Engage in beneficial practices like prayer and meditation;
- Have a reduced exposure to violence and drug-taking behaviour;
- May have had a different upbringing or more supportive parenting;
- May deal with mental health and relationship issues better;
- May more easily find meaning amidst life's adverse events;
- May be protected by 'the grace of God' but this is somewhat harder to validate scientifically.

All of these may play an important part but studies that controlled for factors other than religious belief, like lifestyle and social support, still found that a spiritual life independently protected people from certain problems.

The role that a spiritual life plays in fostering good mental health and the ability to cope with adversity goes partway to explaining why it is also associated with reduced risk for physical illnesses such as hypertension, heart disease and cancer.[14][15][16][17] It is also associated with a longer life expectancy. A population study in the USA over nine years showed that death from all causes was significantly reduced and life expectancy increased – from 75 years to 82 years – for those who attended church regularly.[18] These findings are consistent with other data so if countries with other religious or spiritual traditions did similar studies they would probably make similar findings. Again, these findings could not be explained by lifestyle and social factors other than churchgoing.[19]

Examples of the negative effects of religion are generally more newsworthy in the medical and general press than the positive ones. When, for example, someone does an unreasonable or intolerant thing in the name of religion it attracts a lot of attention. This is not an argument against spirituality but rather an argument against dogmatism, intolerance, or blind-faith unsupported by reason. Furthermore, well documented abuses have been perpetrated by a section of religious communities. It is also seen that some people with psychosis will have religious content in their delusions and hallucinations.

Some say that spiritual experiences are merely due to activation of particular regions of the brain.[20] Indeed, stimulating certain parts of the brain electronically can produce elevated or religious experiences. Activity in temporal lobes of the brain is particularly associated with religious and psychological phenomena including blurring of interpersonal boundaries.[21] In religious and philosophical language, people feel like they transcend their individuality or ego boundaries.

Religious experiences are among the hardest to study because they are so hard to define, isolate and measure. Yet undoubtedly, the beneficial effects of religious practices like prayer and meditation partly explain the enhanced health.

SPIRITUALITY AND CLINICAL MEDICINE

Spirituality has sat uneasily alongside medical science and practice, as medicine has become more technologically and materially focused. Spiritual issues are not often discussed between doctors and patients. Perhaps this is because doctors believe that spirituality has little impact upon physical and mental health, that it is unscientific, or that it is someone else's role to talk about spirituality. Evidence, however, suggests that four out of five patients wish to discuss spiritual issues with their doctors, particularly when they are dealing with a life-threatening illness, serious medical condition or the loss of a loved one. They want their doctor to understand their spiritual beliefs because they think it will affect the doctor's ability to 'encourage realistic hope (67%), give medical advice (66%), and change medical treatment (62%)'.[22]

Gauging a patient's spiritual awareness or exploring the ways in which they search for meaning should be a standard part of a thorough medical history. This is especially so when dealing with mental health issues and major illness. One cannot really be said to know another person without an understanding of their responses to the most important questions that we ask ourselves about life's meaning. The treatment of especially sensitive conditions like depression, not to mention terminal illness, will take place in the dark without an understanding of a person's deepest motivations, fears and hopes.

Broaching philosophical and spiritual issues obviously requires skills and sensitivity on behalf of the doctor, and courage, trust and openness on behalf of the patient. It cannot take place meaningfully and successfully without cultural tolerance and the ability to be non-dogmatic on behalf of the doctor and patient. When done effectively it can facilitate counselling and psychotherapy enormously[23] but each person needs to be allowed to explore issues related to spirituality and meaning in their own way. If a doctor or psychotherapist is not religious themselves it does not relieve them of the responsibility to respectfully open up such discussions where relevant. It is then up to the patient or client to decide how far they wish to take the conversation. Part of inviting discussion in a respectful way is the practitioner taking care not to push a line of thought, whether it is religious or secular. Religious, spiritual or philosophical sensitivities and biases, like political ones, can make discussion divisive and difficult.

If there are significant issues or questions uncovered in a discussion on spirituality then the practitioner is more informed and may be able to direct the patient to other channels to explore further. In-depth questions about spirituality and religion – such as spiritual counselling, or interpretation of scripture or doctrine – should probably be referred to culturally appropriate non-medical experts.

Unfortunately, despite the gathering body of evidence, little if any reference is made to spirituality in current medical education and practice. A physical factor with a similar impact on health would certainly not be ignored, but then we should not be surprised that science is comfortable only with what it can easily measure. A perceived lack of a holistic approach is a central reason why many look outside standard medical practice for their healthcare.[24] In coming generations it will be necessary for medical practitioners to become more aware of the evidence of the effect of spirituality on health.

For many, especially the young, the search for meaning is becoming rarer in the hustle and bustle of modern material life. We pursue meaning and fulfilment via as many paths as there are people on the planet, but perhaps we often search for meaning and fulfilment in places which cannot provide it. Though the search may be honest, if it is misdirected then disappointment, stress, depression and social conflict may be the outcomes. Perhaps these issues will become increasingly relevant for coming generations, as the lack of meaning comes at an increasing cost. A balanced form of spirituality which is not scientifically naïve nor culturally intolerant may be a prerequisite for the mental and material wellbeing of a dispirited community and healing profession.

Known health benefits of spirituality[25] [26] [27]

Mental Health

- Reduced incidence of depression and suicide
- Quicker recovery from depression
- Less depression after major surgery and improved coping with disability, illness and stress
- Reduced substance abuse including of alcohol and illicit drugs
- Facilitation of psychotherapy
- Improved palliative care
- Better physical health e.g. reduced incidence of heart disease and hypertension
- Reduced mortality from all causes and greater longevity
- Improved recovery from cardiac surgery
- Reduced incidence of, and longer survival with, (bowel) cancer
- Reduction of lifestyle-related illnesses

THE SEARCH FOR MEANING

It is a basic human need to search for meaning. It is a prerequisite for growth and understanding. It is the firm foundation upon which resilience and coping ability are built so that we can weather the storms of adversity that come our way. It gives life its richness and direction, and gives us fulfilment.

It is up to each of us to search for meaning in a way which is appropriate to us. We all make meaning whether we are aware of it or not. Even if we vigorously question religious assumptions or dogma, it does not mean that we have rejected the search for, or the possibility of finding, meaning. It simply means that we are seeking it through inquiry, reason and knowledge rather than faith.

To live in a world where there appears to be no meaning, or to encourage others to see the world in that way, is to close down the very thing which makes us human. It severely limits our potential for growth and encourages nihilism. When enough people start thinking the same way, it potentially promotes a similar attitude in the community at large. With an increasing number of people seeing life and the world as meaningless, we should not be surprised to observe the growth in influence of those two companions depression and materialism. The soul-sickness Jung referred to is making itself sorely felt. Thankfully, as all things are cyclical, this state will not endure for long.

4

Exercise

It would be hard to come up with a better strategy for enhancing mental and physical health than regular physical exercise. If the benefits of exercise could be put into a pill and patented then we can be sure that it would be in high demand and would cost us an enormous amount of money. The fact is, however, that it is largely free and the side effects are good.

Wherever possible, lifestyle changes should be first-line treatment for illness, not an afterthought. This is particularly true for preventing disease and managing chronic disease. Obviously, in an emergency situation lifestyle changes play a secondary role until after the condition has been brought under initial control, but lifestyle issues then need to be given attention. After the mind, two of the most important therapeutic tools we have are diet and exercise.

This chapter provides background on exercise and its role in health; subsequent chapters will look at how exercise can be used in the prevention and management of specific conditions.

Exercise patterns in the community

A significant proportion of the community are sedentary, that is, they do not do enough exercise to obtain a health benefit from it. In most affluent countries 30 to 40% of people are classified as sedentary and only 15% do regular vigorous aerobic exercise.[1] A survey on physical activity levels among Australian adults[2] found that 43% were not active enough to achieve health benefits. Some members of the population are particularly likely to be inactive[3] such as women, the elderly, migrants and refugees, those with lower education and socio-economic status, and parents with children under five years of age.

In remote rural areas people are more likely to be sedentary than people in metropolitan areas and regional centres. Overall, walking tends to be the most popular form of exercise. Participation in moderate-intensity exercise is low and more than 70% of adults aged over 25 do not participate in any vigorous physical activity on a weekly basis. Men tend to be more active than women in their leisure time. This may be a reflection of the division of family duties and household work as well as attitude to exercise. Exercise frequency and intensity tends to drop substantially once we are beyond the 18–24 age group and bottoms out among the middle-aged, the 45–54 age group. This is unfortunate because this is the exact time when the risk of heart disease, cancer and other chronic diseases starts to escalate. Although uncommon, over-exercise is also a health problem for some because of the level of stress it places on the body.[4]

People have long been known to become less physically active when they leave school, but there is now an increasing trend for children and adolescents to be inactive. Just 20 to 30 years ago the great majority of children walked to school whereas now this is uncommon.

Exercise and health

There are many ways of expressing the same message. You could say that physical exercise protects us against a range of illnesses. Alternately, you could say that physical inactivity, or a sedentary lifestyle, is a risk factor for a whole range of conditions.

Chronic conditions related to inactivity include:[5 6 7 8 9]

- Heart disease and associated risk factors such as:
  - Metabolic syndrome
  - Hypertension
  - Type-2 diabetes
  - Hypercholesterolaemia
  - Smoking and poor nutrition
- Various cancers
- Mental health complaints such as:
  - Depression

- Anxiety
- Osteoporosis
- Overweight and obesity
- Gallstones
- Cognitive decline and dementia
- Infections related to poor immunity
- Insomnia

Physical inactivity is a major contributor to the burden of disease in the community. Figures indicate that it ranks second only to tobacco smoking as a cause of disability and death in Australia.[10] Figures are similar in other affluent countries; in poorer countries where things like poor sanitation, malnutrition and HIV are more predominant, the contribution of physical inactivity to the diseases of ageing is less of an issue. In Australia, physical inactivity accounts for 6% of disease in males (second highest factor, after smoking) and 8% in females (highest factor) and contributes to approximately 8000 deaths per year. The figures, however, ignore the contribution that physical inactivity makes towards other risk factors like high blood pressure, obesity and other unhealthy lifestyle factors.[11] On the positive side, smokers who start exercising are more likely to give up smoking and people who cease smoking sometimes take up exercise for weight control.

For reasons that are not entirely clear, physical activity has a stronger effect on protecting against illness when it is for leisure rather than work, which means we need to be active for a significant proportion of our non-working hours. We can also add to the amount of exercise we do by increasing our incidental or non-structured physical activity, like taking the stairs, using fewer labour-saving devices around the home and walking to and from work or the train station or bus stop.

EXERCISE AND LIFE-EXPECTANCY

There is a consistent relationship between regular physical exercise and a reduction in the risk of death from any cause over a given period.[12] Everyone can derive the benefit of a longer life, even when exercise is taken up in later in life.[13 14] It has been said, of course, that exercise adds years to your life but the down side is that those extra years are spent jogging!

For a middle-aged person, a significant reduction in mortality really starts to become obvious after about two to three years of regular exercise. This means that we can't go for a walk one day and expect that we have halved our morality risk the next. It's a bit like superannuation: the initial contributions don't seem to amount to much but if we keep contributing then after a while there is a substantial investment that can help to protect us in our old age. When it comes to reducing mortality risk, we need a long-term view. Yet there are many other important health benefits which start to make themselves obvious within weeks of starting to exercise regularly; benefits such as more vitality, better mood and fewer infectious diseases.

EXERCISE AND MENTAL HEALTH

Exercise is a powerful strategy for maintaining mental health and treating mental health problems. It can also help the brain to remain healthy, and preserve mental capacities and memory. These issues will be discussed at length in the chapters on mental health and dementia in Part 3.

EXERCISE, OBESITY AND OVERWEIGHT

Obesity is one of the major health problems affecting affluent countries.[15] It contributes to the risk of developing other conditions and risk factors such as diabetes, high blood pressure (hypertension), high blood fats including cholesterol (hyperlipidaemia), gallstones, gout, osteoarthritis and some cancers. It is said that obesity is associated with 90% of Type-2 diabetes, 20% of hypertension, 32% of cancers and 37% of heart disease in non-smokers. Obesity is linked to a lack of self-esteem, social and work discrimination, cancer, asthma, dementia, arthritis and kidney disease. Lifestyles in affluent countries predispose us to metabolic syndrome. This is made up of a cluster of factors: high blood fats including cholesterol, high blood pressure, high blood sugar (which can lead to type-2 diabetes, heart disease, high blood pressure and fatty liver) and obesity around the trunk.

It has been estimated that the cost of obesity in Australia in 2005 was $1721 million. Of this amount, $1084 million were direct health costs and $637 million indirect health costs due to lost work productivity, absenteeism and unemployment. The cost per year for each obese adult has been estimated at $554.[16] Another estimate suggests that obesity and inactivity in China presently account for over 3.5% of that country's GDP and by the year 2025 will account for over 8.7% of GDP.[17] Such is the cost of growing affluence.

Regular exercise is crucial in the prevention of weight gain and the successful maintenance of weight loss.[18] The prevalence of obesity has been increasing due to a convergence of factors such as the rise of TV viewing and computer use, our preference for takeaway and pre-prepared foods, the trend towards more computer-bound sedentary jobs, increased use of cars and effort-saving household appliances, less emphasis on physical education in schools, and fewer opportunities for sport and physical exercise. It is important to note that the increase in overweight and obesity is due more to physical inactivity than overeating and calorie-rich foods. Bernie Crimmins, an Australian doctor with a strong interest in exercise, suggests that 'our genes have not changed but our lifestyle has – ancient genes, modern lifestyle'. In other words, our lifestyle is changing faster than our genes can adapt.

Median 'screen-time' – time spent in front of the television or computer – for Australians between 10 and 13 years is now nearly four hours a day with boys viewing significantly more than girls on average. This is well above the upper limit recommended by most experts of two hours per day. A high level of screen-time is associated with a more than fourfold risk of physical inactivity, more obesity, a higher risk of Type-2 diabetes and poorer sleep patterns.

Surveys of school children in NSW throughout the 20th century show a steady rise in BMI (Body Mass Index).[19] Interestingly, there is some evidence to suggest that the average calorie intake of children actually fell in the decades leading up to 1970, which may indicate that the increase in BMI had more to do with greater inactivity than greater calorie intake.[20]

The BMI, a widely used scale to compare our weight to the healthy ideal, is calculated by the formula:

$$\frac{\text{Weight (kg)}}{\text{Height (metres)}^2}$$

So a 90 kg person who is 175 cm tall has a BMI of

$$\frac{90}{1.75 \times 1.75} = 29.4$$

A person with a BMI under 20 (19 for Asians) is classified as underweight, between 20 and 25 as a healthy weight, between 25 and 30 as overweight, and over 30 as obese. It is worth noting that we can also have a normal BMI but be 'metabolically overweight', meaning that if we are inactive we tend to have too little muscle and proportionately more fat.

Although being overweight according to the BMI is a predictor of being at risk of various illnesses, there is a more important marker of risk. It is not just excess weight but the pattern of weight distribution which is important. Abdominal or 'apple' obesity mostly around the trunk is associated with greater risk. The so-called 'pear' distribution of fat, mostly around the hips and legs, is less of a problem than the apple distribution. One way to measure which category we fall into is the waist–hip ratio. If this is above 1.0 for women or 0.9 for men then a person is said to have the apple distribution of fat; below these figures would be classified as the pear distribution. So if a person's waist circumference was 97 cm and their hip circumference was 93 cm then the wasit–hip ratio would be $\frac{97}{93}$ = 1.04.

The prevalence of overweight and obesity combined in Australia in 2007 was 74.1% in men and 64.1% in women. The overall prevalence of obesity was 30.0% based on BMI. Waist circumference can also be used as a measure of obesity and 44.7% are obese, based on waist circumference (greater or equal to 102 cm [men] and 88 cm [women]). The prevalence of Metabolic Syndrome was 33.7% in men and 30.1% in women.[21]

How weight loss works

Weight is governed by a simple formula. On one side we have 'energy in' – the calories (or kilojoules) in the food we eat – and on the other side we have 'energy out' – from the physical activity we do and from our body's metabolism. We cannot lose weight unless we expend more energy than we take in. Although people tend to be most anxious about one side of the equation – energy in, or food intake – more attention needs to be given to the other side, energy out.

The main user of energy is our Basal Metabolic Rate, or BMR. It is the amount of energy the body uses just to maintain our body temperature, circulation, the functioning of our nervous system and organs such as the lungs, heart, kidneys and so on. In the same way that a car consumes petrol while it is idling at the lights, our body uses energy for all its basic functions – in fact, 70% of our energy is expended this way. Some people have a faster metabolism than others – i.e. their choke is pulled out further – and they find it much easier to lose weight than those with a slow metabolism. However, there is something we can do to increase our BMR: exercising not only burns calories on its own accord but also elevates our BMR for two hours after exercising.

The next greatest use of energy, 20% of the 'energy out', is from the direct effect of exercise. When we exercise we burn calories as fuel to move the body; heat is produced, too. This is called the Thermic (or heating) Effect of Exercise, or TEE. When we exercise vigorously, the TEE increases significantly, as well as the post-exercise effect on BMR.

The remaining 10% of our energy expenditure comes from the Thermic Effect of Food (TEF). The TEF relates to the fact that digesting food is an energy-consuming process in itself and therefore it also burns calories and raises the BMR. Harsh dieting can be a poor weight-loss strategy for many reasons. Firstly, it is not sustainable because it is not enjoyable and doesn't create a positive and healthy attitude to food. Such diets rarely work in the long term. Secondly, such diets are often nutritionally deficient and unbalanced and therefore are associated with a range of health problems. Thirdly, if a diet is too harsh, the TEF is lost and the BMR drops so the person burns fewer calories overall. These are the body's ways of adapting in times of famine. Additionally, the person may have too little energy to exercise. The reduction in 'energy in' due to the diet is largely offset by the negative effects on energy expenditure.

As we become fitter there is an increase in the levels of enzymes that break down fat stores into fuel to power the body. The body's ability to clear fat from the bloodstream also increases. We begin to burn more fat at higher intensity and over a longer duration. Regular exercise also has the effect of improving insulin resistance – that is, it helps the body to become more sensitive to insulin and to clear sugar (glucose) from the bloodstream. All of the above have benefits for decreasing the risk of Type-2 diabetes and improving cardiovascular health. Because of these benefits, the American Surgeon General recently decreed 'Fitness, rather than fatness, should be targeted when addressing the growing problem of global obesity.'

In many ways, it is better for our health if we are fit but carrying a few extra pounds rather than being our target weight but sedentary. Being overweight and sedentary is associated with a whole range of negative metabolic effects.

MET

The MET (Metabolic Equivalents) is a measure of energy expenditure and gives us a guide to the energy being used in various forms of exercise. It can be used as a guide for how much exercise to do, and for how long. The following table is provided as a rough guide to give you an idea of how strenuous various forms of exercise are and how fast they burn calories. Of course, a heavier person will burn more calories (or kilojoules) per hour than a lighter person.

ACTIVITY	METS	Kcal/hr
Sleeping	1.0	80
Desk work	1.5	110
Driving	1.6	120
Sitting	1.4	100
Walking–3km/hr	2	150
Walking–5km/hr	4	330
Cycling	6	440
Swimming	4	300
Tennis	5	420
Squash	8	600
Running–jog	8.7	640
Running–fast	16.3	1200
Shovelling	5	400

The Exercise Prescription

When we decide to begin exercising or modify our exercise program we need to bear in mind our current level of fitness, health and age. Very strenuous exercise is not to be advised for those who are older, unaccustomed to strenuous physical activity or who have chronic health conditions like heart disease. Very strenuous exercise in a person who is at risk of a heart attack can actually precipitate one rather than prevent it. It is therefore better to take a responsible approach and build up over time. Listening to our body and working with it is an important principle to follow. The body needs to feel like it is working, but not feel like it is being strained by the activity.

The simplest and safest way to start is to begin walking, which is an excellent form of exercise and produces many health benefits. For many people it is not vigorous enough to play a major role in weight control because it doesn't raise the metabolism enough, but it is a good way to ease into exercise. We need to walk briskly enough that we feel that we are working, not just dawdling. Nearly all the health benefits of exercise can be gained with a regular level of activity of about 15 MET/week. This equates approximately with 4 hours of vigorous walking throughout the week.

In general terms, we see greater health benefits the more often, longer and intensely we exercise. But once we reach a certain point, the benefits plateau. The maximal benefits of exercise can be gained with one of the following activities – or a combination of them – spaced regularly throughout the week. Higher levels of exertion will certainly lead to greater endurance and better performance but there are no added health benefits such as a reduction in heart disease or cancer.

- Walking briskly for 3 to 4 hours per week;
- Swimming for 3 to 4 hours per week;
- Playing 18 holes of golf 3 times per week;
- Cycling for 2.5 hours per week;
- Running for 2 hours per week;
- Gardening for 4 hours per week.

At very high levels of exercise there are potential health costs. Intense exercise or over-training stress the body and can predispose us to chronic fatigue, musculoskeletal problems, stress fractures and heart problems, depending on the type of physical activity. Immunity can be positively and negatively affected by exercise, depending on the level of activity. Moderate exercise can protect us against catching an infection, but if we have already caught an infection, vigorous exercise can worsen its severity and duration. Regular intense or prolonged exercise can reduce immunity and over-exercise produces a significant allostatic load, or 'wear and tear'.[22] Elite athletes, for example, often have poor immunity and come down with infections quite readily.

The type, intensity and time we dedicate to exercise has to be assessed in light of what we are trying to achieve. For example, an overweight diabetic who is trying to lose weight will need aerobic exercise like light jogging or cycling, compared to a frail and elderly woman who needs to do weight-bearing exercise, like walking or resistance training, to manage osteoporosis. The needs of a person who has recently had a heart attack will be different again, by starting slowly and building up the frequency and intensity of the exercise over a longer period of time.

Age, sex, socio-economic background, disability, medical conditions, body type and level of fitness all matter. As a general principle, it is wise to start slowly, especially if we are older or have been sedentary for some time. It is worthwhile to seek advice from a suitably trained health professional to put together an exercise program that is right for us.

Non-structured or incidental physical activities are also an important part of exercise. These are everyday activities which add to our overall energy expenditure and improve fitness. Examples of non-structured exercise include:

- Leaving the car at home sometimes and walking or riding a bike instead;
- Getting off public transport a stop or two early and walking the rest of the way;
- Using stairs rather than lifts;
- Getting rid of the remote control for the television;
- Turning off the television altogether;
- Using fewer labour-saving devices.

Not everything related to affluence and technology is beneficial. Our use of labour-saving devices is estimated to reduce our physical activity by about an hour per day.

A pedometer, which measures the number of steps we take, can be a useful tool to help monitor our exercise. One approach is to measure the number of steps we take in a normal day (excluding when we are exercising) and then try to double those steps. There are various programs encouraging people to aim for 10,000 steps per day, which is a good goal to aim for. Heart rate monitors can also provide objectivity in training or guidance for those whose heart health may be a concern.

HEART RATE

How much exercise is enough? How intense does exercise need to be? Basically, we need to get our pulse rate up, which is a sign that the body is working, and we need to do it a number of times per week. The general recommendation is that we raise our pulse to 60 to 70% of its maximum level 4 to 7 times per week for 30 to 45 minutes. Our maximal heart rate can be approximately calculated by subtracting our age from 220. For example, a 30-year-old's maximal pulse rate would be 220 minus 30, which is 190 beats per minute. They should raise their pulse to between 60 and 70% of 190, which is a pulse rate between 114 and 133 beats per minute, and they should do this 4 to 7 times per week for 30 to 45 minutes. A 60-year-old's maximal pulse rate would be 220 minus 60, which is 160 beats per minute; they should work towards raising their pulse to 60 to 70% of 160, which is 96 to 112 beats per minute, 4 to 7 times per week for 30 to 45 minutes. A good way to check how we are going is to stop every five minutes or so to measure the pulse rate and see if we are in the target range. Once we have a sense of how strenuously we need to exercise to be in the target range, we don't need to keep checking our pulse rate so often.

TYPES OF EXERCISE

Different types of exercise – aerobic exercise, resistance training and stretching – provide different benefits. All forms of exercise are useful and play different roles. The body burns fat for low-intensity activity and as the intensity increases, carbohydrate and fat tends to be burned. Aerobic exercise is the best way to burn calories but resistance training is also good for maintaining muscle mass and improving the metabolism of glucose and fat, which also aids weight loss. It is useful to have some of each form of exercise in our weekly routine.

Aerobic exercise

Aerobic exercise, which is mainly aimed at expending energy and increasing aerobic capacity, includes walking, cycling, running and other vigorous activities. We know we are expending more energy when we start puffing. This means that the body is taking more oxygen to burn the fuel to maintain the activity. When introducing aerobic exercise into your routine it is sensible to step up gradually from light exercise to more intense activity. Moderate intensity exercise produces a rise in our breathing rate, light sweating, a healthy glow of the cheeks and a 'healthy tired' at the completion of the activity. We should be able to talk as we are exercising.

If we exercise more vigorously we are not be able to speak easily because of puffing. If we can achieve that higher intensity of activity then we should be encouraged to do so, but only gradually and providing the body seems to be tolerating the increase.

Resistance or weight training

Resistance or weight training helps to maintain muscle tone, stability and strength. It has its own benefits, even for the elderly, in whom it is useful for neurological and orthopaedic conditions and in the prevention of falls.[23] It helps to improve our ability to function in daily life, like getting around, doing housework, gardening and hobbies, and is useful for chronic lung conditions.

It is important to take care and seek guidance before commencing resistance training, so that it plays a positive role for us rather than leading to injuries.

Stretching and balance

Although less energy-consuming and providing fewer fitness benefits, stretching, tai chi, yoga and Pilates have an important role to play, particularly in improving flexibility, balance and function, and, for the elderly, reducing falls. They can help us become more aware of our body and posture, and assist in rehabilitation for a wide range of conditions including stroke and recovery from orthopaedic operations. If you have a medical condition it is important to be guided by a trained therapist, such as a yoga therapist, as there may be stretches and postures indicated for some conditions and contraindicated for others. There are professional bodies that accredit highly-trained yoga, tai chi and pilates therapists. Another benefit, in fact, some would say the most important benefit, is that these practices help to focus and relax the mind. Along with other forms of exercise they can have significant benefits for stress reduction.

Fiatarone-Singh, one of Australia's leading researchers in exercise, has compiled a table (below) of which types of exercise are best for specific health conditions.[24]

Exercise prescriptions

Illness	Recommended exercise
Arthritis	Aerobic
	Resistance
Cancer	Aerobic
Chronic renal failure	Aerobic
	Resistance
Heart failure	Aerobic
	Resistance

Coronary heart disease	Aerobic
	Resistance
Dementia	Aerobic
Depression	Aerobic
	Resistance
Osteoporosis and falls prevention	Aerobic
	Resistance
	Balance
Stroke	Aerobic
	Resistance
Type-2 diabetes	Aerobic
	Resistance

THE BARRIERS TO EXERCISE

If we attempt to get back into exercise we may notice that there are many potential barriers making it difficult to translate that good intention into action. Some barriers are real and some are perceived to be more problematic than they really are. It is important to identify these barriers and to find ways around them. Our healthcare professional can assist us greatly with this.

Lack of time

Considering there are 168 hours in a week, 3 hours per week is not a lot to put aside when weighed against the enormous health benefits. We often manage to find time to work too much, to waste time, to watch television, even to worry, but we find it difficult to allocate time for exercise. Lack of time is often a cover for a lack of motivation. It is always easy to find something else more pressing to do when we want to avoid something. Yet it is also harder to enjoy those other aspects of our life – work, family, hobbies, etc. – if we are not feeling healthy.

We need to critically examine our priorities and use of time and then make time available for exercise. Obviously an exercise routine needs to work in with family and other demands. If, for example, our reason for not exercising is that it is more important to spend time with the family, then we can combine exercise with family time by exercising together. Children need it as much as we do.

A solution for those who are capable of it is to exercise at greater intensity. A shorter but more intense exercise session gives many of the same benefits as a less intense but more time-consuming one. Incidental exercise can be another solution, in that we may be achieving another goal – e.g. gardening – at the same time as we are exercising.

There is evidence that exercising in the morning prior to breakfast is better for fitness and weight control than exercising in the evening. That may not always be possible, so exercise whenever the opportunity is available.

Lack of motivation

To combat lack of motivation it is useful to consciously acknowledge the benefits of exercise and the costs of remaining inactive. For those who respond better to the carrot than the stick, focusing on the benefits may be more motivating. Our healthcare professional should be able to assist us with motivation and ongoing encouragement and will hopefully have the stick and carrot at their disposal.

Playing a team sport, having a training partner or personal trainer, or being involved in community schemes can also assist. Making a financial outlay to a gymnasium can improve motivation in that we at least want to get value for our money.

Much more will be said about increasing our motivation in the chapter 'Changing behaviour' in Part 2.

Lack of money

Many people assume that exercising is an expensive pastime, and indeed there are forms of exercise that are expensive such as skiing, hiring a personal trainer or participating in an activity with expensive equipment. These are significant disincentives for those on limited budgets. It is easy to forget that physical exercise can also be free. Walking is free. Digging in the garden is free. Jogging costs the price of some running shoes. Pools are relatively cheap. When we compare the expense of most forms of exercise with what we are prepared to spend on other forms of leisure activity we find that the argument of lack of finances does not have much clout.

Physical injuries and limitations

The exercise capacity and range of appropriate activities of some people may be limited by injuries, joint problems or chronic pain, particularly in the legs and lower back. If we are troubled by such conditions it is important to seek guidance from a trained healthcare professional when developing an exercise program. Where weight-bearing exercise is a problem then there are alternatives like swimming or bike riding, which use the big muscle groups in the legs but avoid the pounding effect of walking or running. Swimming, although less vigorous than running, can be very rewarding and body-friendly. A suggestion for those who have difficulty with swimming is the use of a flotation device such as a pull buoy, which is placed between the legs and makes swimming a lot easier in terms of staying afloat, as well as giving extra work for the upper body.

Those with back problems should bear in mind that for most forms of back pain physical exercise is an important part of rehabilitation and prolonged rest has a detrimental effect. Seeking advice from a doctor, physio or chiropractor about lifing and back care will be important here.

Weather

This can be an important issue to take into account when exercising but it can also be another cover for lack of motivation. In colder months it is easy to be less enthusiastic about going out of doors and exercising, particularly in the mornings. In the warmer months hot weather can be equally problematic. Choosing the right time of day helps, as does dressing appropriately to avoid cold in the winter or heat exhaustion, dehydration and sunburn in the summer. In the summer, exercising early in the morning or late in the day and choosing to swim or go to an air-conditioned gym can help solve the problem, as can exercising outdoors at the warmest time of day or going to the gym or playing an indoor sport in the winter months.

5

Nutrition

We are – or at least our bodies are – what we eat. Although healthy nutrition is obviously important it is not always easy to know what healthy nutrition is and how to bring it into our life. There are many competing views about nutrition and there is probably no one right way to approach it. This chapter provides some general principles and information intended as a guide rather than the final word on nutrition.

Food as medicine

Many of us are aware that too much sugar can affect our child's behaviour, and predispose our teeth to decay and our bodies to diabetes. We may also know that garlic helps to ward off infections, that ginger can reduce nausea, oily fish helps to keep the heart healthy and that prunes can aid with constipation.

Using food as medicine is one of the oldest strategies for maintaining health and treating disease. The wisdom of using food as medicine is just as relevant today as it ever was. Whether we are a gourmet chef or a toasted sandwich connoisseur, we can all learn some simple ways to improve our diet and therefore our health. In recent years evidence has mounted for the importance of nutrition in preventing a range of medical conditions. For example:

- Folic acid, usually at a dosage of 400 mcg per day, is now a standard recommendation for women before they conceive and during the first trimester of pregnancy. It cuts the risk of spina bifida and other neural tube defects in babies by over 70%.

- The Anti Cancer Council has issued a list of cancer-preventing foods. Their report reinforces the value of cruciferous vegetables such as broccoli, cauliflower and cabbage in the prevention of cancer.
- Foods rich in omega-3 fats, such as fish, walnuts and linseed oil, have been proven to help protect against cardiovascular problems. They also have an anti-inflammatory effect for a number of conditions and are associated with a reduction in the risk of dementia.[1]
- Low glycaemic index foods can be used in the diet to manage and help prevent diabetes.
- Honey-based preparations are outstanding for a variety of skin conditions including ulcers, burns, eczema and infections.

There are some medical conditions, such as coeliac disease, for which the management is almost entirely nutritional. Coeliac disease is a chronic disorder of the small intestine triggered when a person who is genetically predisposed to having a gluten sensitivity eats foods such as wheat, barley or rye. (Oats have also been on the list for coeliac sufferers to avoid but there is some research to suggest that they may be safe.[2]) Full-blown coeliac disease is not very common but lesser levels of gluten sensitivity may be more prevalent than first realised. Some adults may have had coeliac disease for many years which was incorrectly labelled as irritable bowel syndrome. Once diagnosed, if these patients omit gluten from their diet, they will make an almost complete recovery.[3]

Nutrition is now known to be crucial for preventing and managing the major lifestyle diseases such as heart disease, stroke and Type-2 diabetes but unfortunately most doctors receive precious little training in nutrition or using food as medicine. Accordingly it is uncommon to find nutrition entering the conversation doctors have with their patients about the prevention and management of chronic conditions.[4] The *US Healthy People 2010* report has as a target that 75% of primary care physician visits for cardiovascular disease, diabetes or hyperlipidaemia include nutrition counselling. The level of nutrition advice given by doctors is nowhere near that figure. For example, data suggests that only 20% of oncologists provide dietary advice despite the clear relationship between nutrition and cancer. Most of that counselling, if given at all, is limited in terms of content and duration.

Doctors have possibly been slow to recognise the importance of nutrition for a number of reasons including an earlier lack of evidence, poor dissemination of evidence and limited training in nutrition. Doctors sometimes find their time with patients is restricted. They are often keen to spend that time talking about other aspects of treatment as many patients don't comply with dietary advice anyway, because they have a negative perception of healthy food or would prefer to take the easier options of taking a tablet or eating fast food. Also, nutrition is considered an unsophisticated intervention compared to technology and drugs; it is too low key, not dramatic enough, for some doctors. For an oncologist to acknowledge that a change in diet might confer a greater survival benefit than the chemotherapy, for example, would be very confronting.

This has meant that much of the responsibility for providing or reinforcing advice on nutrition has fallen to allied health practitioners including dieticians and natural therapists. It has also meant that sound nutritional advice from other health practitioners is often not reinforced by doctors or, even worse, is sometimes undermined by them.

It seems pretty straightforward that the food we put into our body will affect how our body and mind perform. Unfortunately we often take more care of the oil we put in our car than the oil we put in our mouths. The modern diet of most affluent countries is far from optimal. The National Nutritional Survey in 1995 indicated that as a nation Australians were not eating enough vegetables. As many as 30% of Australian women were iron deficient; it is estimated that 40% of diabetics were currently undiagnosed and that one in three Australians did not have enough calcium in their diet and were at risk of developing osteoporosis. In a 1998 study by Sir Richard Doll, diet was found to be the most significant contributor to cancer risk ahead of smoking, so clearly food as medicine has a vital part to play in health maintenance and management. Despite such data the picture for a large portion of the community has not improved in recent years.

Many of the foods used as medicine are useful in the prevention of a whole range of illnesses. This means that by including or increasing just a handful of foods in your diet you can do a lot to improve your overall health and reduce your risk of falling ill.

Nutrition, if you look in to it deeply, is a vast area and one in which there are many conflicting opinions even among nutritional experts. There will always be arguments about specifics and there is probably no one answer to what is the best diet. Therefore the rest of this chapter focuses on general and simple *principles*, providing some specific advice where possible.

One important principle never to lose sight of is that food is to be enjoyed. It is natural to enjoy food in its own right and also the social interaction that is a part of eating with others. This chapter does not aim to create such a high level of anxiety about food that eating becomes a source of stress rather than enjoyment. Being anxious and preoccupied about food will probably offset many of the nutritional benefits associated with eating a healthy diet. It is near impossible to avoid all foods or additives which might be harmful; what matters is the food choices we make as a general rule. Of course, if we are dealing with a major illness then we may need to be stricter with our nutrition but even then, with creativity and the right attitude, the aim should always be enjoyment rather than long-suffering deprivation.

Although this chapter mainly explores food as medicine, there is the issue of herbal remedies and nutritional supplements such as vitamins, minerals and antioxidants to consider. This is a vast area in itself. Some herbs and supplements clearly have beneficial effects, but there are three things are worth saying about them. Firstly, they will never be a replacement for a healthy diet. Secondly, it is worthwhile to seek advice from a suitably trained health professional or at least a reputable and evidence-based source of information before taking remedies and supplements. Thirdly, avoid exceeding the recommended intake. Simply because a herb or supplement might be good for us does not necessarily mean that more will be better. Sometimes natural supplements and remedies can be dangerous if guidelines are ignored.

A balanced diet

Generally speaking, a balanced diet is a moderate but diverse diet. Although eating healthy foods is the rule, a balanced diet also allows for occasional indulgences. The key is to make a distinction between 'everyday foods' and 'sometimes foods', as Dr Rick Kausman, an acknowledged Australian expert, calls them.

Eating a healthy diet is a way of life. Making dietary changes can be difficult initially, so make progressively small changes that are easy to establish; once they are established it is relatively effortless to maintain them.

BUILDING BLOCKS OF A BALANCED DIET

Food is made up of large building blocks known as macronutrients. These are:

Protein	Lipids: fats and oils (including cholesterol)	Fibre	Carbohydrates (including sugars and starches)

Also important but present in small amounts are the micronutrients:

Vitamins, phytochemicals and vitamin-like compounds (including phytoestrogens, carotenoids and flavonoids)	Minerals (including salt, iron and trace elements like selenium, iodine and magnesium)

A balanced diet incorporates the following combination of these nutritional building blocks:

Fruit, vegetables and juices

Eat a wide variety of fruit and vegetables. Aim to eat at least five servings a day in total, only one of which is a starchy vegetable like potato or pumpkin. This amounts to a total of at least 400 grams per day for the average adult. Up to nine serves a day is even better for your health. Unfortunately there has been a downturn in vegetable consumption, with less than 10% of people eating the suggested five portions of fruit and vegetables daily, according to the Victorian Population Health Survey.

Limit bought fruit juices as they have a lot of natural sugar in them (fructose). Although commercially produced fruit juices may say they contain 'no added sugar' they have a high sugar content if they contain fruit concentrate. Just one serve of most commercial juice contains up to between 10 and 15 teaspoons of sugar. Regular consumption is a significant contributor to childhood obesity even although well-meaning parents are trying to give their children a healthy option. Commercial juices also contain none, or very little of, the beneficial fibre you obtain when you eat fresh fruit. They also provide virtually no value in terms of hydration. Juices squeezed at home are far better in terms of calories and nutritional value.

Carbohydrates

Carbohydrates, in the form of sugars and starches, are a crucial source of energy. Eat good-quality starchy foods as this is your body's primary and preferred source of energy. These include quality breads such as rye, sourdough and wholemeal. Other good sources of starch are pasta, potatoes, sweet potatoes, pumpkins, lentils, cereals and grains such as oats, barley, rice, millet, maize, buckwheat and quinoa.

Sugars are a vital part of our diet but unfortunately we tend to have too many refined carbohydrates in our diet relative to the amount of exercise we do. When a carbohydrate-based food is refined it means that we are often eating a lot of sugar but with virtually no nutritional value in terms of fibre, vitamins or minerals. The sugar has been extracted and the rest left out. These are empty calories. Foods with a high content of refined sugar also have a high glycaemic index (high GI) which means that they lead to big surges in our blood sugar. As a consequence the body has to produce large amounts of insulin to clear the sugar from the bloodstream and over time our bodies become far less sensitive to the insulin – a condition known as insulin resistance. This is an important factor in the later development of Type-2 diabetes.

Fibre

Fibre is the part of fruits, vegetables, grains and beans that our body is not able to digest. During digestion fibre is not absorbed and it helps the flow of waste through the bowel. Fibre, along with good water intake, helps our bowels to stay regular and assists in the handling of fats. Most people would benefit by increasing their fibre intake. Improving fibre intake is best done gradually and by consuming foods such as oats, beans, lentils, nuts, seeds, fruit, vegetables, cereals and grains. Warm porridge or an oat-rich muesli is still one of the best starts to the day that you can give yourself.

Protein

Enjoy moderate amounts of good-quality protein from sources such as lean meat, fish, eggs, beans, lentils, nuts and seeds. It is advisable to eat fish at least twice a week, including one serve of oily fish such as salmon, sardines or mackerel because they are also rich in omega-3 fatty acids. If eating red meat, a maximum of 400 to 500 grams is recommended. Processed meats are the least healthy protein option and increase the risk of bowel cancer significantly.

A diet deficient in quality protein may also be one factor leading us to overeat because the body in part regulates appetite so that we will keep eating until protein requirements are satisfied.

Fats and oils

This is a complex area of nutrition. Not all fats are equal and fats are healthy or unhealthy depending on their type and the amount we consume. Eating a healthy balance of fats is an important part of your diet.

Most people need to eat more foods rich in omega-3 fatty acids such as: avocado, oily fish (salmon, mackerel, sardines, whitebait, herrings and kippers), walnuts, sunflower seeds and flaxseed oil or meal. Omega-3 fatty acids can help prevent the development of cancer – particularly of the breast, colon, uterus and skin – depression and bipolar psychosis, Alzheimer's disease, high blood pressure, pre-eclampsia, diabetes, the eye condition of age-related macular degeneration, menstrual syndrome and postmenopausal hot flushes.[5] The normal Western diet contains less than 50% of the recommended daily allowance (RDA) of omega-3 fatty acids. Note that omega-3 fatty acids are heat and light sensitive and the nutritional content of foods containing omega-3 can be impaired by exposing them to light, cooking or storing them for too long. Another healthy oil to include in our diet is olive oil, which has a range of beneficial fats and is an essential part of the so-called 'Mediterranean Diet'.

Generally we need to reduce our intake of omega-6 fatty acids and saturated fats found in animal-based products such as meat and full-fat dairy. Trans-fatty acids found in many highly processed foods such as pies, doughnuts, fried chips, cakes and biscuits are associated with a higher risk of many illnesses and should be avoided or at least kept to a minimum. Margarine, at one time viewed as a healthy option, often has high concentrations of trans-fatty acids.[6] Saturated fats can be reduced by eating less fast and convenience foods, dairy products and meat, and preferring lean meat when it is eaten. Red meat can vary markedly on the amount of fat it contains. For example, kangaroo is approximately 0.4% saturated fat, lean lamb 4.9% and sausage beef 8.7%.

Water

The other important component of our diet is water. It has no nutritional value in itself but is vital in providing the background against which the rest of our metabolism takes place. Good fluid intake also helps to keep our bowels regular. Many people have a deficient water intake which can lead to chronic tiredness, headaches and other symptoms. It is good to try to drink 1.5 to 2 litres of fluid in a day, at least half of which should be plain water. Sweet drinks provide no hydration benefit and should be avoided. Drinks which have a diuretic effect (making us want to go to the toilet to pass urine), such as alcohol, do not provide much hydration benefit; in fact, one of the main reasons we feel so terrible when we have a hangover is dehydration. Sports drinks contain salts and sugars and are designed for rehydration when exercising vigorously. They are not a good choice as an everyday drink.

Antioxidants

Oxidation is a normal part of ageing, like a piece of apple which browns after it is cut. Oxidation is largely due to the effect of naturally occurring substances called 'free radicals'. Modern living is conducive to producing more free radicals such as having a poor diet, by being inactive and experiencing stress. Antioxidants help to mop up and neutralise free radicals and so are an important part of ageing well and remaining vital. Many foods are rich sources of antioxidants like vitamins C and E, or minerals like selenium.

Food additives

Nearly all processed foods contain various additives like artificial colourings, flavourings and preservatives. Some of these are harmless, some we don't know enough about and some are not at all harmless. For example, a recent study in *The Lancet* found a link between certain artificial colours and preservatives in the diet and hyperactivity in children.[7] As a general rule it is good to avoid additives if possible. If we have health concerns which may be related to food additives it is advisable to see a healthcare practitioner trained in nutrition.

Colour balance

There is great wisdom in the ancient notion of eating a range of different colours in our diet. The colour of food – and here we are talking about the naturally occurring colours of fruits and vegetables – can indicate beneficial vitamins and phytochemicals. Each day, try to eat a balance of different-coloured fruits and vegetables. For example:

Orange and yellow

Yellow or orange foods such as pumpkin, squash, sweet potatoes, apricots and carrots are typically high in beta-carotene. It helps our body to make vitamin A, which is vital for healthy skin, hair and nails, protects against night blindness and helps to activate the immune system.

Green

Green foods such as barley grass, spinach and cabbage are typically high in chlorophyll, which is essential for detoxification, reduction of inflammation and the prevention of bacterial growth in wounds.[8][9] It is also thought to be of benefit for anaemia, possibly because its molecular structure is similar to haemoglobin, which carries oxygen in our blood.

Red

Foods such as tomatoes and red grapes are high in lycopenes, resveratrol and other chemicals which are thought to have a role in protection against cancer.

RECOMMENDED DAILY INTAKE (RDI)

We cannot live without the right amounts of vitamins, minerals and phytochemicals on a daily basis. Eating the Recommended Daily Intake (RDI) of these elements will keep us from having major nutritional deficiencies but many experts recommend a higher intake for optimal health and vitality. For this reason it might be better to think of the RDI in terms of 'minimal daily intake'. It should be said, however, that although something is good for us it does not always mean that more will be better. Some vitamins like A and D can be toxic in very high levels so if taking supplements it is important to observe the dosages recommended on the bottle or seek advice from a trained health professional.

Men tend to need a higher intake of vitamins and minerals than women and the amount we need also varies according to our body size, so a range of figures is provided in the RDI table below.[10] Dietary intake of vitamins and minerals is also affected by the quality of the food, method of cooking and the soil from which it comes, so the figures provided for dietary sources are averages.

Recommended daily intake of vitamins and minerals

Abbreviations

g – gram

mg – milligram (one-thousandth of a gram)

mcg – microgram (one-millionth of a gram)

Dietary element	RDI	Role	Good dietary sources
Vitamins			
Vitamin A	800–900 mcg	Vision, bone growth, reproduction, healthy skin; antioxidant	Sweet potatoes, carrots, cabbage, pumpkin, spinach, capsicum, apricots, cantaloupe, mango, liver, eggs
Vitamin B1	1.2 mg	Conversion of food into energy, growth, heart, nervous system, digestion	Peas, spinach, brussels sprouts, beef, pork, wholemeal bread, nuts, soya beans
Vitamin B2 (riboflavin)	1.2 mg	Energy (glycogen) production and release, growth, production of niacin	Chilli, okra, cottage cheese, milk, yoghurt, meat, eggs, fish
Niacin	14–16 mg	Energy, fat and amino acid production and release, skin, intestines, nervous system, manufacture of DNA	Peas, mushrooms, meat, corn, salmon, swordfish, kidney beans, peanuts, soya beans
Vitamin B5 (Pantothenic acid)	4–6 mg	Energy production and breakdown of amino acids, fats and carbohydrates, manufacture of B12 and haemoglobin (in red blood cells), cell membranes	Sweet potatoes, avocado, mushrooms, yoghurt, meat (especially kidneys and liver), salmon, trout, lentils, broad beans
Vitamin B6 (Pyridoxine)	1.3–1.9 mg	Amino acid production and digestion, insulin and antibody production, allergic response, neurotransmitter production, haemoglobin (in red blood cells) production	Pine nuts, bananas, chicken, beef, mackerel, salmon, sardines, trout, tuna
Vitamin B12	2.4 mcg	Growth, haemoglobin (in red blood cells), nervous system, DNA production, processing fats and carbohydrates	Dairy, kidneys, liver, eggs, beef, seafood; vegans may need supplements

Dietary element	RDI	Role	Good dietary sources
Biotin	30 mcg	Conversion of proteins, fats and carbohydrates	Rolled oats, oysters, liver, egg yolks, sardines, soya beans, peanuts, yeast
Folate	400 mcg (supplement recommended during pregnancy)	DNA production, growth, haemoglobin (in red blood cells), healthy foetal development	Corn, asparagus, brussels sprouts, cabbage, cauliflower, leafy green vegetables, avocado, spinach, oranges, liver, blackberries, chickpeas, wheat germ, rolled oats, kidney beans
Vitamin C (ascorbic acid)	200–300 mg	Collagen and strength of bones, ligaments, blood vessels, teeth, growth, tissue repair, wound healing, immunity, iron absorption, red blood cells; antioxidant	Asparagus, broccoli, brussels sprouts, cabbage, capsicum, parsley, tomatoes, blackberries, grapefruit, guava, kiwi fruit, mango, melon, oranges, pineapple, strawberries
Vitamin D	10 mcg	Absorption and use of calcium and phosphorus, bones, teeth, cartilage, immunity	Contain over 3 mcg per 50–100 g: egg yolks, cod liver oil, salmon, sardines, tuna; we need regular moderate sun exposure to ensure adequate vitamin D levels
Vitamin E	7–10 mg	Protection of vitamin A, red blood cell production, clotting; antioxidant	Wheat germ, prawns, almonds, hazelnuts, peanuts, pistachio nuts, soya beans, sunflower seeds
Vitamin K	60–70 mcg	Blood clotting (can interfere with anticoagulant medications)	Asparagus, broccoli, brussels sprouts, cabbage, carrots, cauliflower, celery, peas, spinach, apricots, grapes, pears, plums; also produced by gut flora in the bowel
Co-enzyme Q10	50–100 mg	Healthy heart, improved blood pressure, healthy blood lipid profile, antioxidant	Red meat, fish, broccoli, cauliflower, nuts, spinach, soy products

Dietary element	RDI	Role	Good dietary sources
Minerals			
Calcium	1000 mg	Bones and teeth, blood clotting, nerve conduction, muscle function	Cheese, milk, yoghurt, parsley, sardines, hazelnuts, canned fish with bones, almonds, tofu; absorption of calcium is poor in vitamin D deficiency
Magnesium	350–450 mg	Bone and teeth formation, nerve conduction, muscle contraction, fat and protein processing, assists in calcium regulation, regular heart rhythm, preventing cramps and reducing the risk of gallstones	Whole grains, artichokes, spinach, wholemeal bread, bran flakes, kidneys, meat, beans, legumes (including peanuts), nuts (Brazil, almonds, cashews), sunflower seeds, tofu
Phosphorus	1000 mg	Bones and teeth	Whole grains, oats, dairy, meat, poultry, seafood, legumes (including peanuts), lentils, nuts (Brazil, almonds, cashews), sunflower seeds
Potassium	4700 mg	Water regulation, acid balance in blood, sugar (glycogen) storage, muscle and nerve function, heart rhythm, kidney and adrenal gland function	Whole grains, potatoes, asparagus, avocado, spinach, tomatoes, bananas, cantaloupe, oranges, meat, broad beans
Sodium (salt)	1600 mg	Water and blood pressure regulation, acid balance in blood, nerve conduction, muscle function	Contained in nearly all foods; most people over-consume sodium especially in processed and convenience foods
Sulphur	Not known	Manufacture of amino acids, carbohydrate metabolism, insulin, connective tissue	Bean sprouts, leafy green vegetables, cabbage, raspberries, dairy, meat (especially liver and kidney), egg yolks, chicken, seafood, legumes, nuts

Dietary element	RDI	Role	Good dietary sources
Trace elements			
Chromium	25–35 mcg	Insulin function	Potatoes, broccoli, green beans, tomatoes, apples, bananas, grapes, oranges, red meat, turkey
Copper	1.2–1.7 mg	Skin, hair and eye pigment; bone, teeth and heart development; antioxidant; nerve function, iron processing	Whole grains, liver, seafood and shellfish, nuts (almonds, Brazil and pistachio), sesame seeds
Fluoride	3–4 mg	Teeth and bones	Fluoridated water; also found in toothpaste
Iodine	150 mcg	Thyroid function	Seafood, sea salt, iodised salt
Iron	8 mg men; 18 mg women (may need more if pregnant or menstruating)	Haemoglobin (in red blood cells) production, muscle function	Spinach, dried apricots, offal, red meat, egg yolks, poultry, sardines, tuna, legumes (soya, broad and kidney beans, chickpeas); vitamin C improves iron absorption
Selenium	60–70 mcg	Immune function, thyroid; antioxidant	Brown rice, wheat germ, wholemeal bread, poultry, fish (tuna), shellfish (oysters), Brazil nuts
Zinc	14 mg men; 8 mg women	Breakdown of fats, proteins and carbohydrates, cell growth and repair, DNA production, wound healing, fertility and reproduction, senses	Cheese, red meat, eggs, poultry, crab, lobster, oysters, Brazil nuts, hazelnuts, soya beans

HOW TO READ FOOD LABELS

The ability to read food nutrition panels and other parts of the label is an important skill to develop in order to make informed food choices. Transparency and honesty in labelling is important but hard to legislate for. Clever marketers often find a way to create an impression which is far from the truth.

The ingredients must be listed on the label in order of quantity by weight, from the most to the least, except for water which can be listed at the end. More detailed information is contained in the nutrition information panel, which lists the nutrient components of the food such as the vitamins, minerals, fats and salt. These are given per average serve and per 100 grams, which allows for easy comparison between different products. How much is okay? As a rule of thumb:

- Salt: A low-salt product contains less than or equal to 120 mg/100 g salt.
- Sugar: A low-sugar product contains less than 5% (5 g/100 g) sugar.
- Fat: A low-fat product contains less than 3% (3 g/100 g) fat. Overall, aim for products that have less than 10% fat (10 g/100 g) and are low in saturated fats. Cholesterol should preferably make up less than 20% of the total fat content. Avoid trans fats altogether.
- Fibre: A high-fibre product contains more than 3 g of fibre per average serve.

Maximising sales of the product is obviously the producer's main aim in labelling. If a claim is made on the label such as '99% fat free', 'good source of fibre' or 'contains vitamin C', then by law the nutrition panel must confirm this. If a food or product makes claims about medicinal properties then those claims need to be backed up by clear evidence.

This means that labellers sometimes try to find creative ways to give the impression that a product is healthy. Beware of deceptively worded statements and other techniques like:

- 'No added sugar': This makes us think that a food is low in sugar when in fact it might be high in natural sugar, like fruit juice concentrate.
- 'No added salt': Such foods may still contain yeast or soy extracts like Vegemite or soy sauce as a way of increasing their salt content.
- 'Reduced fat', 'Reduced sugar' or 'Reduced salt': These foods may still be high in fat, sugar or salt though they are lower by comparison to some other brand or variety.
- '30% more' or '60% less': Such labelling doesn't tell you more or less in relation to what.
- 'Light' or 'Lite': Although it may mean low in fat or sugar, that is not necessarily the case. Light in comparison to what?
- '__% fat free': By expressing fat content this way a product may seem lower in fat than it is. For instance a '96% fat free' product

(such as full-cream milk) is in fact a '4% fat' product, which on a label would create quite a different impression on the shopper.

- 'Cholesterol free': A cholesterol-free product may still be high in fats of one sort or another and the amount of saturated fat – not cholesterol alone – in our diet is more influential on our blood cholesterol level. Note that no plant product contains cholesterol, so if you see a plant product with 'Cholesterol free' on the label, the marketers are simply stating the obvious.
- 'Organic': If you want to buy organic, look for 'Certified' on the label, because this means the product actually has been assessed and approved.
- Endorsements: An endorsement on a label – for instance, by a health organisation – may mean that a product is beneficial in one way – it might be low fat or low sugar – but doesn't necessarily mean that the product is nutritious or helps to prevent other diseases. The commercial implications of such arrangements means they are of dubious value – many health organisations are paid handsomely to give their approval to a product.
- Plain English: If the product description and nutritional information is not in plain English on the label, we have to wonder why the marketer doesn't want us to easily understand it.
- Serving suggestions: Pictures of serving suggestions often appear on labels, enticing us to buy the product, but remember that sometimes these suggestions can enhance or diminish the actual nutritional value of the food.

TASTE

Because of our increasing reliance on processed and fast foods, our palates have tended to become used to their high sugar, fat and salt content. This appetite regulation takes place in specific centres in the brain; they are set to require certain tastes. This means that when we change to a healthier diet, food initially will taste unusual or even be tasteless because we have become so used to sugar, fat and salt. Over time this will change as our palates acclimatise to the subtler tastes in fresh, whole foods. We soon begin to notice that the sugary, fatty and salty foods we once craved taste sickly. Making a dietary change can be very difficult if it is too much too fast, as is often the case with crash diets. Smaller, slower changes are generally easier and more sustainable.

OTHER PRINCIPLES OF A BALANCED DIET

- Eat dairy foods in moderation and choose high-quality products.
- Sugary foods such as biscuits, ice cream, snack bars, sweets, chocolate, cakes and high-sugar yoghurts are for special occasions only.
- Limit your intake of high-fat foods such as high-fat cheeses, butter, crisps, chips, fried food, most cakes and biscuits and cream.
- Cook with garlic, onions and ginger for their medicinal properties.
- Avoid processed meats like hams, salami and sausages in order to avoid nitrates used in their processing.
- Avoid deep-fried foods and charred foods because of their fat content and the carcinogens (cancer inducing chemicals) they contain.
- Choose low-salt foods and use salt sparingly to lower your risk of high blood pressure. Many processed foods have higher levels of added salt than we realise.

Food quality and preparation

Eating good-quality food and preparing it well means that you are optimising the amount of vitamins and minerals you obtain from your diet whilst minimising your exposure to harmful chemicals such as pesticides and herbicides. Many chemicals thought at one time to be safe are later either found not to be as safe as first thought or are dangerous in combination with other commonly consumed chemicals and pesticides. The following guidelines will help you to select good-quality food and prepare it to optimise its nutritional value.

CERTIFIED ORGANIC

Food that is labelled 'certified organic' has been grown without the use of pesticides or herbicides, in soil that has also been free of these contaminants for specific amount of time. Many supermarkets, health food stores and markets stock a range of organic fruit and vegetables but read the labels carefully as they can be deceptive. If a product bears the label 'organic' rather than 'certified organic' it was not necessarily produced in accordance with the principles mentioned above.

Apart from reducing our levels of chemical exposure, organic produce has a higher nutritional content. Organic fruit and vegetables have at least a 40% higher antioxidant content and milk produced according to organic methods has a 90% higher concentration of antioxidants. Organic fruits and vegetables also have much higher levels of minerals, in particular iron and zinc.[11] This is because of a range of factors including better quality soil, a longer ripening period, and the fact that the fruit or vegetables are not grown and sold on the basis of size and appearance irrespective of quality.

WHOLE FOODS

When we choose fresh, unadulterated whole foods we get the best possible opportunity for obtaining excellent nutrients and healing benefits. Numerous studies have shown that taking vitamin and mineral supplements is not nearly as beneficial as consuming good-quality foods high in vitamins, minerals and phytochemicals. Real health benefits are achieved from eating real, whole foods. Whole food contains a vast array of beneficial nutrients, some of which we know about and many of which we don't. Refining or processing a food, or isolating one compound from a food, means that a vast array of beneficial compounds are left out. This may be why many of the herbs which are found to have clinically beneficial effects also have fewer side effects than a pharmaceutical being prescribed for the same reason. The natural product probably contains many bioactive compounds, not just one, and probably also contains many unknown compounds which buffer against side effects.

There have been a number of cases where the benefits of a nutrient have been reduced or eliminated when it has been isolated from the whole food. A case in point is beta-carotene supplementation in the prevention of lung cancer. Foods rich in beta-carotene (as well as other vitamins and minerals) are probably protective against cancer,[12 13] yet trials on supplements of beta-carotene for heavy smokers and asbestos workers concluded that it has no protective effect against cancer and possibly even increases the risk.[14 15] In fact, the beneficial effects of eating fruit and vegetables high in beta-carotene in patients with lung cancer is reduced when combined with beta-carotene supplementation.

Choose wholegrain breads and check labels to ensure any soy products you eat use whole soy beans not soy isolates.

FRESH, LOCAL AND IN SEASON

Choose fresh foods where possible. Avoid canned foods when you can buy the same food fresh. For example, steam whole corn on the cob rather than buying canned corn. Snap-frozen vegetables can contain higher levels of some vitamins than fresh vegetables that were picked unripe, transported long distances and then left sitting in shops or at home for long periods. However, frozen vegetables are usually blanched at high temperatures before being frozen, which can reduce their nutrient content, so fresh really is best if the time from paddock to market is kept to a minimum.

Choose locally grown foods as they are likely to be fresher and in season, and less energy will have been used in transport. For maximising nutritional value, eating food in season is important. This can mean soups and casseroles incorporating root vegetables in cold weather, and more cooling light foods such as salad vegetables in summer. The cost of fruits and vegetables are less when they are in season and the ripening is slower and more natural, meaning that the nutritional value is higher. A lot of things happen to a food between it being picked in the paddock before it arrives on the plate.

From Paddock to Plate

1. Chemicals: pesticides, fertilisers, herbicides	5. Packaging
2. Additives: flavour enhancers, colours, preservatives	6. Transport: more food miles if imported or out of season
3. Irradiation	7. Storage – Time spent on store shelf or in storage
4. Refining, artificial ripening and colouring	

GENETICALLY MODIFIED FOODS

We do not yet know the implications of the genetic modification of foods. The promised benefits of GM foods are yet to be established. Because commercial interests are at stake, those who have invested in genetic modification are likely to exaggerate the benefits and downplay the risks. Labelling laws are still being clarified.

COOKING

When preparing food we want to protect the nutrient content as much as possible. The nutritional value we assume is in a food can be significantly diminished by the time it has been cooked and served. Minimising the amount of heat you use in your cooking can help to preserve the vitamins and phytochemicals. Some principles to keep in mind are:

- Cook vegetables for the shortest possible time.
  - Vitamin C, for example, is destroyed by heat.
  - The cancer-protective effects of broccoli are significantly diminished when broccoli is cooked. Fresh broccoli has approximately three times more cancer-protective constituents than cooked broccoli. Folate, important for brain and nerve function and blood cells, is affected by heat.
  - Light can also diminish the nutritional value of some foods. For example folate (in green vegetables), and omega-3 fatty acids in fish and flax-seed oil are light sensitive.
- Steaming and brief stir-frying are preferred cooking methods. In the winter, cooking a casserole slowly on a low temperature is preferable.
- If boiling, use a minimal amount of water because many vitamins and minerals leach out of food into the water it is cooked in.
- In contrast, the level of lycopenes, which have cancer-protective qualities, is higher in cooked tomatoes than fresh.

What influences our food choices?

Many things affect food choices.[16] Nutritional content and hunger are far from the most common. Getting a better understanding of what drives our food choices can help us to make better and more conscious decisions about what to include in our diet.

- **Personal preference:** Depending on what our mother ate before we were born and on what we were fed thereafter, our tastes for particular foods are influenced and determined through exposure. These become our preferences.
- **Habit:** Much of what we eat has become the product of habit and conditioning. We often eat without thinking about what we eat. We also eat because it is time to eat according to the clock or because it is the designated lunchbreak at work, even if we're not the slightest bit hungry at the time.

- **Boredom and emotional distress:** When we are bored or feeling miserable we often eat to provide some pleasure. Unfortunately, when we are feeling bad and use eating as a way to compensate, then we often get into a negative cycle of overeating and addiction.
- **Ethnic heritage or tradition:** Our culture plays an important role in eating patterns and preferences. It influences what we are exposed to, what food we consider acceptable and what aligns with ceremony, religious tradition and celebration. This can work with and against us. The Mediterranean diet, for example, has a range of health benefits whereas the Australian cultural reliance on meat does not work so well. Many cultures have traditional healing systems which have well developed approaches to nutrition. Examples are the Indian system of Ayurveda, Traditional Chinese Medicine and the use of food as medicine among indigenous cultures.
- **Social interaction:** Dining is an important part of our social life; it is a form of welcome and creates an atmosphere of conviviality.
- **Availability and convenience:** Wide food availability can be a blessing and a curse. Easy access to quality food is certainly a blessing, but the abundance of food in affluent countries means that over-nutrition is an increasingly common problem. Taking half the food from affluent countries and giving it to poorer countries would improve the health of both the developed and developing world.
- **Cost:** Unfortunately many people assume that eating a healthy diet is expensive, but the simple principle of eating fresh fruits and vegetables in season is very low cost. Eating slowly and in moderation is low cost. Avoiding sweet drinks, commercial juices and snack foods that provide empty calories would save huge amounts of money for many households.
- **Time:** In an increasingly busy and time-poor world we often choose food on the basis of whether or not we have the time to prepare a meal. Another assumption is that the only sort of fast food available is junk food. Convenience foods can be healthy. Fruit is fast and healthy. So is rice crackers and hommus. A quick stir-fry of vegetables with a little seasoning and tuna can be quick. There are many excellent books crammed with nutritious recipes for the time-poor and for those with a limited budget.
- **Positive and negative associations:** Our present-day attitudes to foods have historical and cultural associations that may no longer

be applicable. For instance, an over-emphasis on dairy and meat may in part be related to the time when these foods were scarce and they were a sign of wealth and health. Many foods deceptively marketed as being healthy may not be. We may have a positive association with the words 'contains real fruit' and 'no added sugar' on a muesli bar or fruit drink, even though it is loaded with empty calories and has little nutritional value.

- **Values:** Our values, for example being compassionate towards animals or environmentally conscious, can influence what we eat. We might choose to become vegetarians or only to eat meat which is farmed in humane and environmentally friendly ways like free-range chicken.
- **Body weight and image:** Although carrying extra weight at one time was associated with affluence and health, now an unrealistically thin body has become the goal for many young people. This has contributed to a concerning rise in the incidence of eating disorders like anorexia nervosa.
- **Nutritional needs and hunger:** All of the above suggests that we often eat for reasons other than need and we often make food choices based on things other than nutritional value. Unfortunately, often the last thing we consider is what the body needs, when it needs it and how much it needs.

A healthy approach to weight management

CALORIE RESTRICTION

If a little is good then more is not necessarily better, and this is certainly true of calorie intake. The overconsumption of energy-dense foods – that is, food high in carbohydrates, sugars and fats – is associated with poorer health and lower life-expectancy in virtually every way that these can be measured. Calorie restriction, on the other hand, is associated with reduced oxidative stress (producing more free radicals that accelerate ageing), cancer, heart disease and diabetes, and with significantly greater life expectancy.[17][18][19] Calorie restriction does not mean starving ourselves but it does mean gradually reducing the empty calories in our diet. An example of a nutritious diet which is calorie restricted is the Ornish diet. See the chapter 'Cancer' in Part 3 for further information on calorie restriction.

SPECIAL DIETS

There are many diets in the marketplace and they raise their own issues. Many of them have the goal of short-term weight loss but are not necessarily nutritious, balanced, based on sound evidence, satisfying or sustainable. Most weight-loss diets will produce short-term weight loss but within one to two years up to 90% of people will exceed their original weight.[20] Over the longer term, dieting is associated with a cycle of overeating and then restrained eating and can lead to a poor attitude to food. It is also associated with depression and poor self-esteem, rebound overeating, eating disorders and poor body image.[21][22]

There is, however, a place for special diets in the context of dealing with particular health conditions. Coeliac disease or gluten sensitivity is not uncommon and is treated by excluding wheat, rye, barley, spelt, oats and their products from the diet. If you suspect that you may be intolerant to gluten – the major symptoms are sometimes vague but include bloating, a variable bowel habit, abdominal pains, weight loss and lethargy – then seek advice from a trained practitioner, as there is no need to go gluten free if you have no medical reason.

During pregnancy it is important to have a healthy and balanced diet but particularly a good intake of folate and other B-group vitamins, calcium and iron. Calorie intake also needs to be higher, particularly in the latter stages of pregnancy, because a woman is not only eating for herself but also for a quickly growing baby. Women who have not reached menopause need extra iron to make up for that lost through menstruation and a good calcium intake to help prevent osteoporosis.

Vegetarians need to keep up with iron intake and those on a vegan diet may require vitamin B12 supplementation, because it is only found in animal products. Those with food sensitivities will need to exclude those foods from their diet.

6 STEPS TO WEIGHT MANAGEMENT

The best diet is a healthy one that we can maintain long-term and modify according to our differing needs at different stages of our life. For optimal health we should be on the lean side of the healthy weight range or BMI of 20 to 25. That having been said, individuals' metabolism and genetics vary, which makes it difficult for some people to achieve that goal. Being fit mitigates the majority of health problems associated with being a few kilos outside the healthy weight range. An important point to emphasise is that nutrition is only one aspect of a healthy lifestyle. WeightWatchers does offer some advice about appropriate exercise but unfortunately most fad diet programs give almost no attention to this other aspect of healthy living.

Dr Rick Kausman is an Australian expert on cultivating a healthy and sustainable approach to weight management. The following points are adapted from this program; for a fuller description of his approach there are several articles,[23] and the book *If Not Dieting Then What?*[24]

1. **Achievable and sustainable goals:** Most rapid weight-loss programs come to naught within two years. Along the way they can reinforce negative attitudes about food and create a sense of defeatism. It is far preferable to make smaller but healthier changes to nutrition and exercise patterns which can become established and sustained. The weight loss may not be as dramatic but it will prove better in the long run.

2. **Positive attitude towards food:** For many people guilt, depression, fear or shame drive the motivation for dietary change. This does not lead to happiness or self-esteem. Common language around food confirms many unhelpful attitudes. We might say or think we are 'bad' or 'wicked' when we eat a sweet or fatty food. Advertising reinforces such ideas with slogans. Often a break in a rigid dietary routine leads to intense guilt and self-loathing as the pendulum swings forcefully from self-deprivation to over-indulgence. We should respect ourselves whatever our bodily weight might be. Eating is to be enjoyed. Rather than using value-laden words like 'good' or 'bad' it is better to use words like 'everyday foods' and 'sometimes foods'. We can indulge occasionally if we want to and when we do we should enjoy the experience but not overdo it.

3. **Non-hungry eating:** Boredom, obligation, habit, celebration and many other reasons influence when and how much we eat. Sometimes thirst can lead to a hunger-like sensation. In fact, so prolonged has our eating pattern been motivated by things other than hunger that we are out of tune with our bodies and we almost forget what hunger feels like. We also tend to ignore the messages our body gives us about when to stop eating. Recognising, respecting and/or re-establishing our body's inbuilt intelligence about what and when to eat is a vital part of eating healthily and maintaining a healthy weight.

4. **Being physically active:** Weight and energy management is an equation of 'energy in' (food) versus 'energy out' (physical activity).

5. **Body image:** For reasons which make little sense, a modern culture has grown up in film, advertising and fashion which revolves around an unhealthily thin body image. This is an image which a significant number of girls and young women – and an increasing number of boys and young men – see as the ideal body type. Low body weight is associated with a significant number of physical and psychological problems. For those with anorexia nervosa an inability to experience the normal bodily messages associated with hunger or to perceive the body's thinness compound the problem. Cultivating guilt about feeling overweight is as unhelpful as aspiring to an unreasonably low weight. Generally, eating disorders co-exist with other psychological and emotional issues which need to be cared for independent of the eating pattern.

6. **Slowing down:** One of the common experiences in eating these days, particularly with the busy lives we lead, is that we don't often slow down enough to taste and chew the food we eat. As such we significantly reduce the enjoyment associated with eating and we impair the digestive process. Furthermore, we don't have time to register when the body has had enough and will often eat more than the body needs. Eating with attention and slowing down can help to remedy such a problem and is one of the reasons why mindfulness-based activities are so helpful for eating disorders such as binge eating.

Further nutritional advice in relation to particular illnesses will be given in Part 3.

6

Connectedness

Connectedness is a term used in research for the level of connection we feel to the people and social institutions around us. We can feel a connection or lack of connection to family, friends, school, workplace and workmates, and our local community. Other terms used for connectedness and the lack of it are social support and social isolation.

Some creatures naturally lead reclusive lives but human beings by nature are social. Ever since we existed we have tended to gather into hunting and gathering groups and, eventually, when agriculture was developed, we formed geographically fixed communities. These communities have steadily grown into the townships and urban environments which we now know. The point is that our survival and continued productivity depends upon our ability to live and work as one. Because connectedness is so vital to our survival it is deeply etched into our natures genetically, psychologically, socially and behaviourally.

The need for connectedness is evident for communities, eco-systems and individuals. Connectedness is closely related to 'harmony', a word derived from the Greek word 'harmos' which means 'to join'. Harmony is a joining of different parts to enable them to work as a unified whole. The enjoyable and productive effects of harmony, whether it is expressed in a community, orchestra or sporting team, are as obvious as the unpleasant and unproductive effects of disharmony. Disharmony goes by other names in the healthcare setting, such as disease and imbalance. The word 'religion' also indicates the importance of connectedness. It comes from the Latin word 'relegare' which means to 'bind or tie together'. Religion is meant to bring us together and unify us. It is indeed unfortunate that religion is so often used as a means of dividing rather than uniting.

Social isolation is a significant risk factor for illness. It is closely linked to poor mental and physical health, independent of other lifestyle factors.

Connectedness can be expressed and fostered in many ways. This chapter looks at its impact upon health and what it means for different people at different stages in their life. This chapter also examines the use of social support in healthcare through support groups.

Social isolation and stress

Social isolation is painful, so much so that various forms of it are among the top ten stressors, according to widely used scales of life stresses.[1] Top among stressors is the grief of losing a family member. Next come things like getting married and marital breakdown, marital reconciliation and divorce. Conflict at work is also amongst the greatest stressors in people's lives.

Most of us some of the time and some of us most of the time, wish to shun social connection. This is not an indication that connectedness is not part of our nature. It is rather an indication that we find the pain of separation so strong that we sometimes attempt to protect ourselves from being close to others in order to avoid the pain of further separation.

The pain of feeling disconnected is expressed in many ways including physical illness, anxiety, depression, low productivity, substance abuse and domestic violence. We have all experienced the pain of disconnectedness whether it be feeling lonely at a party, being ostracised by a peer group or experiencing family breakdown. Thankfully such experiences are mostly short-lived and when we intelligently reflect upon them we can learn and grow. However, when isolation is persistent and severe it brings a lot of other problems with it.

Social isolation is not the same as solitude. Solitude can be healthy, such as taking time to reflect, enjoying peace in meditation or enjoying being alone on top of a mountain. We can be connected and in solitude at the same time. Conversely, we can be among many people and be socially isolated at the same time because we do not feel at home or that we are relating to people in the way we wish to.

Thus, social isolation is more of an internal state than an external one. It relates to how we feel within ourselves and how we are relating to the people and environment around us.

Social isolation and illness

In medical school doctors learn to take the 'social history' of their patient and it is a very important part of understanding a person's health. Until recent times connectedness has been under-recognised as a causal factor in illness. Our level of connectedness determines not just whether we become ill but how we cope with that illness. Some of the illnesses and problems associated with social isolation include:

- Mental illness and suicide;
- Substance abuse;
- Violence;
- Heart disease;
- Infectious diseases;
- Unhealthy lifestyle;
- Loss of social skills;
- Cognitive decline and dementia.

Although social isolation can contribute to these illnesses it should be noted that illness can also contribute to people becoming socially isolated.

As risk factors, social isolation and socio-economic factors make a major contribution to many of the common physical illnesses which doctors treat.[2][3] They are as important as smoking, being overweight or having high cholesterol. If we express this in a more positive way by emphasising the opposite side of the argument, we can say that social connectedness is protective against all of these illnesses and can therefore be therapeutic.

Sociability, for example, predicts resistance to infection. When 334 volunteers completed questionnaires that gauged their sociability they were then exposed to the cold virus and monitored, and it was found that those who were more sociable were less likely to develop a cold. This was independent of social, demographic and other health factors.[4] It has been found that social and productive activities such as games, day trips, gardening, shopping and community work are as protective against death in the elderly as physical activity. These social activities were found not only to reduce mortality but also to improve memory and cognitive function.[5] The level of social support a person with heart disease has is a major predictor of the course of their disease.[6] Those who are socially isolated are far less likely to survive following a heart attack.[7] Men are three times as likely to die from their heart disease in the following six months if they are socially isolated.[8] The effects are especially significant for the elderly, with their risk of death increasing fourfold after a heart attack if they are socially isolated.[9] The level of a patient's social support should not be ignored in doctors' treatment plans. Being married, having contact with family and friends, group affiliation and church membership have all been found to be protective against a variety of illnesses and are associated with greater life expectacncy. One might argue that these results are not due to the direct effect of connectedness but that being isolated means that a person does not seek or have access to medical care, but these results hold even when all those other factors are ruled out.

If a lack of social connectedness makes us sick then the solution lies in improving social structures, attitudes and community values. If relationships are not valued, if working conditions do not make it easy for parents to spend time with families, and if an increasing number of people are having to bring up children as sole parents, then we are not just breeding problems for the current generation but also for the ones coming after.

Connectedness and mental health

In dealing with the problem of suicide, much attention has gone into identifying risk factors and intervening with people at risk. Risk factors for suicide include:

- Depression and the feeling of hopelessness;
- Guilt;
- Substance abuse;
- Physical illness;
- Bereavement;
- Abortion;
- Previous suicide attempts;

- Living alone;
- Child custody disputes and marital problems;
- Family history of suicide;
- Absence of religion or a sense of meaning;
- Being male.

Risk factors generally come in multiples and when they do they have a synergistic effect. This can make the risk of suicide much greater, unless there are a number of protective factors present. Protective factors are the other side of the coin; they help to nullify or neutralise the effects of risk factors. Always thinking of risk rather than protection is rather symbolic of our community's concentration on illness rather than wellness. One of the most protective factors against suicide, particularly for the young, is connectedness.

A major study on adolescents found that connection to the family and at school offered the most protection not just against youth suicide and emotional distress but also substance use and violence. [10] The effect of having multiple risk factors was shown to be enormous, but for those who had multiple protective factors, even if they had multiple risk factors, the risk was reduced to near normal. The most protective aspects of family connectedness were having a parent present in the house, especially at important times like upon waking in the morning, after school, at dinner and at bedtime. Children and parents doing activities together was also very important. The absence of a parent at home, especially where the child had access to drugs and guns, was associated with a whole range of risky behaviours among adolescents. Of course, a large-scale survey like this is perhaps an arduous and expensive way of finding out the obvious.

An adolescent having an antisocial attitude to life is associated with a range of other problems such as a higher risk of mortality, a 10- to 40-fold increased chance of criminal behaviour, psychiatric problems, dysfunctional relationships and a greater need to use health support services.

Among young people who go to a GP for any reason, over 20% will have thought about suicide in the preceding fortnight. [11] Such statistics, along with the almost ubiquitous risk factors in adolescents' lives, can create a sense of fear in the community and a tendency to overreact to the ordinary changes of adolescence. Communities can amplify a problem by becoming anxious and reactive just as an individual can. In dealing with an important and emotive issue like suicide, especially among adolescents, there is a delicate balance between trying not to let vulnerable youth slip through the cracks because of a lack of attention, and amplifying a problem through becoming preoccupied about it.

Promoting protective factors against youth suicide is a job requiring the cooperation of a great many people and groups in society. Policy makers, politicians and funders need to create conditions which are family friendly and conducive to community building. Researchers need to provide evidence that helps to make the case that community building is a major health priority. Schools need to recognise connectedness as a core aim of education and need to be supported by the education system in realising that aim. Parents need to acknowledge the importance of connectedness and be supported in the community and workplace to make family and community a priority. Healthcare professionals need to identify those at risk and provide support, therapy or referral as appropriate. Health professionals can also play a number of other roles such as:

- Raising awareness about the links between social factors and health;
- Providing encouragement and support to people wishing to improve their 'social health';
- Gaining counselling skills to help people with communication, conflict and relationship issues;
- Being aware of local resources and support services;
- Providing support groups within their practice.

Poverty and social disadvantage

Poverty and social disadvantage have an impact on a person's level of engagement or disengagement in the community and can impact upon their mental health and the level of opportunity they experience. For example, studies that have examined the impact of income, education, health status and life-style risk factors on mortality have found that low income is associated with a three-times increase risk over a given time-frame compared with high income groups.[12] This is not explainable by other factors. Taken as a risk-factor for illness, poverty as significant if not more significant than smoking, drinking, being overweight and inactivity. The reasons are likely to be many and varied but will include the fact that those who are from less affluent backgrounds are more often exposed to occupational hazards, have poor access to health care, have higher work stress, are subject to racism and classism, and have less of a sense of control and self-mastery.

Anger, hostility and social disharmony

In recent years there has been an emerging trend towards the fragmentation of community, workplace, school and family. Although the causes of social disharmony appear complex, beneath the surface there may be some simple themes. People need people. We have a basic need to belong to families and communities and this is reflected in our social institutions, moral codes and behaviour. Not only do we need people, but we have a basic need to get along well with others, but there are many aberrations of this, which can lead to social disharmony.

How we learn to deal with difficult emotions like anger during our upbringing has major implications for the rest of our life. There are two particularly important periods of development as far as emotional expression is concerned – early childhood and adolescence – although the brain will continue to mould itself throughout life depending on how it is used. If a child suffers a lack of warmth and nurturing, important pathways in the brain – particularly from the frontal lobes where reasoning and regulation of emotions takes place, to the emotional centre, in the limbic system – are not laid down properly. A family's warmth and nurturing continue to be important through adolescence because these pathways are still not fully developed.[13] This in part explains why teenagers generally have a difficult time controlling their impulses and empathising with others. Adolescents who develop problems with anger also have a larger amygdala – the fear and stress centre in the brain.[14]

If we don't deal with anger in a healthy way it breeds discord and disharmony, and is one of the greatest enemies of connectedness. There are obviously positive and negative ways of dealing with anger. Communicating in a constructive way is central to a healthy expression and resolution of anger but this is no easy skill to develop. Certainly a step in the right direction is to at least not vent anger in ways that are destructive both for ourselves and others, such as through verbal or physical fights or substance abuse. Waiting to discuss an issue until we or others have cooled down is a useful start – if we have the awareness and self-control to do it.

A commonly promoted message, particularly in the media, is that expressing anger in ways such as hitting a punching bag helps to rid one of it. This approach, however, is not associated with a cathartic effect, despite popular belief. Obviously hitting a punching bag is better than hitting someone, but if practised regularly such strategies are actually associated with increased aggression.[15] This having been said, sport can provide a useful outlet for pent-up emotions, provided the principles of sportsmanship are observed, rather than sport just being used as a vehicle for legalised violence. Team sport can be a very valuable vehicle for learning social skills and ethical principles but unfortunately these goals are increasingly taking second place to winning at all costs.

Anger and hostility have detrimental effects on our health as well as our relationships with others. A group of young adults (18 to 30 years old) were followed up for 10 years to measure the effects of hostility on coronary artery calcification – hardening of the coronary artery – which is a sign of rapidly progressing heart disease.[16] Hostility is a personality and character trait associated with an attitude of cynicism and mistrust, and high levels of anger and overt or repressed aggression. Young adults with high levels of hostility were two and a half times as likely to have coronary artery calcification. Those with very advanced coronary artery calcification were nearly 10 times as likely to have high levels of hostility.

One way that hostility presents itself is in bullying. Children tend to be more open and transparent so bullying is easier to identify in them, but in fact it is common at all ages. In adults it tends to be more concealed and covert. Despite the fact that bullying is common it would be difficult to make a case for it being an expression of healthy psychology. In children aged 11 to 16, studies have suggested that bullies are at least as depressed as their victims,[17] with depression among bullies being four times as common than in the general population. They are far more likely to have suicidal thoughts and psychosomatic symptoms. Bullying, whether it is perpetrated by individuals, groups or countries, rather than being an expression of strength is really an expression of aggression masking weakness and vulnerability. It can be the product of developmental problems such as a lack of warmth and connectedness at home, particularly during childhood.

Love, marriage and connectedness

LOVE

There are many different forms and expressions of love, which fall into three broad categories. These roughly correspond to the three main motivational regions of the brain: the appetite (mesolimbic) centre, emotional (limbic) centre and the higher (frontal lobes) centre.

Love which is largely directed to the physical body and the pleasure derived from it corresponds to the appetite region of the brain. It is no doubt enjoyable and vital to the survival of the species because it drives reproduction. If such a love does not include any higher motive then it is probably worthy of that old-fashioned word 'lust'. When overindulged and divorced from higher motivation then it can lead to infatuation, addiction and possibly contribute to depression, particularly in adolescents.[18][19]

There is the love which might be called 'romantic' and which corresponds to the brain's emotional region. Romantic love is born of a strong attraction to another person which is more than just physical. This is the type of love most commonly represented in movies, magazines and folklore, which portray it as always having a happy ending and as going on forever. Studies into the biology of romantic love, however, confirm what everyone already knows: it does not go on forever.

Romantic love is associated with changes in neurotransmitter receptors reflective of high dopamine activity, which is associated with pleasure, reward and addiction; and low serotonin activity, which is associated with lower mood.[20] Biochemically at least, romantic love is a bit like an emotional roller-coaster ride. It is not so surprising that romantic love causes chemical changes in the body – but the fact that these changes are virtually identical to the changes seen in obsessive-compulsive disorder (OCD) can be seen as amusing, concerning or interesting depending on our perspective. Whether it tells us more about OCD or romantic love could be debated, but the researchers also found that in the case of romantic love our brain chemicals tend to revert back to their original state after an average of six months. One suspects that this is when one finds out if there is more to the relationship than just the initial romantic rush.

The third form of love, which corresponds to the higher reasoning region of the brain, might be called 'Platonic'. Love which is worthy of the name Platonic is that which is of the soul or spirit. It has a transcendent quality about it. In this deeper form of love the body is seen as a superficial and less consequential thing.

A lack of or poor quality of deeper relationships, is associated with poorer mental and emotional health, particularly of adolescents.[21] There have been no studies on the biology of Platonic love but one suspects it would correspond with a state of deep peace and quiet happiness.

Platonic love is about the importance of long-term friendship, companionship and being in a relationship where we feel at one. It is about being able to communicate deeper feelings. Such relationships are deeply healing and probably the most important for long-term mental, emotional and social health, despite the fact that lust and romantic love are a lot more alluring. It is Platonic love which Shakespeare reveres in his sonnets when he refers to true love.

Mind you, a long-term and deep relationship between two partners can encompass all of the three forms of love mentioned above. Romance can embrace physical attraction and romantic love can and should mature over time into a far deeper relationship which embraces deeper ideals, like loyalty, compassion, service and gratitude. We have the potential for all of them within ourselves but unfortunately far too much attention seems to be given to the superficial notions of love.

MARRIAGE

The choice to be single or in a long-term, committed and one-on-one relationship is a profound one. The marital relationship – the most widely adopted model of such a relationship – seems to be the most important that we form in our adult years and is clearly associated with health outcomes, for better or for worse. Marriage figures prominently in the top ten life stressors: losing a loved one, getting married, separating, getting divorced and marital reconciliation. The fact that virtually every culture has fostered the family unit based upon the marital relationship probably tells us that it is written into our biology and psyche at a very deep level and is not easily ignored.

Despite some bad press, it has long been acknowledged that marriage is good for health. Married people have lower mortality rates from all causes, including cancer and heart disease.[22] A review of nearly 300 references indicated that marriage, even if it is only moderately happy, is beneficial for social, mental and physical health.[23] Marriage protects both men and women from health problems, although according to many studies it may be relatively more protective for men than women.[24][25][26] Other studies suggest that relationships have a greater impact on women's health than men's, while work has a greater effect on men's health.[27]

Greater companionship and equality in decision-making in a marriage has a strong positive influence on women, but not so much on men. The positive effect of marriage on the health of men is partly related to the improvement it brings to men's lifestyles, hygiene and health habits. This is fairly obvious when we look at most married men who have been left to their own devices for a few days.

Marriage acts as a buffer for stress and protects against depression and other mental health problems.[28] After the initial transition into married life, overall it has a positive effect on coping and emotional health.[29]

A happy marriage is a lot better for our health than an unhappy one, and if our relationship is under considerable stress it is no protection against illness. An unmarried person is likely to be happier and healthier overall than an unhappily married one.[30] In one study it was found that of a variety of psychological and social factors, the single best predictor that a woman would relapse into depression was one question: 'How critical is your spouse of you?'[31] Living with someone who constantly undermines our self-esteem is not conducive to self-development and empowerment. The level of confidence in a relationship is important to understanding links between marital distress and depressive symptoms, especially in women.[32] A lack of confidence leads to ongoing anxiety, instability and insecurity.

When we recall marital conflict, it raises our blood pressure and induces many of the effects of the fight or flight response.[33] This effect is more pronounced in women. It can contribute to high allostatic load – wear and tear on the body – if it is prolonged.

Women with heart disease have a threefold higher chance of relapse and death over the following five years if they continued to live in a stressful marital or other cohabiting relationship.[34]

Marriage status also effects our immunity. Recent bereavement, as we might expect, is a significant risk factor for death from a whole range of causes.[35] Recent bereavement is associated with poor immunity and response to immunisation whereas having a happy marriage is associated with better immune function.[36] Recent separation or divorce is associated with a significant increase in the chance of death from infectious disease, such as a sixfold increased chance of death due to pneumonia.[37] This gives substance to the common belief that an elderly person is more likely to die soon after their partner. There can be even more significant immune problems during marital separation.[38][39]

Marriage can also affect disease progression, severity of symptoms and how well we cope with chronic fatigue syndrome,[40] acute and chronic pain,[41] and cancer. Its effects on these conditions can be either negative or positive, depending on how happy our marriage is. It has also been found that 'social support in the form of marriage, frequent daily contact with others, and the presence of a confidant may all have protective value against cancer progression.'[42]

Getting marital counselling can have a range of positive effects and not only on emotional health. There are even improvements in sperm count for infertile couples who receive cognitive-behavioural therapy (CBT).[43] It can also assist with blood pressure control.[44]

Social support in healthcare

Social support can be provided in the healthcare setting in a number of ways. Firstly, many people, particularly the elderly, find attending a healthcare practitioner as beneficial from the perspective of social interaction, reassurance and comfort as it is from a medical perspective. In a more formal sense, the most common way that social support is built into healthcare is through support groups, group therapy and group-based education.

Support groups are built on a few basic principles although it would be true to say that there is no one way to run a support program. An important principle is that the participants have a common bond, whether in terms of having the same medical condition or confronting the same life issue. They are most often run by health carers and counsellors but many successful groups are run by the participants themselves. Support groups can provide participants with access to information, skills and services. They can also provide a safe place to share concerns, insights and the celebration of breakthroughs. Support groups can be confronting for some people and for them one-on-one support may be more appropriate.

Accessing information is one of the most important reasons that patients seek support. Studies have suggested that the community ranks the most important information sources are doctors, family members, nurses, friends, the Internet, other medical personnel and other patients, in that order. Patients rate nurses, other medical personnel, and support groups as most important while family members of patients tended to be more satisfied with the Internet.[45] The Internet is becoming an increasingly common means of accessing support and information although it does have its risks, particularly for children. Whether the internet is an adequate replacement for actual human contact is unclear. It probably is not, but it may play a beneficial role nevertheless, particularly in people reticent to speak to healthcare professionals. For example, successful mental health and eating disorder programs have been delivered via the internet.[46] Furthermore, it can be a cost-efficient way of delivering services to people who would otherwise not be able to access them.

Social support is also gained in an informal way through our daily social interactions, job, studying in a class, being a member of an organisation or club and by being a member of a family. When we are dealing with any health issue we should draw upon these social connections.

7

Environment

The first law of ecology is that everything is related to everything else.
Barry Commoner – a respected environmentalist in the
early days of the environment movement.

What do the following patients have in common?

- A 14-year-old boy performing poorly at school;
- A 68-year-old ex-smoker living in an inner-city suburb who has a persistent cough;
- A 77-year-old woman living alone who has a hip fracture;
- A 67-year-old Vietnam War veteran who has depression and malaise.

The answer is that all of these cases involve an environmental issue of one sort or another. The 14-year-old boy has had an ongoing low-level lead exposure due to heavy metal residues in the soil where he lives. The 68-year-old ex-smoker has a significantly increased risk of chronic airway disease and lung cancer because he lives near a major freeway entrance. The 77-year-old woman has an increased risk of hip fracture because of social isolation, immobility and lack of sun exposure, which all predispose her to osteoporosis. The 67-year-old Vietnam veteran was exposed during the war to the defoliant Agent Orange.

Environment is so ubiquitous, so much a part of our day-to-day experience, that it is easy to overlook its effects on our health and wellbeing, despite the high level of publicity and public debate about environmental issues such as climate change and pollution.

Environment impacts on us in two ways: directly – such as the impact of drought on agriculture and water quality; and indirectly – such as the impact that drought has on the social cohesion and mental health of farming communities. This chapter explores the physical elements of the environment – earth, air, water, light and space – and the social, emotional and intellectual environments we create for ourselves. It explores the various ways in which environment impacts upon health, and how we can personally foster a healthier environment.

Why do we need to know about the environment?

It is important for everyone to know about the environment. Why?

- Unhealthy environments contribute to many illnesses; equally, healthy environments can help protect us from illness or aid recovery.
- Policy decisions about environmental issues significantly impact upon our lives. It is now a prominent public and political issue which is hotly debated.
- We can influence our own environment by voting in elections, or by becoming active in the environmental movement or at a local level by taking care of our own backyard and neighbourhood. To do so, we need to be well informed.
- We are all citizens breathing the same air, drinking the same water and being affected by the same issues.

What is 'the environment'?

The most obvious way we define the environment is in relation to the physical elements. In classical times it was thought of in terms of Air, Earth, Water, Fire and Space.

These elements are represented today in the environmental issues of soil quality; exposure to chemicals in our air, water and soil; energy consumption; climate and sun exposure; food quality; the sounds we are surrounded by; and space and urban crowding.

We can also think of environment in other, more subtle ways, such as our domestic, social, cultural and intellectual environments.

These, consciously or unconsciously, etch themselves deeply into our character, thinking and behaviour. Consider, for example, how much of an effect being in a crowd of fellow sports fans has on our emotions, sense of identity and how sociable we feel. A casino is a carefully constructed environment designed to encourage a kind of hypnotic mindlessness and timelessness. Everything from the incessant tinkling of coins in poker machines, to the absence of windows and clocks, is designed to capture our attention and condition us to keep gambling. A garden or park can induce other responses, cultivating peacefulness, refreshment and open attention. A health clinic can be set up to convey health messages and inform people. A supermarket checkout with various items on display is designed in such a way to encourage impulse buying. A library, with its quiet atmosphere and partitioned desks, is designed to encourage studiousness and concentration, and to remove distractions. A restaurant can be designed in such as way as to heighten a social buzz or romantic intimacy.

Whether we are aware of it or not, environment has an impact upon us everywhere we go. Some examples of the impact and importance of environment will be explored but there is much more to find out from government and non-government sources.[1]

AIR

Air quality can be a problem anywhere, but it tends to be most problematic in highly urbanised areas. The main sources of air pollution are motor vehicles and industry. Currently 10% of vehicles run on diesel but this 10% of cars produce 80% of fine-particle air pollution. This pollution is the type that finds its way deep into the lungs and contains the highest proportion of harmful chemicals. And the number of diesel vehicles on our roads is rising because of their fuel economy, so although there are gains by reducing greenhouse gas emissions these are offset by pollution. Vehicle emissions have been reduced, but levels are still too high and diesel is still being subsidised.[2] Living on a busy main road that carries heavy transport is a significant risk to health. A study in Europe found that among children under four years old, up to 6.4% of deaths were attributable to outdoor air pollution. Acute chest infections from indoor air pollution accounted for 4.6% of deaths.[3]

It is not just living in a city which increases the risk of becoming ill from air pollution; it matters even more where one lives within that city. Living on a main road is associated with a greater risk of heart disease, chronic lung conditions like asthma and cancer (particularly lung cancer) than living in a side street. Living near a freeway entrance is even worse.[45]

Air quality in the home is also important. There are concerns about some synthetic building materials like formaldehyde used in building materials and furnishings. There are also issues about mould and lack of ventilation. The so-called 'Sick Building Syndrome' has proved difficult in terms of determining how important or common an issue it is but it would seem prudent to give attention to issues like ventilation, dampness, neutral light and building materials in the design of our houses.[6]

Air quality at work also matters, as the spate of asbestos-related cancers indicates. And it is not only health that is affected by poor indoor air quality; work performance and satisfaction can be affected by indoor air quality in the workplace.[7]

Living or working in close proximity to smokers places one at significantly higher risk of all the illnesses to which the smoker is prone, including lung cancer.[8] Depending on how often they are exposed to cigarette smoke, how good the ventilation is and their genes, the non-smoker's risk can be as much as half that of the smoker. Changing the environment can work for everyone; for example, making a place smoke-free not only helps to improve the health of non-smokers but also helps smokers to give up smoking.[9]

WATER

In Australia, 72% of water is used for agriculture but unfortunately much of it in very inefficient or wasteful ways. Growing crops which require high water consumption – such as cotton or rice – on land that is not naturally suited to it not only risks wasting water but also puts the land at risk through salinity and soil degradation. Over-irrigation disrupts river flows, causing the build-up of silt at river mouths and other problems which have a range of environmental 'flow-on' effects, including salinity, soild degradation and loss of river vegetation.

Dry-land agriculture through choice of crops – plants that grow well in dry climates – and watering methods, like drip-irrigation – whether for home gardeners or farmers – offer the most environmentally friendly options. Also important will be the use of rainwater tanks and using grey water in the home and garden.

Chemical- and fertiliser-polluted runoff from farms makes its way into wetlands, the ocean and water catchments, where it causes problems for the people and wildlife who consume that water. This in part explains why waterways have become less viable and increasingly choked with algae. An example of a group of chemicals that affect people are Environmental Endocrine Disruptors (EED), which include many pesticides, herbicides and fungicides used in agriculture. Their chemical structure is like human hormones and therefore they interfere with our natural hormone function. For example, if a man has the EED diazanon in his system he is 10 times more likely to have a low sperm count and infertility.[10] We can be exposed to EEDs through farm work such as spraying crops, eating crops that have been sprayed with EEDs, and drinking contaminated water. Therefore the safe handling of such chemicals, or even rejecting their use at all through organic or biodynamic farming practices, provides important protection.

SOUND

Ambient sounds in the environment can have a positive or negative effect on mental and physical health. Chronic high noise exposure is associated with the same physiological effects as stress. For patients in hospital, excessive background noise is a common problem and it tends to go on night and day. As just another indication that sometimes hospitals are far from the healthiest environment we could invent, this noise exposure is associated with higher stress, decreased wound healing, sleep deprivation and stress on the cardiovascular system.[11] A study on over 4,000 middle-aged patients who were admitted to hospital found that annoyance with daily environmental noise was associated with a significantly increased risk of heart attack.[12] Such noise levels are commonly found in many work environments. Schoolchildren exposed to elevated noise levels have significantly poorer attention spans and adapt less well to social situations. They also show an increased level of opposing behaviour in comparison with other schoolchildren.[13]

We know from experience how much of an effect sound can have. Music, for example, can engender powerful memories along with all manner of associated emotions. Advertisers know that music can engender major changes in mood, thought and behaviour within moments. The therapeutic aspect of music has been acknowledged for thousands of years. The philosopher Plato saw it as being of the utmost importance and as having great potential to do good or harm. 'Musical training is a more potent instrument than any other because rhythm and harmony find their way into the inward places of the soul on which they mightily fasten,' he wrote in *The Republic*.

In contemporary times music has been used clinically for a wide range of health problems. From current evidence it seems that music has great potential as a form of therapy in itself and as an adjunct for dealing with symptoms like pain and stress.

Therapeutic effects of music

- Relaxation, pain and symptom management for a variety of chronic diseases [14] [15] [16]
- Reduction of cardiac reactivity and improvement of cardiac performance [17]
- Reduction of anxiety[18] and physiological stress [19]
- Improvement of cognitive function and memory in the elderly, [20] young adults [21] and children [22] [23]
- Improvement of mood and mental clarity[24] [25]
- Improvement of mood, and cardiac and respiratory function for critically ill patients [26] [27]
- Brain wave (EEG) changes and reduced cortisol in depressed adolescents associated with less stress and better mood [28] [29]
- Increased empathy in children [30]
- Enhanced immunity [31]
- Increased melatonin levels [32]

Music can have positive and negative effects. Classical music, such as Mozart, and slower or more melodious music have the most beneficial effects. Interestingly, playing this type of music in high-risk urban public spaces has reduced crime rates. Jazz has been associated with many positive effects. Happy and bright music can improve mood and vitality levels. There are many very ancient forms of contemplative music from East and West such as the Gregorian Chant, Shakuhachi flute and some Indian ragas which are beneficial, especially in reducing anxiety and improving focus.

On the other hand, harsher, faster and more aggressive music has a range of negative effects on body and mind. When exposed to fast-tempo music children have shown increased aggressive behaviour.[33] Particular personality types are drawn to corresponding music types.[34] Music such as grunge rock is associated with increases in hostility, sadness, tension and fatigue, and decreases in caring, relaxation, mental clarity and vigour.[35] A taste for heavier rock or heavy metal music predicts 'suicidal thoughts, acts of deliberate self-harm, depression, delinquency, drug taking and family dysfunction'.[36] This was confirmed by studies looking at the long-term prevalence of self-harm and attempted suicide. There was a strong association between Goth subculture and a high prevalence of self-harm (53%) and attempted suicide (47%) in a 'dose–response relationship' meaning that the more a person listened to Goth music, the stronger the association was.[37] Punk and Mosher music was also problematic but less so. The explanation is a combination of people at risk choosing certain sorts of music, and the music and cultural environment promoting certain sorts of thought, mood and behaviour. Music with 'degrading sexual lyrics' is associated with a much higher chance of undertaking risky sexual behaviours.[38]

It is important not to judge or condemn any particular type of music, and censorship is certainly a very delicate topic in modern liberal society. Nevertheless, we can 'prescribe' music for ourselves which has the therapeutic effects we want. We can be more conscious of the emotional and physical effects that music has on us. At least we will then be better able to consciously choose those forms of music which produce the physical, mental and emotional effects which we wish to cultivate.

One should remember that regular exposure to loud music and sounds, and even occasional exposure to very loud sounds, can cause long-term hearing loss and tinnitus (ringing in the ears). It is important to wear ear protection when you know you are going to be exposed to loud sounds.

There is much we can do to improve our sound environment. We can, to a large extent, choose what sorts of sounds and music we wish to have in our environment and at the same time reduce the impact that intrusive sounds have by being mindful of our response to them.

SPACE

The effect on health of urbanisation is double-edged. There are the benefits of access to healthcare, sanitation and food, and of having ready contact with people. Then there are the problems of over-crowding and increased pollution, social deprivation, crime and stress-related illness. In less-developed countries, urbanisation also opens the door to diseases prevalent in the West, including high blood pressure, heart disease, obesity, diabetes and asthma.[39] Urban populations in low-income countries have double the rate of communicable diseases like HIV and TB compared to non-urban populations.[40] Closed spaces, especially when poorly ventilated, are also an excellent breeding ground for infections.

How we use space within a building has a significant impact upon us. A small space or low ceiling can create a sense of feeling cramped, especially if there is no natural light or windows or doors to the outside, as in many workplaces. Public spaces, urban design, town planning and the design of gardens and streetscapes can add an enormous amount to the utility and enjoyment of where we live. Apart from their natural beauty they can also make it easier for people to meet and socialise. The wide open spaces found in natural settings, whether in the country or seaside, can have a particularly beneficial effect and we should try to make time for such outings on a regular basis.

CLIMATE

Probably the largest environmental issue confronting us at the moment is climate change. It is undoubted that the climate is changing, and at a faster rate than anyone had predicted. There is no debate that humans are contributing to that change. The exact mechanisms behind climate change and the question of what we should do in response are hotly debated, but the debate is clouded by political and economic agendas, making it difficult to gain a balanced view of the facts before us. Some of the effects of climate change are predictable, others not. Some of the likely effects include an increase in the number and severity of extreme weather events such as droughts, floods and storms, loss of species and biodiversity, rising sea levels due to the melting of the polar ice caps and loss of cultivatable land.

This will likely lead to economic hardship, particularly in the long term, a greater incidence of bushfires due to hotter, drier weather,[41] dislocation of populations and the breakdown of communities, mental health problems and the spread of diseases borne by mosquitoes.

As individuals acting by ourselves there is little we can do about climate change. If we act together as a community there is much we can do about it. To minimise the impact of climate change we need to reduce our reliance on fossil fuels that put carbon dioxide into the atmosphere, producing the greenhouse effect; and we need to nurture and protect trees, which take up carbon dioxide. The trees are the lungs of the planet and it almost seems like the planet has emphysema nowadays. Simple measures we can take are:

- Turn off unnecessary lights, use low-voltage lighting and energy efficient bulbs such as compact fluorescent bulbs;
- Choose energy-efficient appliances;
- Reduce unnecessary driving and drive a fuel-efficient, smaller car;
- The use of biofuels is contentious – they may be more environmentally friendly but contribute to food shortages;
- Build energy-efficient housing;
- Use evaporative air conditioning and minimise the use of refrigerative air conditioning where possible;
- Install an energy-efficient hot water service.
- Use an energy provider who invests in renewable energy sources;
- Invest in renewable energy at home such as solar energy;
- Plant trees and give your support to the creation of green spaces, especially in urban areas;
- Be environmentally conscious when shopping – opt for bio-degradable, earth-friendly products with minimal or recycled packaging;
- Reuse and recycle;
- Be an advocate for environmental issues politically and in your local community.

Sadly, Australia and the USA are world leaders, on a per person basis, in the production of greenhouse gases. Unfortunately, the thinking in some circles has been that it would be economically detrimental to limit greenhouse gas emissions but the simple truth is that a failure to adequately care for the environment will have a far more detrimental economic effect and for a much longer time. We cannot afford not to care for the environment.[42]

SUNLIGHT

Sunlight gets a lot of bad press. It may well be that promoting an important health message – avoid sunburn or excess sun in order to reduce the risk of skin cancer, cataracts and ageing of the skin – has been taken too far according to an increasing number of experts in the field.[43] The message should be to avail ourselves regularly of the right amount of sun exposure, not to avoid the sun entirely. Health promotion campaigns to reduce the incidence of sunburn have been very successful, but probably too successful in that the message is almost solely driven by issues related to the skin.[44] Surprisingly for a sun-drenched country like Australia, we are now seeing problems like bone and other diseases related to low sun exposure.[45] While it is important to avoid sunburn or excess sun exposure it is also important to have regular moderate doses of sunlight.

Much of the health benefit of sunlight comes from the fact that our body uses UV radiation from sunlight to make the active form of vitamin D, which is important for bones, a healthy heart and immune system, and for defences against cancer. We are unable to get as much vitamin D as we need from diet alone.

A healthy recommendation for sunlight exposure, which will keep vitamin D levels high, is 10 to 15 minutes of sunlight falling on most of the body on a day with a UV index of 7, which is an average sunny day not in the height of summer. On a day when the UV index is higher or lower, or less of the skin is exposed, we need to adjust the amount of time we spend in the sun – for example, 20 to 25 minutes would be required if the UV index was 3 and if less of the skin was exposed. For that period of time the skin needs to be free of sunscreen because it absorbs UVB radiation before it enters the skin. An SPF8 sunscreen reduces the capacity of the skin to produce vitamin D by over 95%[46] and an SPF15 sunscreen reduces the capacity by over 98%. Those with fairer skin need to take care with sun exposure as they have a higher risk of sunburn. People with illnesses such as SLE or taking some medications can become sensitive to sunlight and also need to take extra care. In summer months the sun is strongest around the middle of the day so avoid prolonged sun exposure two to three hours either side of midday (or 1 pm during daylight saving).

Sun-derived vitamin D can be supplemented with vitamin D supplements and foods rich in vitamin D. This is particularly important for those who:

- Find it hard to get adequate sun exposure such as the frail and elderly;
- Live in colder climates, particularly in the winter months;
- Have darker skin (melanin, the skin's natural pigment, filters out UV radiation).
- Have their skin covered for cultural or religious reasons;

- Have health conditions such as MS which respond well to vitamin D supplements.

The benefits of sun exposure

Sun exposure has been found to help prevent or treat:

- Coronary Heart Disease
- Cancer
- Mental health problems
- Rickets, osteomalacia (bone softening and deformity) and fractures
- The skin condition psoriasis
- Multiple sclerosis
- Diabetes

Source[47]

Coronary heart disease

The number of deaths from heart disease[48] is higher in colder months, as are people's cholesterol levels.[49] It has also been found that having a higher-than-average level of vitamin D in our body is associated with more than a halving of the risk for heart disease[50][51] and helps in the management of high blood pressure.[52]

Cancer

It is episodic sun exposure causing sunburn, rather than regular moderate sun exposure, that increases the risk of malignant melanoma. If anything, regular moderate sun exposure probably protects the skin from melanoma. But there is more to the sun and cancer story than just melanoma. A study on the potential benefit of regular moderate sun exposure yielded some interesting results.[53] It estimated that due to insufficient UVB and vitamin D, each year 50,000 to 63,000 people in the US and 19,000 to 25,000 people in the UK die prematurely from a range of cancers. Vitamin D deficiency from inadequate sunlight, diet and supplements cost the US an estimated US$40–56 billion in 2004. On the other hand, the cost of diseases due to excess sun exposure was estimated to be US$6–7 billion.

In a population study, it was found that our chance of dying from a number of cancers increases the further away from the equator we live because it means we get less sun exposure.[54] In areas of low sun exposure, such as in cold climates, the risk of breast, colon, ovary and prostate cancer, non-Hodgkin lymphoma and another eight other cancers was nearly twice as high as in high-exposure areas, such as in warmer climates.[55][56] The authors predicted that 'many lives could be extended through increased careful exposure to solar UV-B radiation and more safely, vitamin D supplementation, especially in non-summer months.'

Mental health

It is a normal phenomenon that mood and energy levels become lower in winter months. It is probably nature's way of conserving energy at a time when, historically, food supplies might have been limited. But there is a more serious condition than the winter blues: Seasonal Affective Disorder (SAD), which brings a significantly lowered mood and is due in a large part to receiving less sun exposure in winter.[57][58] A low level of sun exposure is also related to an increased suicide risk.[59][60]

If a lack of sunlight has a negative effect on depression then it has also been shown that sunlight can be therapeutic. 'Dawn simulation' – treating patients with light that simulates dawn – was significantly more effective than 'bright light therapy' and placebo in the treatment of depression.[61] Mental health may be affected in other ways by low sun exposure with some data suggesting that there are higher rates of schizophrenia among those who have inadequate sun exposure.[62][63]

Bone problems

Increasing vitamin D, through sunlight exposure, diet or supplements, protects against rickets and osteomalacia for children and fractures, particularly in the elderly.[64][65] One review concluded that sunshine is also a cornerstone of prevention of osteoporosis, the age-related thinning of the bones and the higher risk of fracture they are prone to.[66]

Psoriasis

Ultraviolet light, from natural and artificial sources, is a well-established treatment for psoriasis, an inflammatory skin condition. However, care must be taken as there are other inflammatory skin conditions – such as dermatitis and SLE – which can be aggravated by sun exposure.

Autoimmune diseases

A large part of the variation in the incidence and relapse rate of multiple sclerosis has to do with the level of sun exposure.[67][68] The overall incidence of MS in Australia varies six- to seven-fold from Queensland

– low rates – to Tasmania – high rates. In tropical countries MS is nearly unknown and becomes more common further from the equator.[69] In one study, over an 11-year period the mortality rate from MS for people who already had the disease was nearly halved if they got regular sun exposure at home.[70] If they also had regular sun exposure in their work then their chance of dying was approximately one-quarter of those who didn't. Australian data has also shown that regular sunlight exposure reduces the chance of developing MS in the first place.[71] Tasmanian studies show that higher sunlight exposure between the ages of 6 and 15, particularly to winter sun, reduced the risk of having MS in adult life to approximately one third.[72] Although the mechanisms are yet to be fully understood, vitamin D and psychoneuronimmunology (PNI) may play important roles. The potential for using sunlight as therapy for MS is yet to be tested but MS patients would be best advised not to wait for the research to catch up. Many MS sufferers can overheat easily and so taking care with sun exposure on hot days is important.

There seems to be a relationship between inadequate sun exposure, inadequate vitamin D and Type-1 diabetes, which is an autoimmune condition (as distinct from Type-2 diabetes, which is related to diet and exercise). A population study found that a low number of hours of sunshine exposure correlated with an increased likelihood of a child developing diabetes; again, as with MS, there is a strong geographical variation in Type-1 diabetes cases.[73] There is increasing evidence that vitamin D plays an important role in helping to prevent and treat a whole range of other autoimmune disorders – such as rheumatoid arthritis and inflammatory bowel disease – because of its anti-inflammatory effect.[74][75]

SOIL

In Australia 5.7 million hectares are affected by salinity or are under imminent threat. That figure is estimated to grow to 17 million hectares by the year 2050. Salinity degrades land available for agriculture as well as the integrity of water supplies. Soil acidification affects 29 million hectares and that figure is projected to reach 55 million hectares by 2050. Land that is affected by salinity or acidification is far less productive. Land clearing and the soil erosion that results from it is another well-known problem that can reduce the land available for agriculture.

Many detergents contain high levels of chemicals, salt and/or phosphates, which means that recycling grey water from washing machines and kitchen sinks by using it to water the garden can be unhealthy for the soil, making it less productive and fertile.

Soil which has become depleted of trace elements such as selenium or the right balance of organic matter and micro-organisms produces crops of depleted nutritional value. Hence, caring for and replenishing the soil is an increasingly important practice for the farmer or home gardener.

Land which has been polluted with chemicals and heavy metals such as lead, for example from unclean landfill, will remain that way. Living on that land can expose people to those chemicals and metals. This is of particular concern in children, for whom lead exposure can delay learning and cause ADHD (attention deficit hyperactivity disorder).[76][77]

ELECTROMAGNETIC FIELDS (EMF)

There is considerable evidence that electromagnetic fields (EMFs) are associated with a range of health problems, in particular, cancer in children.[78] It is all but impossible to avoid exposure to EMFs as they are a part of the natural as well as the manmade environment. Exposure to manmade EMFs can be due to our close proximity to high-voltage powerlines, and use of mobile phones, computers, microwave ovens and other appliances.

There has been a lot of conflicting evidence about the use of mobile phones and increased risk of brain cancer, some studies showing a link and others showing none.[79][80][81][82] If there is an increased risk then it is associated with long-term, frequent use of a mobile phone, holding it up to the same side of the head each time. As to whether we should or should not use a mobile phone, there is not enough evidence to say definitely no, so it is an individual choice we must make, depending on how we measure risks versus benefits.

The use of household appliances like televisions and computers does not seem to be associated with health problems related to EMFs (but there are other health problems related to a high level of 'screen time' such as inactivity, weight problems and, for high television use, cognitive decline). Although appliances like microwave ovens, hairdryers and electric blankets produce EMFs the level is probably low enough that it is not a major health concern; they do not seem to be associated with an increased risk of cancer or other significant illness.

It is becoming increasingly evident that living in close proximity to high-voltage powerlines is a health issue, particularly for children.[83] It has been implicated in a high incidence of cancer, especially leukaemia, and has a negative effect on the body's production of melatonin,[84] which is an important hormone for immunity, sleep and protection against cancer. The safe distance to live from high-voltage powerlines is at least 300 metres.

Creating a healthy environment

How do we create a healthy environment around us? We can do a lot to create a physical and social environment that will help nurture the things we wish to cultivate in ourselves. We can create an environment that fosters a sense of peace, the appreciation of beauty, creativity, fun or privacy. Equally, we can create an environment, knowingly or unknowingly, that fosters unrest, negative emotions, laziness or isolation.

In order to create a quality environment it is important to become aware of the current environment we have created for ourselves. This is simply an aspect of mindfulness. Strangely, we are often quite oblivious to the environment which we have chosen for ourselves and the messages it sends. So first, we need to ask ourselves a number of questions about the environment we live in.[85] When we look around at our environment, does it:

- Make people feel welcome;
- Give a sense of balance, relaxation, wellbeing and comfort;
- Promote interaction between people;
- Nurture physical health (e.g. good ventilation, sunlight, a comfortable temperature);
- Remind us of what is most important to us;
- Promote stimulation, creativity, inspiration and beauty?

Once we know where we need to make improvements, there are some basic principles to follow:

- Use objects and images which are symbolic of principles, things or people we value, like plants, artwork, photos and memorabilia. Also use objects and images which inspire us.

- Ensure there is enough natural light.
- Choose colours which complement the purpose of the room. Pastel colours can be more calming; red and other bright colours can be energizing. For example, most emergency departments are now painted in pastel colours to help calm patients, whereas many retail outlets will use bright colours to attract attention.
- Reduce excess or harsh ambient noise and choose soothing or stimulating music (depending on the purpose of the room) or natural sounds like birdsong or water.
- Clean air is important. If you live in a very polluted place use air filters; otherwise, ensure good natural ventilation. Choose heaters carefully – some gas heaters can leak, and unclean filters and ducts can produce dusty air. Avoid some building chemicals and dust.
- Keep a balanced temperature and choose environmentally friendly heating and cooling systems.
- Arrange seating to allow easy interaction between people and to put them at ease.
- Fill our homes with company which brings out the qualities we wish to cultivate in ourselves and which enhances our mood, attitude, healthy habits and social support.

Once we have given attention to the home environment it might be worthwhile to also look at our work environment and see if there are possible changes that can be made there. It's also worth asking ourselves whether we have enough time in natural environments – like the seaside, forests and parks – to help renew and refresh us.

Part 2
Putting the Pillars into Practice

This part of the book looks at some of the principles of health promotion, behaviour change, goal setting and motivation. Using the information in Part 1 as a guide, we can use these principles to transform knowledge into action. The principles can be applied to a wide range of lifestyles and situations. Together, Part 1 and Part 2 are like the bedrock upon which the advice about specific medical conditions in Part 3 is built.

8

Changing behaviour

Changing behaviour is easier said than done – this is rather obvious to anyone who has tried to do it. It is particularly difficult to change a behaviour:

- Which has been ingrained for a long time;
- Which involves an element of addiction;
- Where the environment is working against the change of behaviour;
- When we are not clear about our goal and how to get there; or
- When we have a mixed motivation for making the change.

Behaviour is deeply rooted in our attitudes, biology, skills and insight, and is modified by the environmental influences around us. Unfortunately, most of the time, we doctors think it is enough to provide some information and make a medical case for behaviour change, but this is of limited benefit. For instance, doctors telling smokers that smoking is bad for their health and providing some medical reasons increases the annual rate at which they quit from about 1% to 2%. What is missing is 'enabling strategies' that encourage us to develop the insights and personal skills we need to take medical information and make the next step into action. When enabling strategies are provided then information is far more effective. In the case of smokers, quitting rates can be improved to around 30% or higher.

Behaviour change skills, motivation, empowerment, health coaching principles, the behaviour change cycle and goal setting are the subjects of this chapter. These topics are at the core of health promotion and health psychology, and can help us to set and achieve goals based on the Essence principles.

Autonomy

Being able to successfully change our behaviour, and maintain that change, requires more than just being given some information by a health expert. As Professor S L Syme, Emeritus Professor of Epidemiology at the University of California, Berkeley, who did much of the early research into heart disease risk factors, said, 'if you want people to change . . . behaviour, you can't do it with proclamations from the top down by experts. Experts need to learn a new way of being an expert, to empower people to participate in the events that impinge on their life.'

One famous study that Syme and his colleagues conducted, the 'Mr Fit Study', suggested that a perceived lack of control is a central factor in the development of heart disease or cancer. Gaining a greater sense of control is consistently associated with better health outcomes.

When we meet with a stressful life event, if we have control over the event – or control over our attitude and reaction to it – we have relatively little disturbance or 'dis-ease' as a result. It doesn't matter whether we are measuring immune function, blood pressure, digestion, brain activity or anything else: a lack of control is associated with significant and prolonged stress and disease. Over time, this begins to leave an indelible mark on our health. For example, in a study of over 800 employees who were followed up for 25 years, high job demands combined with low job control led to more than a doubling of the risk of dying from heart disease compared to workers who didn't face such strains.[1]

Another word for control is 'autonomy', which means 'self-government'. Different regions of the brain equate to different drives and motivations; basically, we have reason, emotion and appetite. Nearly two and a half thousand years ago, Plato said: 'The just man sets in order his own inner life and is his own master . . . and is at peace with himself.'[2] The order Plato spoke about was related to reason balancing and tempering emotion and appetite; in modern parlance we would call it appetite regulation and emotional regulation. So although we aspire to have self-control we do need to consider which part of the self we are going to be controlled by.

An important question is, 'Are all expressions of autonomy healthy ones?' If not all national governments are good then the same might be said of people. Which part of the 'self' would we like to be governed by?

For thousands of years wisdom traditions from virtually every culture – East or West – have suggested that the way to foster enlightened autonomy is to be guided by the rule of reason, supported by positive emotions like compassion, empathy and courage. Together, these are meant to temper the appetites (pleasure, food, money and sex, to name a few). This enlightened sense of autonomy is associated with harmony of mind, body and environment. It is developed from early in life through education, patience and practice.

The control we most commonly recognise in ourselves in modern times is the uneasy balance between tensions and counter-tensions. We know what it is like to be ruled by fear, anger or misunderstanding. This goes on even when our rational mind tells us that there is nothing to fear, that the anger won't help the situation, or that we have jumped to a wrong conclusion. The more we try to 'stay in control' the more we tend to get caught in a cycle of suppression and overreaction. This tug of war between tension and counter-tension is accompanied by stress, anxiety, and conflict, both internal and external. Consequently, our communication is strained, we either make decisions rashly or we procrastinate, our perspective is biased, and we feel manipulated or try to manipulate others. We could hardly call the decisions and actions we make while in this state autonomous in the true sense of the word.

If we think that our lack of freedom has more to do with what is going on around us rather than within us then we are missing the point. Freedom is not just a state of having no limitations or restraints put on our behaviour. It is an inner state. Self-awareness, mindfulness or emotional intelligence – whatever we want to call it – is a prerequisite for personal empowerment and effective action.

Health education which is aimed at giving information but ignores self-empowerment and self-governance is nearly useless in producing sustained behaviour change and better health outcomes. But strategies that empower people also need to be supported by the right environment. A doctor might provide someone with all the information and skills they need to quit smoking, but their efforts to quit will be undermined if they're subjected to a constant barrage of cigarette marketing and always exposed to smokers at work and at home. If we want to increase our level of exercise then living in a safe area with good facilities and parks makes it much more likely to happen. No matter what behaviour change we wish to make, choosing and enhancing our social and physical environments carefully is both a community and individual responsibility.

Health Promotion[3]

Because health is dependent on so many factors – the 'determinants of health' – promoting health, whether it is of individuals or communities, needs to take many factors into consideration. Health is affected by our socio-economic status, our social supports, the level of education we receive, our employment (or the lack of it), and our physical environment. Health will be modified by our personal health behaviours, our upbringing, the access to health services and our culture as well as our gender and genetic inheritance.

To put this into a practical context, the road toll among young males is a major indictment on our community. It is largely contributed to by alcohol abuse and speed. Helping young males avoid binge-drinking, drink-driving and speeding requires attention to the attitudes and skills of young males. These are not necessarily easy to change at a time in life when there is a confluence of circumstances like a feeling of immortality, over-confidence, and a still rudimentary ability to control impulses. All this is taking place at the same time as they are attaining new-found freedoms. Most cope with this well, but many don't. Success in reducing the road toll for young males can be greatly assisted by things such as legislation (laws on alcohol consumption and drink-driving), changes to alcohol advertising, increasing the price of alcohol, and social marketing aimed at changing attitudes to drink-driving. It also requires providing alternatives to, firstly, drinking excess alcohol (e.g. making water available in clubs and pubs) and, secondly, driving while drunk (e.g. providing adequate public transport). These strategies work and save a huge amount of social, emotional and economic waste. For example, since 1989, the Transport Accident Commission has saved the Victorian community more than AUS$4 billion. Road fatalities have gone from over 1000 to approximately 300 over a time when the population has nearly doubled and the number of cars on the road has trebled. It has also been done on a relatively small budget when weighed in the balances with the costs saved.

A population approach is far more cost-effective than treating individuals. This is well illustrated in the reduced rates of many infectious diseases through immunisation. Illnesses such as measles are uncommon now. Polio is rare but still around. Smallpox has all but been eradicated.

Major Health Promotion successes in Victoria have included:

- Tobacco control;
- Reducing road trauma;
- HIV/AIDS control;
- Skin cancer prevention.

Now less than 17% of adults smoke whereas the figure was around 75% among males 50 years ago. The effects of this change will be increasingly felt in coming generations. In the mid 1980's the number of new HIV/AIDS cases per year in Australia was over 2300. Now that figure has dropped to around 700 per year. Skin cancer rates – most importantly the rates of malignant melanoma – have dropped in recent years. This is largely due to the weekend sunburn rates falling by 60% in Victoria between 1988 and 1998. Changing the Australian culture to view sunbaking in a different light has taken generations.

VicHealth figures suggest that, per life-year gained, smoking prevention costs approximately 1/500th as much as treating lung cancer. The treatment for AIDS in Australia in 1993 cost over $46,000 per life-year gained whereas it only costs $185 per life-year gained when the money is spent on preventing HIV infection. Unfortunately, there is also money to be made by some segments of the community in marketing things like smoking, alcohol and unhealthy foods. There is also a big market in promoting pharmaceuticals rather than preventive strategies. Hence, much health promotion is a marketing war vying for the hearts and minds of the community, and there is no greater prize in this regard than influencing the young in our community.

According to the experts, successful Health Promotion is dependent on a number of factors.

1. HAVE GOOD BACKGROUND DATA AND INFORMATION

Not only do we need to know things like which health problems are prevalent and who they affect, but it is also important to know how effective any interventions or programs are. Thus unbiased research, data and evidence are vital.

2. CLEAR AND SENSIBLE POLICY, LEGISLATION AND REGULATION

The policies of organisations and political parties set the agenda. They can also support or undermine any attempts to implement effective strategies. Positive examples of using legislation to enhance health, some of which were given above, include tobacco, alcohol, speeding and the wearing of seatbelts.

3. QUALITY COMMUNICATION

Communicating well with the community, and advocacy to policy-makers on behalf of the community, can make or break health promotion initiatives. Communication also includes education, enhancing motivation, changing attitudes, improving cooperation, and the provision of practical information about services.

4. WELL TRAINED AND DIVERSE PROFESSIONALS

It goes without saying that you need well trained healthcare workers to see that initiatives are well planned and effectively delivered. Those involved with implementing health promotion are not just doctors and nurses but include those providing counselling, screening, marketing, education, business support, sporting bodies, those involved with the arts, police, media and local government.

5. ENCOURAGING COMMUNITY INVOLVEMENT

Health promotion is implemented through the community, by the community and for the community. Without community engagement, inspiration and support any initiative will be bound to be far less effective and will waste resources.

6. POLITICAL SUPPORT AND FUNDING

Without ongoing political support and funding even the best ideas in the world will come to little. An important aspect of the success of health promotion initiatives is that the political and financial support does not become politicised in a way that it undermines the job that is there to be done.

Motivation

Our reasons for acting the way we do are often unseen by us and therefore unexamined. As such, habits and assumptions rule. Being able to understand our competing motivations for our behaviours is an important first step in being able to change them. Often we don't look at the pros and cons for continuing to follow a particular line of action. At least if we examine the pros and cons then our choices will be more conscious and we will have less reason to feel put upon if we suffer the negative consequences of an unhealthy behaviour.

As an example, if we eat an unhealthy diet, consciously or unconsciously we are doing so for a number of reasons. We might have assumed that:

1. Diet is not an important health issue;
2. An unhealthy diet is less expensive than a healthy one;
3. It tastes better;
4. It would take too much effort to change;
5. It takes too much time to prepare healthy food.

If we examine these assumptions a little more closely then they may not stand up to scrutiny. We may:

1. Learn that we are increasing our chances of getting cancer, diabetes or heart disease;
2. Realise that healthy food can cost less than buying fast food or pre-packaged food;
3. Discover that we can be creative in the kitchen and use recipes that bring out the good tastes in healthy food;
4. Realise that the effort we make now will be outweighed by the hardships we will face when we become ill;
5. Come to see that it can take a lot more time to heat a pre-packaged pizza than it takes to pick up a piece of fruit and a handful of walnuts, or a healthy dip and rice crackers.

It can be a useful exercise to sit down and examine all the costs and benefits for maintaining a given health behaviour or changing it. The following table – which breaks down the costs and benefits of starting a regular exercise routine – is an example that we can follow for any health issue that is important to us, such as quitting smoking, learning to manage stress, reducing fat and sugar in our diet, and so on.

The next step is to look at some of the things standing in the way of change and consider how valid or fixed they are. We might think that we are too tired to make the effort to exercise, but is the actual reason that we are tired all the time because we are not exercising? If we reflect for a moment we might remember that when we did exercise more regularly, although we felt tired at the end of it we had a lot more energy overall. If we are concerned about injury then we might need to choose a form of exercise suitable to our current age and level of fitness. What was appropriate at 20 years of age is not necessarily appropriate at 60.

Costs and benefits of starting regular exercise

	Changing behaviour (regular exercise)	Not changing behaviour (no exercise)
Benefits	More vitality	Comfortable
	Better mood and less anxiety	Easy
	Weight control	Time for other things
	Less likely to become ill from:	
	• infections	
	• heart disease	
	• cancer	
	• dementia and others	
	Social interaction	
	Greater endurance	
	Sense of achievement	
	Less pain	
	Better concentration	
Costs	Some financial outlay, depending on type of exercise	Low vitality
	Out of comfort zone	Lowered mood and greater anxiety
	Requires effort	Weight problems
	Time taken from other things	More likely to become ill from:
	Might injure oneself	• infections
		• heart disease
		• cancer
		• dementia and others
		Have to take time away from other things for being ill
		Financial costs of being ill
		Less social interaction
		Poorer concentration and performance
		Sense of not taking on challenges

We can go through this process for any of our obstructing ideas and assumptions. If we do this in a creative and unbiased way we are likely to find that there are few or no valid reasons for not making the healthy change, and a lot of spurious assumptions sabotaging it. Having gone through the process then we should just sit with our deliberations and see whether it is worth changing our behaviour or not. If we make the decision not to change at least we can be clear about why we are staying the way we are. Going through this process with a GP or life coach can be very helpful.

The cycle of behaviour change

A model which outlines the steps we go through in changing behaviour has been developed, and is widely used in healthcare and psychology. Although it was initially applied to quitting smoking it can be applied to any behaviour we can think of. The steps in the process are shown in the diagram below.

The Prochaska DiClemente cycle of behaviour change

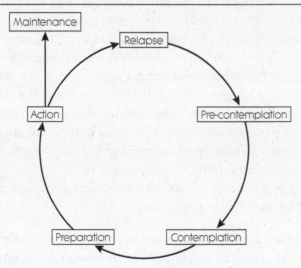

The model shows that we go through different stages in making a change in behaviour. The cycle begins even before we first think about making a change and goes on until the new behaviour becomes established.

When we are considering a behaviour change it is important to firstly reflect on what stage we are up to in the cycle. The art is to move through the stages in order, beginning from where we are now, and in a way that suits our needs and motivations.

1. Pre-contemplation: This is before we have even begun to think about changing our behaviour. At this stage, for example, a female smoker goes to the doctor with a cold but has no thought of giving up and has not made many connections between her smoking and her health (or the health of her child if she becomes pregnant). No change is possible in this stage.

2. Contemplation: Here we first start to think about changing our behaviour. Many healthcare campaigns are aimed at raising our awareness to make us think, and change our emotions and attitudes. We can spend a short time in contemplation (seconds) or a long time (years or even decades) before we change our behaviour. It can be a difficult stage because of all the competing motivations. In our example above, the doctor mentions that smoking is contributing to the woman's tendency to get colds and is putting her at risk of other illnesses. This is an opportunistic way to bring someone into the contemplation part of the cycle, in that the doctor waited for the opportunity to present itself to address the issue of smoking. Sometimes the trigger can be more proactive and structured, for example, when a doctor screens all patients for smoking.

In the contemplation phase it is important to really examine what motivates us. When someone – whether it a healthcare practitioner, friend or family member – encourages us to change our ways, the motivations they suggest need to be relevant to us. For example, concern about lung cancer or heart disease may not seem important if our female patient with a cold is 25 years old, but saving money, improving her sporting performance and attractiveness to the opposite sex, and preventing wrinkles might be.

At this stage we can be supported with further discussion, information, reading materials and other aids.

3. Preparation: In this stage we put things in place to help ensure we change our behaviour successfully. In the case of our example, she accesses some information about how to stop smoking by phoning the QUIT Line, tells her family and friends that she is setting a quit date and makes a list of the places she should avoid when she stops smoking. A lack of preparation can lead to us lapsing back into our old behaviour.

4. Action: Now we are taking action and implementing our new behaviour. In the case of our example, the woman has thrown away her cigarettes and is no longer smoking. For those of us starting an exercise routine, this is the stage when we have got our runners on and have taken our first walk or jog around the block.

A supportive environment is very important here if the behaviour is to be maintained. The tendency to revert to our old, unhealthy behaviour is strongest in the initial stages. Like going uphill, it takes effort to change our behaviour and it is easy to roll down again if we lose focus.

5. Relapse: This can occur at any time and with some habits we can relapse a number of times until we achieve lasting change. It is useful to see relapses not as failures but as learning opportunities. If we have reverted to our old behaviour, it will have been for a reason. Perhaps we lost focus; perhaps we began to kid ourselves that the old behaviour wasn't really an issue any more; perhaps we didn't pay attention to the environments we put ourselves in. The important thing is not to dwell on perceived failure but to learn what caused the relapse so our future attempts have a greater chance of succeeding. To dwell on failure will sap energy and dishearten us unnecessarily. To learn something useful is to make something good out of an otherwise negative situation.

When we relapse we are back at the start of the cycle until something stimulates us to contemplate the behaviour again. Getting back to action could take as little as one minute or as long as many years. It will be up to us.

6. Maintenance: This is where behaviour change becomes long term. The initial difficult stage of establishing the behaviour has passed and we now find that the new behaviour takes very little effort to maintain.

This does not mean that the game is over. Sometimes complacency can bring us unstuck here. For example, our former smoker is at a party and thinks, 'I'll just have one cigarette. It won't matter.' The next thing, she has reactivated dormant thought patterns and neural pathways; they re-establish themselves quite quickly and soon she is back at the doctor, once again a smoker suffering from a cold or bronchitis. Commonly, stress can lead to relapsing into an old behaviour. If a habit was once deeply entrenched it can return with a very surprising level of force, even after many years.

SMART goal setting

When we decide to make a healthy change we need to think about setting goals which will help us to succeed. To set unrealistic goals can be discouraging and defeat us early in the process. We need to be SMART about setting goals, an approach that is widely used and can be applied to setting any type of goal. SMART usually stands for specific, measurable, attainable, realistic and timely, but in this version, attainable is replaced with 'attractive'. Having an attainable goal is all-important but here that objective is covered under the heading of 'realistic'. So, to me, SMART goals are:

1. Specific;
2. Measurable;
3. Attractive;
4. Realistic;
5. Timely.

1. SPECIFIC

A goal is harder to attain if it is vague or ill defined. For example, one might aspire to a goal of 'exercising more', but what does that mean? How much more? How often? What type of exercise? If a goal is not specific then we never really know whether we are achieving it or not. A specific exercise goal would be something like: 'I plan to walk around the park – 3 kilometres – four evenings per week.' It is specific in terms of the type of exercise, the duration and the frequency.

2. MEASURABLE

If we have specific goals it is easy to measure our progress in an objective fashion. Without measurement we can easily feel like we are getting nowhere even though we are making progress, or think we are achieving things we are not. Setting measurable goals can provide encouragement, in that we can appreciate the progress we're making, or it can give us a reality check by making it clear that we are not putting in enough effort. Starting with a measurable goal enables us to modify our goal if we need to: to step it up a little or cut it back. Taking the goal mentioned above, we might find that we have been able to walk only three times, not four, because we are so busy with work and family commitments. We can then decide whether we need to increase our effort or perhaps modify the goal if it is unrealistic. On the other hand, we may be covering that ground easily four times a week and barely puffing, in which case we can set ourselves a new, more ambitious goal.

3. ATTRACTIVE

If a goal is not attractive or enjoyable then we won't maintain it in the long term. If we choose a form of exercise that we really don't enjoy – say, running – then we won't continue past the point when our initial enthusiasm to get fit has died down. We either need to find a way of making running attractive to us – perhaps by running with friends or in beautiful parks – or choose a different form of exercise. We can realise a number of goals in one activity, such as increasing social interaction at the same time as we are exercising – perhaps a team sport that includes running or a different sport altogether such as swimming or cycling. It is best to choose exercise which we enjoy, is appropriate to our age and fitness, and which suits our life situation. A noisy gymnasium might be unattractive for an older person, or a sport that requires expensive equipment might not be right for someone with a limited income. Goals can be health related but the SMART model is applicable to any goal we set ourselves. There are a number of things that can make a goal 'attractive'. It can be because we find an activity pleasurable that we find it attractive, but equally we can find a goal attractive but the means of achieving it may not be. We may wish to achieve a certain career but may not find the effort, sacrifice and study along the way all that pleasant. To persevere, however, can help us to develop a great deal of character and resilience in a way which taking the pleasant option would never have done.

4. REALISTIC

If a goal is unrealistic and not achievable we virtually ensure a sense of failure and discouragement, even if we have made great progress. For example, if we haven't exercised for years, a goal to run 5 kilometres every day is unlikely to be achievable. When we can't meet the goal, we may feel like a failure, and this can discourage us from exercising at all.

A realistic initial goal may be modest but a month later when we have achieved it we can set a new, slightly higher goal. A month later we can revise it again. Through setting a series of realistic goals this way, we can end up achieving a goal that would have been unrealistic at the beginning.

Some people with high confidence and a resilient sense of self can benefit from intentionally setting very high, even unrealistic, goals. They thrive on the challenge. So long as the goal is not dangerous, this can be a valid way of improving performance, for those with the personality and attitude to suit. For them, not meeting a high goal is not a sign of defeat but a motivator to rise to a challenge and make further effort.

5. TIMELY

Giving a goal a specific time frame rather than leaving it open-ended can increase our focus and maintain our motivation. For instance, if we aim to be fit enough to compete in a fun run six months from now it can help us to keep training regularly and not become complacent. A time frame helps us make our goal specific and realistic, helps us map our progress and provides incentive.

SMART GOAL-SETTING ACTIVITY

You might now like to set a SMART goal for yourself. For it to have meaning it needs to be a goal that really matters to you and that you desire to implement. The goal might relate to:

- Exercise;
- Change of diet;
- Weight control;
- Study;
- Learning a skill;
- Getting over a phobia;
- Renovating your house;
- Practising meditation.

BASK

Any time we learn something it will generally relate to behaviours, attitudes, skills and knowledge. Simply thinking that knowledge or information is going to change behaviour is a false assumption most of the time. The most powerful way to change behaviour is through a shift in emotion and attitude – supported and directed by knowledge, of course. In quit smoking advertising throughout the community, increasing knowledge is only a secondary aim: the primary aim is to make a negative emotional and attitudinal association between smoking and wellbeing.

BASK is an acronym for:

- Behaviour: What we do;
- Attitudes: What we believe;
- Skills: What we can do;
- Knowledge: What we understand.

Interventions can be directed at any or all of the above dimensions. A program, like the Ornish program – which is described in detail in the sections on heart disease and cancer in Part 3 – is a good example of a program containing all of these aspects contained in BASK. That is a large part of why it is so successful. Interventions not directed at the right aspect of BASK will tend to be ineffective. For example, it is little use giving knowledge where there is an attitudinal problem which needs to be dealt with first. The knowledge will not translate into action while that barrier is in place.

Journal keeping

Keeping a journal is a powerful way of following our progress, gaining insight and reinforcing behaviour change. A variety of studies suggest that keeping a journal is therapeutic in itself, particularly for dealing with emotional issues. University students who kept a journal about significant events in their lives showed improved immune function and fewer doctor visits for infectious diseases throughout the high-stress periods of the academic year.[4]

Expressing thoughts and feelings in a journal helps us to come to a state of understanding and objectivity about stressful and important life events. For a journal to be of real use it needs to be about events and issues that are important to us. Simply writing about what we had for lunch might be useful as a food diary but it is not going to lead to much transformation.

9

Using the Essence program

This chapter discusses ways in which the Essence principles can be applied personally, by groups and in education. The principles can and should be adapted to suit different needs in different contexts; being creative in applying Essence to our lives increases our enjoyment.

The Essence program for individuals

Some people reading this book will be well and wishing to stay that way. Some will have a minor health issue and would like to prevent it from becoming a major one. Some will be dealing with a major health issue and either trying to recover or at least to cope better with it.

The other parts of this book provide the guidance on what sorts of changes are helpful. Being able to make and maintain those changes will be the real task. Any of us who have tried to make healthy changes in our life understand that it is one thing to know what we should do but it is quite another to be able to do it.

Sometimes we have an epiphany and our resolution to make changes in our life is deep, clear and direct. This type of resolution is generally successful. Sometimes the resolution is not so deep, clear and direct, and when our initial flurry of enthusiasm dies down we find ourselves in two minds. Soon we feel the burden of the changes we made; we become resentful for what we think we are missing out on; and the temptation to go back to business as usual creeps up on us. If we have experienced a true epiphany and know with utter conviction that we are ready to make wholesale changes to our life, we might be ready to take on a whole range of ambitious goals at once, such as eating healthier, exercising more, practising mindfulness and stopping smoking. However, it is generally far better to make small changes and take time to establish them before introducing new ones, rather than to take on big ones and then criticise ourselves for what we perceive as failure.

There are a number of ways we can incorporate the seven pillars of wellbeing into our life:

1. We can prioritise the seven pillars and take one on at a time;
2. We can progress through the seven pillars from top to bottom;
3. We can take on elements in a piecemeal fashion according to our health and lifestyle needs;
4. We can establish mindfulness-based stress management first as a foundation upon which to build other changes.

If focusing on one pillar at a time it is a good idea to decide on an amount of time to dedicate to each one before moving on to the next. For example, we might like to address one per month. This gives us time to establish and reinforce the changes we have set for, say, exercise, before trying to make changes in, say, nutrition. In this way we are looking at a slow, steady but deep change. Establishing a change over time also allows us to start to enjoy the benefits of the change, which increases our momentum to make subsequent changes.

USING A JOURNAL

Keeping a journal can help us to set goals, gauge our progress, identify challenges and insights, and record questions we might want to explore further. It can also help facilitate health and lifestyle changes being made under the guidance of a doctor, counsellor or life coach.

THE SUPPORT OF FAMILY AND FRIENDS

Family and friends can be instrumental in reinforcing healthy change – or sabotaging it. Encouraging family and friends to take on their own Essence goals can help enormously. That way it becomes part of our daily conversation and is integrated into daily life much more effectively. We might like to establish a routine of walking with our son or daughter in the mornings. We might make a family decision not to buy sweet drinks in the weekly shopping or to reduce the family's television watching. We might join a health club with a friend. Sharing a commitment with others makes a world of difference.

GUIDANCE AND SUPPORT FROM A HEALTHCARE PROFESSIONAL

We benefit enormously when our doctor, counsellor, life coach, natural therapist or other healthcare professional takes an active interest in the Essence principles.

To integrate the Essence elements into our healthcare, we can use this book to supplement the health advice we are already receiving from healthcare professionals, or we can make an arrangement with a healthcare professional to address each of the seven pillars sequentially. When working through the book with a healthcare professional it is useful to:

1. Re-read the background information;
2. Negotiate a goal or goals related to each pillar as we move through the program;
3. Discuss and have a clear understanding of the behaviour change strategies;
4. Have regular follow-ups to monitor progress – perhaps fortnightly;
5. Present our insights, challenges and questions from our journal to our healthcare professional;
6. Acknowledge our gains and revise our goals as we go.

Some health professionals may not have the time, motivation or skills to implement the program – for instance, we might be having treatment for cancer from an oncologist who is too busy to go into our lifestyle issues and other aspects of our healthcare at length. Even so, that specialist can still, through the subtle and overt health messages they give us, be a powerful supporter of change – or they can undermine it. They can reinforce healthy change by encouraging us and pointing us in the right direction for more information, resources or additional healthcare professionals.

If we find ourselves under the care of a healthcare professional who doesn't offer encouragement or, even worse, undermines our legit-imate efforts to integrate lifestyle and self-care into the management of our health, then we have a decision to make. Do we access their expertise in their particular area and cease to mention other healthcare issues to them, or do we look for a different healthcare professional with a more holistic approach?

Even better, you may find a healthcare professional who runs the Essence program for groups within their practice.

The Essence program for groups

In groups we learn from others' insights as well as our own. Realising that other people are dealing with the same issues that we are helps us to overcome the isolation and self-criticism which are so common. Although our struggles feel personal they are really part of the wider struggle of humanity to learn, grow and overcome suffering.

A support group may have its own agenda – for instance, to provide support for those with a particular condition such as diabetes or multiple sclerosis – or it might be specifically designed to work through the elements of the Essence program.

A group focused on the Essence program can be an enormously useful addition to the treatment that clients or patients are receiving at a healthcare practice and can help support the advice being given by the healthcare practitioners. When a practitioner becomes known for running such groups, other healthcare practitioners outside the practice may also wish to refer their patients.

If the person who is planning to lead the group is unfamiliar with working with groups, they would find some training in group facilitation skills useful. Working with groups is very different to dealing with individuals. Being able to keep the conversation open, draw people out, value each individual's contribution, create an atmosphere of safety and keep everyone focused on the task are all skills the group leader needs. Training courses are available in how to run support groups.

For health practitioners, although it seems like an additional time burden, taking a course for a group will actually save an enormous amount of time at the same time as delivering a more powerful intervention than could be delivered to individuals in a consultation setting. Mind you, there may be times when an individual needs to follow up the course with some individual attention.

A suggested plan for an eight-week program is provided at the end of this book in Appendix 2. Although the program can be run with a group of any size, a group of 10 to 15 is likely to offer a nice balance between having enough people to give the group adequate energy and input, but being small enough that each person has the opportunity to speak each week. Each participant should be allowed time to speak each week, but they also should not feel pressured to speak if they don't want to. At the outset, practical decisions need to be made about what time and day of the week the group will meet, the venue, the cost of the course, and what support materials other than this book will be used, such as other readings, websites or audio visual aids.

The group should take a structured and systematic approach to the program so that participants are clear about where they are up to at any given time. Each week, group members need to be clear about the homework tasks they are setting for themselves, and then follow up on their progress the next week.

At the commencement of the course, some ground rules need to be laid for the group. Such rules could include the need for respect, attentiveness when others are speaking and confidentiality. These help to remind people of important principles that can be taken for granted, and also creates an atmosphere of safety and care.

It is important to practise what we preach, especially in the case of group leaders. Practising what we preach helps group leaders to always remember how difficult it can be to implement healthy change. As a result they empathise more, avoid taking the moral high ground and communicate more authentically. People who practise what they preach are also more able to help someone else through the barriers they're facing, because they have probably had to negotiate them too. We do also need to acknowledge that we are all a 'work in progress', meaning that none of us is perfect. So when we feel that we have not been a good example to the group it can be useful to remember the motto 'If you can't be an example, at least you can be a warning.'

The group leader should avoid the temptation to talk too much or to turn the group meetings into a series of lectures. This turns the course into mere information rather than an exercise in self-development. There is an art in being able to draw people out and that is crucial, because it is when people speak that most learning takes place. When participants speak of their insights, questions and challenges in relation to how things *are* it carries much more weight than when the facilitator tells people how things *should be*. The word 'education' comes from a Latin word, 'educare', meaning 'to draw out'. Education is not about 'stuffing in'. One way of training oneself in this is to practise asking questions so that the group gives you the answers.

There is no such thing as failure when it comes to personal growth and learning. Failures are just learning opportunities awaiting recognition. Self-sabotaging behaviours, with which we are all familiar, only take place in the absence of understanding. We sometimes think that we understand an issue or the need for a lifestyle change, but still we make errors. This means that we have not yet *fully* understood, because if we fully understood we would not do things to our own detriment or the detriment of others. Once we see what is truly going on, failure becomes insight. If a person comes to understand an important principle through a so-called failure, they should see that this is *success*. The aim of the group is to increase each member's awareness. With awareness comes understanding and with understanding comes change. Defusing self-criticism and self-blame in the group will help to maintain an atmosphere of safety, within which we can really begin to see what is happening. Self-criticism distorts our view.

Each participant in the group needs to find their own level and set their own pace. The issue is not so much whether we are taking large steps or small ones but which direction we are moving in. If group members offer and receive acknowledgement and praise for their progress and insights it will help to build enthusiasm and confidence.

The Essence program is a way of life and does not come to an end at the completion of the course. The course is about laying the foundations, receiving support and learning skills to take away from the course and use in our lives. When participants stay in touch with each other at the end of the course it can help reinforce those ongoing efforts.

The Essence program is designed to be educational, to work as a preventive strategy, and to be an intervention for mild to moderate health issues. Group members will occasionally bring up more major health concerns, and although providing encouragement and pastoral care, it may not be appropriate for the group leader to become the group members' doctor or therapist. Anyone suffering from a major health illness may need to be encouraged to seek personalised medical treatment or counselling. The same applies when the Essence program is taught to groups at schools and universities.

The Essence program in education

SCHOOLS

The Essence program is of just as much relevance to children as it is to adults and it can be adapted to school curricula for children of any age. With younger children the general principles and practical behaviour change aspects are emphasised, with less focus on the details. With older children more explanation can be provided to help them understand the principles better and raise their interest. For senior secondary students the program can be integrated with subjects like biology or physical education. The information and skills in the Essence program are important aspects of self-care and they help students sustain a high level of performance when the demands increase in the latter years of secondary school.

Elements of the Essence program can be integrated into the school culture in many ways:

- Increasing the number of healthy food choices at the school canteen;
- Making physical activity part of the daily school schedule;
- Regularly doing mindfulness exercises at the start and end of classes;
- Putting up health promotion posters and making reading material on healthy living available to students;
- Promoting a healthy attitude to sun exposure rather than emphasising total avoidance of the sun;
- Building a sense of community within the school and a connection between the school and the outside community;
- Promoting simple stress management strategies in class.

Educating and engaging the parents can also help children to apply what they learn at school.

HEALTHCARE STUDENTS

It is strange to think that health issues such as those covered in the Essence program are generally not core curriculum for healthcare students. It makes little sense to train healthcare providers in the technological and scientific aspects of their craft but not prepare them personally to meet the rigours of a demanding career or provide all the skills they need to help patients make lifestyle changes for the good of their health.

One of the few places in Australia where medical students receive this kind of training is Melbourne's Monash University, where Essence is the foundation of the Health Enhancement Program. It is provided to help students enhance their own self-care and improve their performance, and to lay good foundations for future clinical practice.

The students at Monash receive a series of eight lectures covering all the major aspects of Essence, in a scientific and clinical context. Without receiving such lectures it is easy for students to think that a program such as Essence is in some way a marginal aspect of their education and has little relevance to their future role as healthcare professionals. Nothing could be further from the truth. An increasing number of patients feel that they have to go to non-medical health practitioners for information that they should be getting from their doctors.

As important as the lecture series is, weekly small group tutorials where the students discuss the Essence principles and how to apply them to their own lives are even more important. Students are encouraged to actively question and not blindly accept what they are being taught. At the end of the day it will always be a personal choice how much of the program a student wishes to take on. Monash's data suggests that over 90% of students personally apply the Essence principles, including mindfulness practices on at least a weekly basis.

Theory by itself is not the same as application. The experiential component is important to help assimilate and deepen learning. Learning about the theory and biomechanics of skiing, for example, is pale by comparison to the experience of being on the ski slopes. The students often find it hard to apply the Essence principles to their lives even when they understand their relevance and the evidence behind them. They might, say, recognise the benefits of exercise but still find it hard to exercise regularly. This is important because it helps students to one day empathise with their patients who will be receiving advice from healthcare professionals but having trouble translating it into action.

In the tutorials students are invited to speak about how they have gone with their weekly homework tasks, along the lines of the eight-week course outlined in Appendix 2: Students are invited to share as much of their personal experience as they feel comfortable to, all the while respecting the fact that some students will not wish to share of themselves in this way. The students come to value each other's openness, just as the members of a support group do. This helps to break down the isolation that makes it hard for some students to cope at university.

In tutor selection the main criterion is that the tutor is a trained healthcare professional with clinical experience in stress and lifestyle management. They also need to have a personal commitment and enthusiasm for the content of the course. They will be leading by their example as much as by their knowledge.

Another important aspect of integration into health practitioner education is to ensure that content is examinable. Assessment, understandably, drives learning for many students. For this reason, tutorials will need to be well standardised and remain on track so that one can be confident that the core material being examined has been adequately explored by each tutorial group.

HEALTHCARE PRACTITIONERS

Many healthcare practitioners who have been practising for some time will find that their undergraduate education did not fully prepare them for guiding patients through health and lifestyle changes, so the eight-week program outlined in the Appendix 2 could be useful for them, too. Even a one-off seminar on the Essence principles would raise their awareness and direct them to further reading. It is certainly advised that practitioners learn about the Essence model and apply it to themselves before applying it in their practices with patients.

Part 3
The Essence of the Prevention and Management of Chronic Illness

This part of the book looks at how the seven pillars of wellbeing can be applied to specific medical conditions and health issues. Advice is given for preventing or managing these conditions, for example foods for asthmatics to include in their diet or exercise suggestions to help prevent cancer. This section of the book therefore relates to the Essence of managing asthma, or the Essence of managing cancer.

It is important to note that the Essence approach to managing health conditions is intended to enhance – not replace – conventional medical management. Having full and open conversations with our doctor and other health professionals is important in helping find the overall management plan that is right for us as individuals. There is no 'one size fits all' when it comes to health.

10

Heart disease and stroke

Education

Cardiovascular disease (CVD), mostly made up of heart disease and stroke, is an important condition to know something about as it is the most common cause of death in affluent countries. Nearly 30% of people will die of heart disease and another 15% from stroke. CVD is commonly seen as a disease of Western lifestyle because it is associated with the 'benefits' that come with affluence, such as an abundance of food, physical inactivity and stress.

CVD is largely caused by atherosclerosis, popularly known as 'hardening of the arteries'. This is when fat deposits in the lining of the blood vessels cause thickening, inflammation, ulceration and eventual blockage of the blood vessel. When the blockage is severe and prolonged enough it can lead to death of the tissue which that blood vessel supplies.

TYPES OF CVD

Heart

Partial blockage of a blood vessel leading to the heart reduces the amount of oxygen-rich blood reaching it, resulting in the chest pain called angina. The pain is typically in the centre of the chest, may radiate down the left arm or into the neck, and settles with rest. Exertion and emotional stress are common triggers for angina because they increase the oxygen requirements of the heart. Complete blockage for long enough, however, will lead to a heart attack. This is known by doctors as an acute myocardial infarction (AMI). 'Myo' means muscle, 'cardial' is the heart and 'infarction' is death. During a heart attack, the heart muscle is starved of oxygen to the degree that cells begin to die. The pain is like angina but more severe, does not settle with rest and is commonly associated with sweating and nausea. A heart attack can cause the heart to go into a dangerous and irregular rhythm known as cardiac arrest, causing a profound drop in blood pressure, cardiac shock and death. This is why people are admitted to hospital for monitoring after a heart attack. Women and the elderly often have different heart attack symptoms to the typical picture, making it more difficult for patients and doctors alike to recognise a heart attack among them. Their symptoms are less 'classical' as the pain can be located in a different place (for example just in the arm, or in the back), can just present as an indigestion-type experience, and sometimes it can even be 'silent', meaning that a small heart attack can sometimes produce little or no pain.

You will hear healthcare professionals use the terms coronary artery disease (CAD), ischaemic heart disease (IHD) and coronary heart disease (CHD) for cardiovascular disease in vessels leading to the heart. It can sometimes be confusing to hear all these terms being used, but they are essentially different names for the same thing.

Brain
When the blood vessels affected are those which feed the brain it is called cerebrovascular disease. Temporary blockage which quickly clears leads to a Transient Ischaemic Attack (TIA). This produces symptoms similar to a stroke – such as loss of speech or paralysis of an arm or leg – but resolves itself generally within hours.

Complete blockage can lead to death of a part of the brain and this is called a stroke. (Stroke can also be caused by bleeding into the brain due to a burst blood vessel – this is known as 'haemorrhagic stroke'.) A stroke causes disability according to its extent and which part of the brain is affected. A person can die from a large stroke but most strokes are not fatal and a person may slowly recover a lot of their lost function over a number of months. Numerous very small strokes over a period of years can produce a type of dementia called 'multi-infarct dementia'.

Legs
When the vessels affected are the ones feeding the legs then it is called peripheral vascular disease (PVD). Partial blockage can lead to

claudication which is calf pain during exertion such as when walking, or even at rest if it is severe. Complete blockage can lead to gangrene of the toes or feet. Diabetics and smokers make up the vast majority of cases of PVD.

Other organs
Other organs in the body can be affected by CVD such as the kidney and bowel. If the blockage is severe it can lead to poor kidney function or even death of part of the kidney or bowel.

RISK FACTORS

A number of risk factors can predispose a person to CVD. Most of them are related to lifestyle and are therefore reversible.

Reversible
- Physical inactivity
- Overweight and obesity, particularly obesity around the trunk
- High blood pressure (hypertension)
- High cholesterol and other blood fats (hyperlipidaemia)
- Poor nutrition
- Poor mental health and social factors, e.g.:
  - Chronic depression
  - Chronic anxiety
  - Chronic life and work stress
  - Social isolation
  - Social disadvantage and poverty
  - Lack of control or autonomy
  - Personality factors such as a high level of anger and hostility
- Diabetes
- Smoking

Irreversible
- Increasing age (although the speed of ageing can be slowed)
- Being male
- Family history of CVD
- Post-menopause for women

CVD is a largely preventable, and even reversible, illness given the right lifestyle approach. The Essence principles are central to the prevention and management of CVD but this does not mean that we should ignore conventional medical management. It is important to have risk factors like high blood pressure and blood fats and sugars regularly checked and managed appropriately. In the case of a heart attack or stroke it is also important to be able to read the signs and seek medical attention urgently. Emergency care can help minimise damage, monitor for complications such as dangerous heart rhythms and reduce the risk of dying.

The National Heart Foundation can provide further information on CVD or we can speak to our doctor.

Stress management

When we are stressed our nervous system is activated to fight or fly what is perceived to be a threatening situation. If extreme, this can trigger a heart attack or stroke, particularly in a person already at high risk. The effects of such stress on the heart are shown in the figure below.

When our nervous system is frequently activated this way over a prolonged period it:

- Places a lot of wear and tear on the heart and blood vessels;
- Can increase risk factors like lack of exercise and poor diet;
- Predisposes us to other risk factors like high cholesterol, blood pressure and blood sugars.

Effects of stress on the cardiovascular system

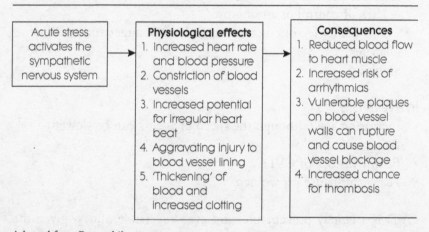

Adapted from Rozanski[1]

Our autonomic nervous system has two halves: the sympathetic nervous system (SNS) which is about activation and which is responsible for our racing heart rate, muscle tension and tremulousness during the fight or flight response; and the parasympathetic nervous system (PNS) which is about rest and maintenance. In positive emotional states, such as humour or compassion, these two aspects keep each other balanced and in check, the SNS activating and stimulating, with the PNS helping to protect the system from the damaging effects of over-activation.[2] In negative emotional states such as anger and fear these two sides become unbalanced, with the SNS taking precedence. This partly explains why anger is a common trigger for a heart attack. To illustrate, over one in six heart attack patients reported feeling significantly angry in the one to two hours beforehand. Acute anger more than doubled the risk of having a heart attack.[3] Stroke is also closely related to anger. Men who express more anger have double the chance of having a stroke; the risk grows to sevenfold for men who both tend to be angry and have a previous history of heart disease.[4] There is also an increased risk of stroke for those with chronic anxiety, panic disorder[5] and depression.[6] On a more positive note, reducing anger, anxiety and depression helps to reverse the risk.

The term 'vital exhaustion' is used to denote the long-term effects of over-activation of the SNS and can be gauged by a person's response to the statement 'At the end of the day I am completely exhausted mentally and physically.' When we overreact to daily events we not only feel stressed but we also feel depleted of energy. In one study, if a man said that the abovementioned statement accurately described his typical day-to-day experience, he was nine times more likely than the average male to die from a cardiac event over the following 10 months. Even three and a half years later, his risk was still three times higher.[7] In another study, patients who had just had coronary angioplasty – a procedure to re-open a blocked coronary artery – were followed for 18 months and it was found that the risk of those with vital exhaustion having another cardiac event was tripled.[8] It is important that anyone who believes they might be experiencing vital exhaustion has a thorough medical check-up. It may pick up another health condition leading to tiredness such as anaemia, a thyroid problem, depression or even, uncommonly, cancer. If those things are excluded as the cause of tiredness then it is time to take appropriate steps to moderate our demands and make time for self-care.

Unfortunately it has taken a long time for the conventional healthcare system to recognise the importance of managing stress and cultivating good mental health in the prevention and management of heart disease and stroke. It is probably the most important factor to deal with because it has an impact on all the other risk factors.

To give an indication of how important it is there is consistent data[9][10] linking chronic depression, anxiety, work stress and social isolation to an increased risk of heart disease and faster rate of progression. Another study[11] found convincing evidence that depression, anxiety, personality and character traits – principally anger and hostility – social isolation and chronic life stress contributed significantly to CVD.

Perhaps one of the most obvious stressors is an alarming event such as an earthquake. On the day of and for a few days after an earthquake there is a spike in the number of heart attacks. Other, less dramatic, stressors can also trigger cardiac events.[12][13] Among workers, more heart attacks and strokes occur on Monday mornings than any other time in the week whereas weekends are associated with far fewer.[14][15][16][17][18] Many find that that work makes them angry, and anger more than doubles the risk of having heart attacks.[19] Now, the practical answer may not be to quit one's job or stay at home on Monday, but changing one's job, or at least one's attitude to work, is helpful.

Another option for managing stress may be to take a vacation but the evidence on this is a little mixed. Although some studies suggest that regular vacations reduce the risk of having a heart attack by nearly 30%,[20] other studies suggest that there are more heart attacks on the first two days of vacation particularly when travelling by car or staying in a tent or mobile home.[21] Also be warned that major football games also increase the risk of cardiac events. Men have a 28% increased risk of heart attack when their home team loses.[22] In England on 30 June 1998, the day they lost to Argentina in a World Cup penalty shoot-out, and for the following two days, the risk of being admitted to hospital for a heart attack increased by 25%.[23] The figures were even more startling for the World Cup in Germany in 2006. On days when the German soccer team played there were over three times as many heart attacks among men and nearly twice as many among women.[24] So if your team is down in a close game then do something quickly: turn off the TV, meditate, do some cognitive therapy, or be philosophical.

Although being unemployed is associated with a higher incidence of heart disease, so too are long working hours, especially under high pressure. The effects of over-employment can be as harmful as under-employment.[25] Low job control, often associated with low socio-economic status, and ongoing work stress produce the biochemical and physiological changes which make heart attacks more likely.[26 27 28]

The way our body reacts in anticipation of a stressful event – measured by a spike in blood pressure or adrenaline levels – is a good predictor of the risk of stroke. For example, men who had a large increase in blood pressure in anticipation of an exercise stress test were nearly twice as likely to have a stroke over the following 11 years.[29] If the men were poorly educated then the risk was three times as great.

Thinking about all the ways in which stress can increase the risk of heart attack and stroke is enough to make us stressed even if we weren't before. The most important thing to remember is that this increased risk is reversible. A review of 23 studies on the effects of psychological and social support in the management of heart disease clearly showed major reductions in disease progression and the number of deaths if people had psychological and emotional support included as a part of their management.[30] Compared to those who were given psychosocial support, those with no such support were 70% more likely to die from their heart disease and 84% more likely to have a recurrence. The researcher's conclusion was unambiguous. 'The addition of psychosocial treatments to standard cardiac rehabilitation regimens reduces mortality and morbidity, psychological distress, and some biological risk factors . . . It is recommended to include routinely psychosocial treatment components in cardiac rehabilitation.'

This can be illustrated by a study into the effects of stress management on those with heart disease.[31] In this study people with heart disease were divided randomly into three groups. All patients received the usual medical management but one group also had a physical exercise program and another group a stress management program. Both programs ran over 16 weeks. When patients were followed up for five years they found that those who had the exercise program had a 32% reduction in heart attacks and deaths due to heart disease; those who had the stress management program had a 74% reduction. They also were far less likely to need cardiac surgery like bypass operations. The main factor distinguishing the stress management group from the others was a reduction in overall distress and, more significantly, a reduction in hostility.

Meditation is also being investigated as a treatment for CVD and a way to reduce risk factors. A series of studies on the effects of

Transcendental Meditation (TM) over four months found a significant reduction in blood pressure[32][33] and a reversal of atherosclerosis over the following nine months.[34] The improvements were not attributable to changes like diet and exercise. Nine months' practice translated into reductions in the risk of heart attack by 11% and of stroke by 15%. In another study on the seven-year effects of TM on the elderly,[35] it was found that the TM group had a 23% reduction in the risk of death from any cause, a 30% decreased risk of death specifically from CVD and a 49% decreased risk of death from cancer.

Spirituality

Spirituality is an important part of many people's ability to deal with stress, depression and hostility. In most of the studies in the field, spirituality is measured by recourse to an easily quantified marker like whether or not a person attends religious services. Regular attendance at religious services reduces biological signs of stress (allostatic load) and probably as a result CVD risk factors such as blood pressure, waist-to-hip ratio, blood fats, diabetic control, cortisol and adrenaline levels.[36] The effect is much more prominent among women. Among people who regularly worship there is also a lower level of inflammatory markers in the blood relevant for CVD (such as C-reactive protein and fibrinogen).[37]

Reviews of the research suggest that religious attendance promotes better health including a reduced risk of heart disease,[38] although some studies have raised doubts about whether this effect is independent of lifestyle and social factors.[39] The beneficial effect of religious involvement on CVD risk is probably due to a combination of lifestyle, social support, better emotional health in terms of coping with anger and depression, and the effect of practices such as prayer and meditation.

Exercise

Inactivity results in a one and a half to twofold rise[40] in the risk of CVD. Physical exercise protects the heart in a number of ways over the long term:[41]

• Improvement in blood fats;

- Better blood flow and reduced clotting;
- Improved blood glucose level and improved action of insulin;
- Reduced blood pressure (especially when exercise is combined with weight loss);
- Improved function of blood vessels;
- Reductions in inflammatory markers which predispose to heart disease.

This all adds up to a slowing of the progression of atherosclerosis and a lowering of the risk of heart attack. Being fit also helps in case one does have a heart attack. The risk of death from a heart attack is halved if the person has recently been involved in regular, moderate physical activity. Although regular exercise over the long term clearly reduces the chances of having a heart attack, very vigorous physical exertion, particularly in those not fit for it, increases the risk by three and a half times.[42 43 44] It is therefore important, especially if older, unfit or

Table 1 Comparison of aerobic and resistance exercise

Variable	Aerobic exercise	Resistance exercise
Bone mineral density	↑	↑ ↑ ↑
Body composition		
Fat mass	↓ ↓	↓
Muscle mass	↔	↑ ↑
Strength	↔	↑ ↑ ↑
Glucose metabolism		
Insulin response to glucose challenge	↓ ↓	↓ ↓
Basal insulin levels	↓	↓
Insulin sensitivity	↑ ↑	↑ ↑
Serum lipids		
High-density lipoprotein (HDL) or 'good fats'	↑	↑
Low-protein lipoprotein (LDL) or 'bad fats'	↓	↓
Resting heart rate	↓ ↓	↔
Blood pressure		
Systolic	↓ ↓	↓
Diastolic	↓ ↓	↓
Physical endurance	↑ ↑ ↑	↑ ↑
BMR	↑	↑ ↑

↑ increased; ↓ decreased; and ↔ neglible effect

Adapted from Braith Stewart[45]

unaccustomed to regular exercise, to initially take things gently and build up slowly.

The Women's Health Initiative Observational study looked at over 70,000 postmenopausal women[46] and found that the faster their walking pace, the lower their risk of heart disease. The message here is to firstly get moving, and then get moving more quickly within our capabilities.

Most of the emphasis has tended to be placed on aerobic exercise – the sort of exercise which makes us puff – but other forms of exercise also provide excellent benefits. The risk of heart disease is reduced further by nearly a quarter if weight or resistance training is included in one's exercise routine as well as aerobic exercise. The table on page 195 gives a comparison between the health benefits of aerobic and resistance training.

Heart failure is the most common reason for hospitalisation in people over 60 years of age. Traditionally, bed rest was advised for heart failure or, at best, doctors gave very guarded exercise advice for fear of worsening the patient's condition. We now know that a graded exercise program results in better vitality, reduced disability, fewer symptoms and better quality of life.[47] In heart failure patients, exercise also results in improved blood flow, reduced enlargement of the heart, improved cardiac output, improved function of blood vessel linings and better function of the ANS.[48] [49] The recommended exercise intensity for heart failure patients is 50 to 70% of their maximum heart rate, which is 'walk and talk' level. If we have heart failure and can't talk while we walk then we need to slow down a little. For those who become breathless very easily when they walk, resistance training may be a better option initially. Resistance training may also be the preferred option for those who have a low threshold for angina.

Physical inactivity increases the risk of stroke threefold.[50] Physical activity helps by improvement in the clotting profile – thinning the blood[51] – and reducing blood pressure[52] and inflammation,[53] all of which add up to a reduced risk of stroke. Drug treatments for high blood pressure do not have the other beneficial effects of reducing clotting and inflammation. Regular exercise can reduce blood pressure in those with hypertension by 6 to 7 mmHg – say from 155 to 148 – or reduce the chances of developing high blood pressure by about 25% in those at risk.[54] Exercise has a beta-blocker-like effect in reducing the pulse rate. It also reduces weight and each kilogram lost reduces the blood pressure by 1 mmHg on average.

Exercise causes particularly beneficial changes in blood fats. What matters is not just how much fat we have in the bloodstream but the types of fats and the ratio between them. Exercise increases the High Density Lipoproteins (HDL); these are the 'good fats'. Diet and exercise together reduce the Low Density Lipoprotein (LDL) – the 'bad fats' – better than diet alone.[55] When those with high cholesterol who are on lipid-lowering drugs take up exercise and adopt a healthy diet they may be able to stop or reduce their dosage. Even those who do take up exercise but still require lipid-lowering medication reduce their risk of CVD by exercising, regardless of their lipid levels and the effects of their medication.[56]

Metabolic syndrome is a cluster of symptoms associated with the affluent lifestyle: high blood fats, blood pressure and blood sugar, and obesity around the trunk. In *The Annals of the New York Academy of Sciences* it was concluded, 'The way to prevent and combat this burden is by regular exercise.'[57] Resistance training is particularly helpful in metabolic syndrome because it helps to build muscle mass which is like a 'metabolic sink' for blood fats and glucose.

Although it is far better not to smoke at all, smokers who exercise have a lower risk of developing CVD than sedentary smokers. Importantly, smokers who commence exercise are more likely to give up smoking and make other healthy lifestyle changes. Exercise is also a good way to control the weight gain that often comes after quitting.

Nutrition

Food is directly involved in many of the risk factors for heart disease, such as high blood pressure, overweight and obesity, diabetes and high blood fats. Many of the dietary principles for reducing CVD are similar to the principles for preventing other diseases. Obviously an important first step is to work towards a healthy weight. The National Heart Foundation[58] recommends a diet which is:

- Rich in fruit and vegetables;
- Rich in wholegrain cereals and cereal products;
- Low in saturated and trans-fatty acids;
  - Common sources of saturated fats are animal products such as butter, meat fat, beef, lamb, chicken skin and full-cream dairy foods;
  - Trans-fatty acids are common in baked and processed foods like pastries and biscuits;

- Low in added salt;
- High in dietary fibre.

The role of excessive salt[59] in high blood pressure is well known. This is a case where a food that was once traded as a valuable commodity is now cheap and used far too liberally in our Western diets. Check labels carefully and where possible avoid foods with salt added. Read the labels on breads as these often have high levels of salt added. It takes a little time for the palate to acclimatise to a diet with less salt in it, so be patient.

Several clinical trials have shown the effectiveness of dietary treatment to lower blood pressure, which in turns helps prevent heart attacks and strokes. One well-known trial[60] studied a diet rich in vegetables, fruit and low-fat dairy foods and which included fish, poultry, whole grains and nuts, with reduced portions of red meats, fats and sugar. Beverages and alcoholic drinks were limited to no more than two drinks per day. After a year this diet lowered systolic blood pressure by 11.2 mmHg.

The following foods are considered to be heart friendly.

OILY FISH

Oily fish[61] such as salmon, tuna, mackerel and sardines are associated with lowered CVD risk because the omega-3 fatty acids they contain lower cholesterol, improve blood vessel elasticity, and 'thin' the blood making it less likely to clot and block blood vessels. In a study of 22,071 male American physicians, those who consumed fish at least once a week had a 52% reduction of sudden cardiac death compared with those who ate fish less than once a month.[62]

Of all the treatments for high blood fats, fish oil is clearly better than any pharmaceutical in reducing deaths. In a review of 97 trials on blood-fat-reducing agents the most effective therapy for cutting deaths from all causes and cardiac deaths was omega-3 fatty acids;[63] they were clearly more effective than statins which were the most effective pharmaceutical. Omega-3 fatty acids should therefore be the preferred first-line treatment for high blood fats. Omega-3s are also preferable to drugs in that they are readily available, cost less and any side effects they have are good ones.

Omega-3 fatty acids are also found in flaxseed oil, walnuts and avocadoes.

SOLUBLE FIBRE

Dietary fibre helps to lower cholesterol, which in turn lowers your CVD risk. Good sources of fibre are fruit, vegetables, beans and grains, e.g. oats, peas, lentils, chickpeas, baked beans, soybeans, apples, strawberries, citrus fruits, barley and psyllium. Studies have shown that seven or more grams per day of psyllium reduces LDLs – the 'bad' cholesterol – by 5 to 15%. This, however, is quite a large quantity of psyllium to take.

COENZYME Q10 (COQ10)

Coenzyme Q10 (CoQ10) is an antioxidant found in high concentrations in red meat. Its levels are highest in grass-fed wild animals such as reindeer and kangaroo but it is also found in fish, soybean oil, sardines and beef. Studies[64] have indicated that CoQ10 is useful for people who have suffered heart failure[65] because CoQ10 improves the efficiency of energy production in the heart muscle.[66] For athletes CoQ10 also improves recovery and endurance.

In a healthy diet red meat can only be consumed in moderation, 400 to 500 grams per week in total. CoQ10 supplements of between 50 and 150 mg have been shown to have beneficial effects for hypertension and heart disease.

FRUIT AND VEGETABLES

Antioxidants in fruit and vegetables offer protection against heart disease. They are also important sources of folate, which helps lower the blood levels of the amino acid homocysteine, which appears to be linked to an increased risk of heart disease. People who eat at least five servings of fruit and vegetables per day have a 26% reduced chance of having a stroke.[67] Pomegranate juice, which contains antioxidants (soluble polyphenols, tannins and anthocyanins), may help to slow atherosclerosis. Cardiac patients who drank 240 ml of pomegranate juice a day showed a reduction of stress-induced ischaemia (reduction in blood flow to the heart).[68] Goji berry juice is a particularly rich source of antioxidants.

LEGUMES AND SOY

Soy foods and legumes have been shown to lower LDL (bad cholesterol) levels, especially in people with high blood cholesterol levels.

NUTS

Nuts, especially brazil nuts, can protect against heart disease because they are good sources of magnesium and magnesium-rich foods can promote a normal heart rhythm, lower triglycerides (a type of fat) in the blood and contribute to lowering blood pressure. They are also a great source of omega-3 fatty acids. However, nuts can also contribute to weight gain so a small handful of good-quality, fresh, raw, unsalted nuts a day is adequate.

TEA

Some evidence suggests that the antioxidants in tea can help prevent the build-up of fatty deposits in the arteries, and that it may act as an anti-blood-clotting agent and improve blood vessel dilation to improve blood flow.

ALCOHOL

A moderate intake of alcohol – no more than two drinks a day for men or one drink a day for women – is possibly associated with reduced risk of heart disease. Some types of alcohol, such as red wine, may contain additional protective factors like antioxidants, although this is still being researched. A high intake of alcohol increases blood pressure and tends to increase triglycerides, increasing the risk of heart disease. Moderate alcohol intake increases the HDL level in the blood and this helps clear other fats from the body.

FOODS RICH IN VITAMIN E

Some studies indicate that vitamin E acts as an antioxidant, helping to protect against LDL or bad cholesterol. Good sources of vitamin E include avocadoes, dark green vegetables, vegetable oils and wholegrain products. It is better to eat foods containing vitamin E rather than take supplements, which do not have the same protective effects.

GARLIC AND ONIONS

Allicin, a compound in fresh garlic, has been found in some studies to lower blood cholesterol. Garlic also has an anti-platelet activity which helps to thin the blood in a similar way to taking low-dose aspirin. Onions have been found to be beneficial too.

GINGER

Ginger has an anti-platelet action so it helps to thin the blood which, if your arteries are narrowed by atherosclerotic deposits, can help to prevent heart attack or stroke.

MEDITERRANEAN DIET

Adherence to the Mediterranean diet is associated with a 27% lower death rate among those with CVD, independent of their nationality.[69][70] This diet follows many of the principles mentioned above as well as using olive oil as the preferred cooking oil and salad dressing.

Connectedness

People in higher socio-economic groups are more likely to make healthy lifestyle change.[71] Those from lower socio-economic groups are far less likely to make such changes, perhaps because of the lack of autonomy they have in their lives. According to the Whitehall studies into work and social status on heart disease, 'giving employees more variety in tasks and a stronger say in decisions about work may decrease the risk of coronary heart disease.'[72] A US taskforce looking into predictors for CVD found that job dissatisfaction and unhappiness were stronger predictors than the usually accepted risk factors.[73]

Marriage, an extended network of friends and family, church membership and group affiliation have been associated with a reduced CVD risk.[74] Social disadvantage and social isolation are predictors of CVD and also of a poor outcome after having a stroke. 'Lack of social support may contribute to poorer outcomes due to poor compliance, depression and stress,' according to a study in the journal, *Neurology*.[75]

Our risk for CVD in later life may also be affected by our social and emotional circumstances early in life, as illustrated by a study[76] looking at childhood loss. The effects of relationships early in life affect how we respond to stressors later on. For example, if we lose a parent in childhood or have poor family relationships, when we deal with a stressful task as adults we show increased SNS activation: higher blood pressure and increased adrenaline and cortisol levels.

We must also remember that our social circumstances have a profound effect upon other lifestyle factors, like whether we exercise or not and our use of healthcare resources.

Environment

Environment can impact upon CVD in many ways. Living in an urban environment with heavy air pollution significantly increases the risk of CVD.[77] Chronic noise exposure can be a stressor and studies have suggested that living in a noisy environment increases the risk of heart disease, mostly among those who tend to be annoyed by noise.[78]

We are exposed to various chemicals at home and work which can increase the risk of heart disease. These include arsenic,[79] environmental endocrine disruptors (EEDs), pesticides,[80] lead[81] and mercury.[82] Those who are concerned about their exposure to chemicals should see a doctor trained in occupational and environmental medicine. On the other hand, our environment can work for us. Employees who experience a 'just' work environment had a 35% lower risk of heart disease than other employees.[83] Regular moderate levels of sun exposure are associated with a reduced risk of CVD, probably because it increases our level of vitamin D.[84]

Environment can also be conducive or not conducive to healthy lifestyle. Having access to attractive and safe parks, for example, increases the likelihood of being physically active. Our social environment at work or home, and the advertising we are subject to, have their effects.

The Ornish program for heart disease

Dean Ornish is a US cardiologist who, in his student days, suffered from the stress and poor health which is common among medical students. He took up yoga and meditation and changed his lifestyle, with great results. This had a profound effect upon him and when he became a cardiologist he was determined to measure the effects of such an approach on people with heart disease. Few other doctors took him seriously and he had to lobby for many years to get funding for a clinical trial into the effects on heart disease of the Ornish program, which is based on yoga principles. It serves as an excellent model for holistic care. Although the Ornish program was not derived from the Essence program it addresses all of the elements.

In medical school doctors tend to be taught that CVD is not a reversible disease and so medical management is mostly aimed at slowing its progression. The Ornish program[85] was the first demonstration that, given the right conditions, CVD is a reversible illness. Importantly, the program improved patients' quality of life as well as producing better clinical outcomes.[86] In the first landmark study on the program published in the *Lancet*, people with already well-established heart disease were divided into two groups. One, the control group, had conventional medical management only. The other group had the same medical management plus the Ornish lifestyle program. The program consisted of:

- Group support;
- Stress management including meditation and yoga;
- Low-fat vegetarian diet;
- Moderate exercise;
- Quitting smoking.

Over 12 months, the frequency, duration and severity of angina in the patients in the Ornish program significantly improved, and angiograms demonstrated that their arteries had become less blocked. Most patients who received conventional care alone slowly deteriorated but, interestingly, a few patients in this group also improved. It turned out that they had made major lifestyle changes of their own accord. In both groups, the more effort the person put into making healthy lifestyle changes, the greater the improvement in their condition. If a person went through the Ornish program but did not apply it afterwards in their day-to-day life they derived no benefit.

The cost of the Ornish lifestyle program is a great deal less than for bypass surgery yet has superior results. In the US at the time of the initial research – in the early 1990s – the Ornish program cost around US$3,900 for a live-in seven-day retreat, weekly support group and various resources. The average cost for bypass surgery at the time was US$40,000. By 1993 the average cost savings were US$58,000 per patient because patients who went through the Ornish program were less likely to be admitted to hospital, have heart attacks, need bypass surgery or require increases in medications.[87] Ornish observed that the program enhanced the patients' mental health and ability to cope with stress, and that this greatly contributed to their good outcomes and healthy lifestyle change. Indeed, poor mental health and high stress are predictors of relapse into an unhealthy lifestyle.[88]

Following up the study participants five years later showed that the health of the two groups had diverged even further.[89] The Ornish group had continued to reverse their disease: they reported less severe symptoms and their angiograms showed even less artery blockage. The other group had nearly two and a half times as many major cardiac events over the five-year period.

Insurance companies are understandably very interested in promoting the Ornish program but, unfortunately, some elements of the medical profession have been slower on the uptake and some even quite hostile to it. As Dr Steven Horowitz, a leading US cardiologist, was quoted in *Business Week* magazine in 1993, 'it is almost medical malpractice' not to offer the Ornish program to patients. The fact that studies such as Ornish's are not more often funded and the results not more widely promoted raises some interesting and controversial questions about funding healthcare services, medico-legal issues and priorities. How long can we afford to put low-cost and effective programs with only good side effects as last priorities, and high-cost and less-effective treatments with so many undesirable side effects as first priorities?

11

Cancer

Education

Cancer is a very real risk, with one person in three being affected before the age of 75. As a cause of death it is closing in on heart disease. But cancer is an entirely different disease to cardiovascular disease. Firstly, it is not one disease but many, all with differing causes and treatments. Secondly, cancers vary enormously in how aggressive or life-threatening they are. Although we dread receiving a diagnosis of cancer, many cancers are not life-threatening, and even if they are, early diagnosis and treatment can improve the outcome. Thirdly, because cancer includes such a wide variety of conditions, some have been extensively researched and others have not. Despite all we know, cancer largely remains something of a mystery.

It is important to understand the generic Essence principles, which are largely the same whatever the cancer, and not be overly concerned about the gaps in information on particular types of cancer. Although most research data referred to in this chapter relates to the more common cancers, the same rules are likely to apply for other types.

WHAT IS CANCER?

In the most general sense, cancer is a disease in which cells:

- **Divide at a rapid rate.** Cells normally obey hormonal and other messages from the body about when to divide and how fast. Cancer cells multiply far beyond what they should and do not respond to the body's messages to stop.

- **Live far longer than they should.** All cells have a regulated lifespan. It can be a relatively short time – days for the cells lining the gut – to many years – for brain cells, for instance. Because of genetic changes, cancer cells often don't seem to know when to die.
- **Don't obey the normal boundaries.** Cells in the body are meant to stay within well-demarcated boundaries and not go into other tissues. Cancer cells press on or invade surrounding organs, causing loss of function and destruction of healthy tissues. Cancer can spread through the body to distant sites via the bloodstream and lymph vessels, and can spread directly to nearby tissues. Cells which have spread to distant parts of the body are called 'secondary cancer' or metastases; the original site is called the 'primary cancer'.
- **Consume considerable resources but have no useful function in the body.** Cancer cells are hungry cells but they produce nothing useful. When cancer is advanced, this consumption of energy can leave the rest of the body depleted – thin and weak or, as doctors call it, 'cachectic'. Thus weight loss is often a sign of advanced cancer.
- **Are no longer a part of the 'self'.** Cancer cells change and mutate over time until they resemble less and less the original tissue from which they came. This means they are no longer recognised by the body as part of the self. If the immune system can recognise cells as cancerous they will attack them as if they were foreign tissue.

Cancers can be largely divided into two groups: solid and blood-borne malignancies. Solid means that the cancer forms a solid lump or mass which, depending on its site, can be felt or seen on an X-ray or scan. The blood malignancies, like leukaemia, form in the bone marrow and other blood-cell-producing tissues like lymph glands.

WHAT CAUSES CANCER?

The body produces cancer cells on a regular basis and so there is an ongoing battle in our bodies between cancer cells being produced and our body's defences. Whatever increases the risk of cancer cells being made or reduces the body's defences to cancer will increase the risk of developing a more advanced cancer. There is no one factor by itself which can be implicated; it tends to be the interplay of a range of factors like genetics (e.g. family history), chemical exposure (e.g. smoking), lifestyle (e.g. diet and exercise), mental health (e.g. chronic stress and depression), social circumstances, environment (e.g. asbestos or radiation exposure), chronic inflammation (e.g. chronic hepatitis or inflammatory bowel disease), poor immunity (e.g. AIDS) and many others. There are undoubtedly many potential risk factors that we don't know about. We could be lucky and have many risk factors but not get cancer, or have few but still contract the disease.

Whatever the interplay of causes, it is generally thought that one way or another, a range of genetic mutations and switches are activated which starts the disease going. As has been mentioned the body makes cancer cells on a regular basis but, through a range of defences, stops the cancerous cells in their tracks before they cause any noticeable illness. This is called 'tumour surveillance'. Things which lower our bodily defences – such as depression or unhealthy lifestyle – or which increase the number of cancer cells that the body is making – such as smoking – can push the balance in favour of the cancer cells and thus allow a cancer to slip through the safety net. A cancer will often have been growing for a number of years before it is obvious or causes a symptom which brings it to the attention of the patient or doctor.

STAGES OF CANCER

Cancers are generally staged according to their level of spread and how aggressive or mutated they are. Staging categories vary according to the cancer type, but the most common staging is:

Stage 1: small lump but no spread.
Stage 2: larger lump but still no spread.
Stage 3: some local spread to surrounding tissues.
Stage 4: advanced; spread to distant sites.

Staging is important because the treatment and prognosis will vary accordingly. Obviously if a cancer is treated in the early stages the outcome will tend to be far more optimistic. Hence, it is not just the primary prevention of cancer which is important through healthy lifestyle, but also the secondary prevention through early detection and screening. There are many forms of screening for cancer such as breast self-examination and mammography for breast cancer; faecal occult blood testing for bowel cancer, in which a stool sample is examined for blood; digital examination and PSA (a chemical called Prostate Specific Antigen) testing for prostate cancer; chest X-ray for lung cancer; and pap smears for cervical cancer. You should speak to your doctor about whether any form of cancer screening is appropriate for you given your family history, age and lifestyle.

CANCER TREATMENTS

Different cancers will respond to different treatments. The most widely used conventional cancer treatments tend to fall into three categories, sometimes unflatteringly referred to as:

1. **Slash:** This refers to surgery, that is, either cutting out the tumour or trying to minimise its impact upon the body by, for example, taking pressure off the brain or unblocking the bowel.
2. **Burn:** In radiotherapy X-rays can be used to kill some tumour cells even when deep in the body.
3. **Poison:** In chemotherapy substances are administered which are poisonous to dividing cells. The dose is measured so that it most affects rapidly dividing cells – the cancer – but doesn't overly damage healthy cells which also divide at a fast pace, for example blood and gut cells and hair follicles. Hence, it is the immune and digestive systems and hair that bear the brunt of many of the side effects of chemotherapy. There are also longer-term effects of chemotherapy such as memory loss and, strangely, an increased risk of some cancers.

There are other forms of therapy being developed such as hormonal treatments, adjuvant therapy, vaccines and immunotherapy. Some promising treatments derived from plant-based products are also being researched. Some therapies are aimed at prolonging survival and others are aimed at soothing symptoms caused either by the cancer itself or the treatments being administered. Many complementary therapies such as acupuncture, massage and meditation have been found to be useful for symptom control and improving quality of life.

It is beyond the scope of this book to detail all cancer therapies; suffice to say that if diagnosed with cancer it is important to have full and open conversations with everyone on the team helping to manage the cancer. Such a team could include oncologists, surgeons, general practitioners, counsellors, social workers, nurses, and other allied health – such as physiotherapists or occupational therapists –

and complementary medicine practitioners. Other important sources of information include the Anti-Cancer Council, media data bases such as PubMed (www.ncbi.nlm.nih.gov/sites/entrez) or respected websites.

It is important to ask the questions we want answered and to press our healthcare professionals until they are answered to our satisfaction. If we do not find the answers and resources we need then it is important to seek a second opinion. It is also vital that we feel as empowered and involved as we wish to be in our cancer management. Our therapeutic team also plays an important role in helping us not to make a poor decision regarding our cancer care. A poor decision could be anything from declining a clearly beneficial conventional treatment to undertaking a line of therapy with considerable side effects and little prospect of cure. Cancer patients and their families are often vulnerable and can be taken advantage of by practitioners favouring exotic and sometimes harmful or very expensive treatments which have no reasonable prospect of benefit. There are examples of both complementary and conventional treatments which would come under this category.

This having been said, if we feel obstructed, undermined or disempowered in our cancer management; if we are told there is nothing we can do for ourselves; if we are told that lifestyle doesn't matter or that there is nothing outside of conventional medicine which can help us, then we need to have a serious think about finding another practitioner. Quality information and respectful and open lines of communication are much needed so that neither practitioner nor patient makes uninformed decisions, and so that the patient's outcome is optimised. The Australian Senate inquiry in 2004 into the management of cancer clearly indicated that the 'cancer establishment' should be doing a far better job in this regard.

CANCER PREVENTION

Following a review of decades of research into the prevention of cancer[1] the World Cancer Research Fund (WCRF) made a series of 'Recommendations for Cancer Prevention'. The following points are adapted from that list.

1. **Be as lean as possible without becoming underweight.** Weight gain and obesity increase the risk of a number of cancers. Maintain

a healthy weight through healthy nutrition and regular physical activity to lower cancer risk.

2. **Be physically active for at least 30 minutes every day.** There is strong evidence that physical activity protects against cancer. Regular physical activity is also vital for maintaining a healthy weight.

3. **Calorie restriction: avoid sweet drinks and limit energy-dense foods particularly processed foods high in added sugar, low in fibre or high in fat.** Energy-dense foods are high in fats and/or sugars and generally low in nutrient value (vitamins, antioxidants, minerals, etc.) and increase the risk of obesity and therefore cancer.

4. **Eat more of a variety of vegetables, fruits, whole grains and pulses such as beans.** Evidence shows that foods containing dietary fibre may protect against a range of cancers, particularly bowel cancer, and help to protect against weight gain and obesity.

5. **Limit red meat – for example, beef, pork and lamb – to less than 500 g per week, and avoid processed meat.** There is strong evidence that a high intake of red meat and processed meats are causes of bowel cancer and probably other cancers.

6. **Limit alcoholic drinks to two for men and one for women a day.** Any consumption of alcoholic drinks can increase the risk of a number of cancers.

7. **Limit consumption of salty foods and food processed with salt.** Evidence shows that salt and salt-preserved foods probably cause stomach cancer. Processed foods, including bread and breakfast cereals, can contain large amounts of salt.

8. **Don't use supplements to protect against cancer.** Research shows that some high-dose nutrient supplements can affect our risk of cancer but it's best to opt for a balanced diet without supplements.

9. **It's best for mothers to breastfeed exclusively for up to six months.** Breastfeeding protects mothers against breast cancer and babies from excess weight gain.

Stress management

The mind and emotions affect every aspect of our physical being and this has important implications for cancer medicine. There is a scientific field which looks at the links between psychological and social factors and cancer, known as psycho-oncology.

There is clear evidence that better mental and social health is associated with better coping and quality of life for cancer patients. But the role of mental and social health in the causation and progression of cancer remains controversial amongst conventional cancer specialists. Because there are so many factors potentially affecting cancer doubt often exists as to how much of a contribution psychological factors make.

Of all the emotional factors that potentially impact on cancer, depression is probably the most important.[2] An authoritative review[3] by a world-renowned expert in the field, Professor David Spiegel, concluded that chronic and severe depression is probably associated with an increased chance of getting cancer but the evidence was strong that depression predicts more rapid progression once a person has cancer.[4] The longer the depression has existed, the greater the risk factor it is for getting cancer.[5] The risk is nearly doubled, independent of other lifestyle variables, and is not related to any particular cancer.[6 7 8]

Poor coping, distress and depression have been linked in some studies to poor survival for cancers including liver and bile-duct,[9] lung,[10] breast,[11] and bowel cancer, and malignant melanoma.[12] Some studies have not confirmed a link.[13] Having a good general quality of life is associated with better survival for a variety of cancers.[14 15 16 17] The perceived aim of treatment influences survival. Anger influences it.[18] Minimisation, where a person minimises the importance or impact of the cancer, influences survival.[19] Minimisation is not the same as denial; it reflects an ability to adapt or to see the illness in a larger perspective. Cancer patients who are married also tend to live longer.[20] Some of the reasons behind these observations will be described later.

If psychological and social factors play a role in the cause and prognosis of cancer then the important question in many cancer patients' minds is whether psychosocial interventions like group support, relaxation, meditation and CBT produce better coping and mental health, and therefore better survival chances. Unfortunately there are very few completed controlled trials examining the survival outcomes of such therapies. It is notoriously hard to get such research funded and many oncologists are dismissive of this field of research. A number of the studies which have been done have shown a significant improvement in both quality of life and survival time, but others have not.[21] We must therefore try and dig a little deeper beneath the surface in these studies.

The most noted and first study of its type was done by Professor David Spiegel who studied women with metastatic (advanced) breast cancer. Half the women received standard medical treatment only; the other half received the standard medical treatment plus took part in group support focused on improving their ability to express their emotions and some simple relaxation and self-hypnosis techniques.[22] The support group learned to cope much better but for the first 20 months there was no difference in the survival outcomes of the two groups, however after that the women in the support program began to show an advantage. Their average survival time almost doubled, from 18.9 months to 36.6 months, compared to the women who didn't have a support program. Ten years after the study, three of the forty women who had received support were still alive but none in the group that had received standard medical treatment alone were alive.

Another study looked at the outcomes for 68 patients with early-stage malignant melanoma.[23] One half received the usual medical care; the other half had the usual medical care plus six weeks of stress management training. When they were followed up after six years, cancer had recurred in only seven of the 34 patients who had received stress management training, almost half the rate of the other group, in which 13 of 34 had recurrences. Far fewer in the stress management group – three people – had died compared to the other group, 10 of whom had died. In this study, immune function was also followed. Originally the two groups were comparable but the stress management group had significantly better immune function six months into the study. We know that melanoma is one of the cancers which is aggressively attacked by the immune system's NK (Natural Killer) cells and the immune-enhancing effect of the stress management program probably contributed to the major difference in survival rates. The immune system, monitoring for any cancer spread, was able to deal with it before the cancer had a chance to grow. Ten-year follow-up still shows a positive effect on survival rates, although this has weakened a little over time.[24] It may be that people lose motivation and 'booster' stress management programs may be required to maintain the therapeutic effect.

Other studies have also yielded promising results in terms of survival for cancer of the liver[25] and gastrointestinal tract[26] and lymphoma.[27] A 2007 follow-up study on gastrointestinal malignancies like stomach and bowel cancer showed a clinically and statistically significant survival benefit in a hospital-based psychotherapeutic support program delivered to individuals rather than in a group. Over twice the number of patients who received support were alive at 10 years compared to those who didn't.[28]

There are six trials which have not shown an improvement in cancer survival rates from mental and social health programs.[29][30][31][32][33] One of these trials was an attempt to replicate the Spiegel study but the results showed that despite some improvements in mental health and quality of life there was no significant effect on survival. Another study on group support for advanced breast cancer survival showed that the intervention did prolong survival time in the support group compared to the control group (24.0 months compared to 18.3 months) but this difference wasn't statistically great enough to be sure that the difference was not a chance finding. The support program did however help to treat existing and prevent new depressive disorders; reduce feelings of hopelessness and helplessness, and trauma symptoms; and improve social functioning.[34]

Therefore, in summary, of the six trials not showing longer survival, three have shown a positive effect on mental health and the other three have not. Of the six trials that showed a positive effect on survival they all showed improved mental health as a result of the intervention. So the trend seems to be that where the psychosocial intervention has marginal or no long-term benefit on coping, mood or quality of life it tends not to translate into longer survival. If the support program produces a significant and enduring improvement in coping, mental health and quality of life then it tends to have a 'side effect' of improving survival. Nine out of 12 studies have followed this rule so far.

Support programs vary enormously in content, duration and delivery so there are many questions left open for future research.[35] What sorts of programs work best? Who should they be run by? What is the optimal duration for such a program? What are the essential ingredients? What advice should a doctor give to a patient regarding this area? To what extent does compliance affect the outcome? Does having a residential component, where participants live in at a retreat centre for 5–10 days, improve outcomes?

It is likely that it is not just a matter of being in a program which is protective but also the level to which a person participates in it and lives by it. In one study it was found that a high level of involvement in the program was associated with better survival; there was no benefit from just 'going through the motions'.[36] One paper suggested that programs of 12 weeks or longer were more likely to be effective.[37] Those which use meditation and foster positive emotional responses including humour and hope are more likely to be successful. Although programs need to take into account that patients' personality traits and coping styles differ, there is mixed evidence on whether traits such as 'helplessness',[38] [39] 'fighting spirit' and 'optimism'[40] affect survival. A number of studies suggest they do, but other studies throw that into doubt.[41]

SURVIVAL MECHANISMS

If improving mental health does indeed have survival benefits then the potential mechanisms explaining that longer survival are worth considering.[42] The original belief in psycho-oncology circles was that the main explanation for why the mind affects cancer outcomes is the link between the mind and our immunity. Immunity may explain some of the benefits of stress management for some tumours – such as malignant melanoma or cancers like cervical cancer which are caused by viruses – but it does not explain them all. The immune system may play a less important role for cancers which are primarily caused by chemical injury such as lung cancer. Many cancers do not wear their mutated antigens on their surface and therefore the immune system cannot recognise and attack them.[43] Following are some key points to consider:

1. The stress response;
2. Genes;
3. Immune suppression;
4. Melatonin;
5. Angiogenesis;
6. Compliance with treatment;
7. Improved lifestyle.

1. The stress response, cortisol and inflammation
When we are stressed or depressed the body pumps out high levels of cortisol which not only affects the body's defences but also accelerates cancer cell replication. High cortisol levels associated with chronic

stress have been found to be associated with poor prognosis for cancer patients.[44][45][46]

The body also pumps out other chemicals which mediate the stress response such as cytokines, including interleukins, which stimulate inflammation. Part of the role of these chemicals is to accelerate cell replication and stimulate new blood vessel growth (angiogenesis) — which is good when the body is trying to repair itself after a fight with a tiger, but not so good for cancer. They can stimulate tumour growth, almost like a fertiliser makes the grass grow. Chronic inflammation is not a good combination with cancer. Even the inflammation associated with surgery has been shown to increase the growth of tumour metastases at distant sites via these hormones[47] so it is important for cancer patients only to have surgery if it is really necessary. Reducing stress hormones such as the ones mentioned above[48] and inducing hormones associated with well-being and relaxation like melatonin may be part of the reason why stress reduction and psychosocial interventions help cancer survival.[49]

Other chemical mediators in the body can suppress cancer growth and even induce cancer cell suicide. The ability to change the activity of such chemical mediators may in part explain why cognitive-behavioural therapy, meditation, stress management, things that reduce inflammation, calorie restriction and aerobic exercise prolong the healthy life span of humans. They affect molecular mediators including interleukins and especially melatonin.[50] That stress management and social support programs reduce stress hormones[51] and induce hormones associated with wellbeing and relaxation like melatonin may be part of the reason why stress reduction, and mental and social support programs help cancer survival.[52]

Some immune mediators (such as TNF-alpha) can kill tumour cells and have anti-tumour effects. We now know that many tumours are dormant through a balance between cell division, cell death and the body's defences.[53] Upsetting this balance may explain why the occurrence and recurrence of cancer often follow traumatic events that were not well dealt with.[54] It may be more accurate to say that emotional disturbance is a contributing factor accelerating a cancer's growth rather than it being the cause of cancer.

2. Genes

We can have a genetic predisposition to cancer but our DNA also has protective cancer suppressor genes. Our psychological state affects our genetics. It has been shown that stress impairs the repair of genetic mutations[55] and produces oxidative damage to DNA. For example, in experiments on workers, a perceived high workload, stress and 'impossibility of alleviating stress' are all associated with high DNA damage.[56 57] Personality factors are linked to higher DNA damage, especially a tendency toward tension and anxiety in the case of men and a tendency toward depression and a feeling of rejection in women.[58] A low level of closeness to our parents during childhood or bereavement in the previous three years is also associated with greater DNA damage. Psychological stress affects the ability of immune cells to initiate genetically programmed cancer cell suicide.[59] The ability of the body to repair DNA is commonly suppressed in cancer patients and this is a potential marker of cancer susceptibility.[60]

Oxidative stress due to psychological stress and a low intake of dietary antioxidants may both be crucial factors in the evolution and progression of cancer.

3. Immune suppression

Stress causes suppression of immune cells, in particular NK (Natural Killer) cells. This leads to reduced defences and poor cancer surveillance for some cancers.[61]

4. Melatonin

Melatonin, which is a naturally occurring hormone that regulates our body clock and is also a powerful antioxidant, also has a number of beneficial effects on genes and immunity which have important implications for cancer.[62] Melatonin supplements have been associated with 34% lower cancer recurrence rates and better cancer survival.[63 64]

Melatonin has beneficial effects on immunity[65] and ageing,[66] and also has anti-tumour effects. It slows cancer cell replication, helps to switch off cancer genes, and inhibits the release and activity of cancer growth factors previously mentioned.[67 68]

Because melatonin regulates our body clock, sleep is intimately linked with melatonin levels and therefore with cancer progression.[69] This may partly explain why things that decrease our melatonin levels, such as doing shift work or working in the airline industry, may also be risk factors for cancer.[70] Body-clock alterations commonly occur in cancer patients, with greater disruption seen in more advanced cases. Emotional and social factors, pain and other symptoms associated with cancer can interrupt our sleep rhythms. Taking care to enhance sleep is a vital part not only of coping with cancer but also helping to improve cancer defences and prognosis. (For more advice on improving sleep, see Chapter 2, 'Stress management', in Part 1.)

Poor mental health is associated with low levels of melatonin. Healthy lifestyle and stress reduction increases melatonin. Helping the body to stimulate its own melatonin has many beneficial effects, but more is not always better. Those who wish to take supplements should seek medical advice first, as at high doses it can actually have negative effects on mood and immunity. There are plenty of ways to stimulate melatonin ourselves, without supplements, as we can see in the following table.

What boosts and lowers melatonin

Melatonin is stimulated by:
- Meditation[71][72]
- Subdued lighting after sunset
- Calorie restriction
- Exercise
- Foods rich in calcium, magnesium, vitamin B6; foods rich in tryptophan (e.g. milk, spirulina, seaweed)
- Relaxing music

Melatonin is inhibited by:
- Stress
- Drugs such as caffeine, beta-blockers, alcohol and sedatives, especially before bed
- Inactivity
- Electromagnetic radiation
- Working night shifts
- Jet lag
- Excessive calories

Sources [73][74][75][76][77]

5. Angiogenesis

Angiogenesis is the process in which tissues make new blood vessels. It is a vital process for tissue repair but also for the growth of tumours, as solid tumours can only grow into other tissues because they are able to lay down new blood vessels.

Certain types of cytokines (the signalling chemicals produced by the body which we encountered above in the discussion on the stress response) mediate the process of blood vessel growth. One particularly important one is vascular endothelial growth factor (VEGF) and in cancer patients high levels of this cytokine are associated with a poor prognosis. The stress response increases the level of VEGF. Cancer patients who report higher levels of social wellbeing – and less stress – have lower levels of VEGF, a good prognostic sign. Feelings of helplessness and worthlessness in cancer patients are also associated with higher levels of VEGF.[78] Other studies have found links with depression.[79] It is known that cancer patients with depression have high levels of the hormones that stimulate angiogenesis compared to cancer patients who are not depressed. Tumours in stressed animals showed a markedly increased network of blood vessels and higher levels of the angiogenesis hormones.[80]

6. Compliance with treatment

It may be that cancer patients with better mental health – due to things such as stress management and social support – improve their outcomes by complying with treatment better and utilising more avenues of therapy.

7. Improved lifestyle

It is known that those who feel better psychologically find it easier to make healthy changes in other parts of their lives such as diet or exercise which improves outcomes.

MINDFULNESS AND CANCER

A lot of work is going into measuring the effects of mindfulness programs on cancer patients. For example, a study[81] has been done on the effects of MBSR on quality of life, stress, mood, hormonal and immune function in early-stage breast and prostate cancer patients. The patients were given an eight-week MBSR program including relaxation techniques, meditation and gentle yoga, and were encouraged to practise daily at home. The patients, who were followed for 12 months, showed significant and consistent improvements in symptoms of stress; their levels of the stress hormone cortisol decreased, a good prognostic sign; and their physiological markers of stress such as high blood pressure were reduced, as were their pro-inflammatory cytokines, which (as has been mentioned) can stimulate cancer cell growth. The program gave patients an enhanced quality of life and fewer stress symptoms.

Much more work needs to be done but the signs are looking increasingly positive that MBSR will have a proven place in cancer management. This would confirm what many patients intuitively sense and have found to be true in their own experience.

Spirituality

Cancer, more than most illnesses, raises the prospect of our own mortality. As such it is often a catalyst for looking at our life and reconsidering what is of importance. Indeed, 80% of people wish to discuss spiritual issues with their doctors when confronting life-threatening illness. Cancer can therefore be a powerful stimulus for personal growth, but for many it leads to an emotional implosion unless they receive adequate support. Spirituality is relevant for cancer patients because of its relationship to better mental health, coping with adversity, enhanced social support, healthier lifestyle and greater life expectancy.

There have been precious few studies on whether spirituality or religion protect against cancer. The only well-performed trial found a significantly lower incidence of bowel cancer, and longer survival in those who got bowel cancer, among those with a religious dimension to their lives.[82] These effects couldn't be explained by other risk factors.

On a more general level, another study found that social and physical functioning were significantly improved and distress was reduced if a person had meaning in life.[83]

A related question is whether the various forms of 'distant healing' can assist cancer patients. A review[84] showed that there was some evidence, albeit a little sparse and inconsistent, to suggest that forms of healing including therapeutic touch, faith healing and Reiki may be helpful in reducing pain and anxiety, and improving function like movement and mobility. Grander claims – such as tumour regression through prayer, therapeutic touch and faith healing – are mainly anecdotal and have not been rigorously investigated or proven.

Exercise

The evidence is becoming clearer that regular moderate exercise helps to prevent a whole range of cancers and prolongs survival for those who already have cancer. Reviewing a vast body of evidence, the World Cancer Research Fund has declared that physical inactivity is clearly a risk factor for cancer.[85]

For example, over thirty studies have shown that physical activity reduces colon cancer risk.[86][87] It also protects against the development of precancerous bowel polyps. The reduction of bowel cancer risk for those who exercise is around 50%.

A large-scale Norwegian study in the *International Journal of Cancer* showed a 30% reduction in the risk of breast cancer in women who exercise regularly, particularly in those under 45 years of age.[88] This was confirmed in a recent analysis of the Nurses' Health Study.[89] Another study[90] looked of 75,000 post-menopausal women between 50 and 79 years of age and showed that those who walked briskly for 1¼ to 2½ hours per week reduced their breast cancer risk by 18%. Those who exercised 2½ to 10 hours per week reduced their risk by 22%. A past history of strenuous exercise at age 35 or 50 was associated with a breast cancer risk reduction. The Norwegian study also showed a reduced risk of lung cancer in women who exercise, independent of whether they smoke or what kind of diet they have.[91]

The possible reasons why exercise is protective against cancer include:

- Effects on prostaglandins and other modulators of inflammation that can stimulate cancer cell growth;
- Antioxidant effects;
- Maintenance of a regular bowel habit and reduction in bowel transit time which helps minimise risk of bowel cancer;
- Protection against obesity (a risk factor for cancer) and contribution to better overall energy balance;
- Encouragement of other healthy lifestyle changes like better diet;
- Improvements in mental health and depression;
- Improvements in immune function;
- Stimulation of melatonin.

Studies have shown that exercise not only helps prevent cancer but can improve patients' survival rate after a cancer diagnosis. For example, a study of almost 3000 women with stage 1, 2 and 3 breast cancer, who were followed up for 18 years, found that the women who walked for three to five hours per week (equivalent of 9–15 MET) had half the chance of death than those who didn't.[92] This was confirmed in a study of a different group of women with breast cancer over a nine-year period, in which regular exercise was associated with a 44% reduction in death rates.[93]

In a study on almost 48,000 men, within 14 years approximately 3000 had developed prostate cancer. Many prostate cancers are very slow growing and not life threatening but some become aggressive and can advance rapidly. In this study, in men older than 65 who exercised regularly, the risk of getting aggressive prostate cancer was one-third that of men who didn't exercise.[94]

A study following more than 500 patients with bowel (colorectal) cancer for over five years found that the risk of death was halved in those with stage 2 and 3 bowel cancer if they exercised regularly.[95]

The above findings could be contrasted with the outcomes of chemotherapy. Most clinicians and patients think that chemotherapy improved survival more than it does. The world's leading cancer journal, *Clinical Oncology*, reported, 'It is very clear that cytotoxic chemotherapy only makes a minor contribution (2%) to (5-year) cancer survival. To justify the continued funding and availability of drugs used in cytotoxic chemotherapy, a rigorous evaluation of the cost-effectiveness and impact on quality of life is urgently required.'[96] If the benefits associated with exercise could be attributed to a chemotherapy drug or other cancer treatment it would be a world breakthrough and would probably cost about $70,000 a year to receive.

In addition to helping prevent cancer and improve survival rates, exercise also helps to manage many symptoms common among cancer patients. It leads to reduced fatigue and greater vitality, greater quality of life, reduced emotional distress, greater physical strength[97] and reduced chronic pain.[98] Exercise reduces pain because it increases endorphins, our body's natural painkillers; has positive effects on mood; relaxes muscles; improves immunity and has an anti-inflammatory effect.

If cancer patients are more informed about the benefits of exercise they will be motivated to do it. It should be a part of the management plan for preventing or treating any cancer. But if taking up exercise, we need to listen to the body and have respect for our age and current level of fitness. Exercising to the point of exhaustion is not useful.

Nutrition

What we eat clearly contributes to our risk of developing cancer but researchers are still trying to sort out which foods protect, which increase risk, and how much is optimal. Overall, a poor diet increases cancer risk probably by 30%.[99] [100]

One point to stress about the following information is that although most studies look at just one food group or one type of cancer, the same principle is likely to hold for other cancers. As a general rule, if a food has been found to be good (or bad) for one cancer it is likely to be good (or bad) for other cancers as well.

Oxidation is a part of the ageing process. It is largely mediated by what are called 'free radicals' which are chemicals that are produced in the body as a normal part of daily life. Free radicals damage other molecules in the cell, including DNA. Antioxidants help to mop up excess free radicals and slow the ageing process. A healthy diet with nutritious food prepared in such a way that it preserves its nutritional value is most protective and principally it is dietary antioxidants that reduce cancer risk. Although there is evidence that some antioxidant supplements, such as selenium, can have a protective effect, the best protection against cancer is a healthy diet rather than a deficient diet plus supplements. This was illustrated by a study on breast cancer which showed that eating vegetables and, even more so, fruit contributed to a decreased risk of breast cancer. 'These results indicate the importance of diet, rather than supplement use . . . in the reduction of breast cancer risk,'[101] the researchers concluded. The greatest role for antioxidant supplementation may be in helping to reduce the negative impact of radiotherapy on cancer patients.[102]

Lowering total calorie intake, otherwise known as calorie restriction, helps to reduce the risk of cancer and a range of other illnesses, and it significantly increases longevity. A 20% or 30% reduction in calorie intake from the average diet was shown to be enough to reduce cancer incidence by 30% and 40% respectively. A 40% reduction in calorie intake may decrease the incidence substantially further to near zero.[103] [104] According to the World Cancer Research Fund (WCRF):

> *Sweet drinks, such as colas and fruit squashes can . . . contribute to weight gain. Fruit juices, even without added sugar, are likely to have a similar effect. Try to eat lower energy-dense foods such as vegetables, fruits and whole-grains. Opt for water or unsweetened tea or coffee in place of sugary drinks.*[105]

A trial on nearly 2500 women with breast cancer found that a low-fat diet led to a 24% reduction in the recurrence of cancer and a 19%

improvement in survival beyond five years.[106] Again, if this effect was associated with a drug we would all have heard about it.

The WCRF recommendation is that there is no guaranteed safe amount of processed meat such as bacon, ham, salami, corned beef and some sausages to include in our diet. No matter how small our intake, processed meat cannot be ruled out as increasing cancer risk, particularly bowel cancer.

Red meat probably also increases the risk for a range of cancers other than bowel cancers[107] and we should limit our total intake to less than 500 g of cooked red meat per week (including pork), which is equivalent to about 700 to 750 g raw. Poultry is probably less problematic, and eating fish two to three times a week is probably protective. If eating meat, where possible it is preferable to buy certified organic and free range. The hormones, antibiotics and chemicals used by many commercial meat producers may be more damaging to our health than is currently known.

SUPER FOODS

A miracle food for cancer has not been discovered but many foods have been identified that contribute to cancer prevention and treatment. Below are some of the super foods – but remember that it is the consistent intake of a balanced, varied and healthy diet which is best, not just focusing on one food item and expecting it to have some miraculous effect. The American Institute of Cancer Research estimates that if the only dietary change made was to increase the daily intake of fruits and vegetables to at least five servings per day, cancer rates could decline significantly. For example, women with breast cancer are much less likely to have recurrences if they eat the five or more vegetable servings per day.[108] A study found that women who had a high intake of fruit and vegetables had a 43% reduced risk for breast cancer recurrence.[109] Researchers working on a study of diet and cancer have shown that 'Protective elements in a cancer-preventive diet include selenium, folic acid, vitamin B12, vitamin D, chlorophyll and antioxidants such as carotenoids (alpha-carotene, beta-carotene, lycopene, lutein, cryptoxanthin).'[110] Organic produce is clearly superior because of its higher concentration of important vitamins, minerals and antioxidants.

Cruciferous vegetables

Cabbage, broccoli, brussels sprouts, kale, watercress, bok choy, turnip and cauliflower[111] are part of the cabbage or cruciferous family. These are not the most popular vegetables, particularly among children, but they are real heavyweights when it comes to preventing and stopping the spread of cancer. In a study involving almost 48,000 people over a 10-year period, those who ate five or more weekly servings of cruciferous vegetables, especially broccoli and cabbage, had half the risk of developing cancer than those who had one or fewer servings per week. Other studies confirm their protective effect, for example, those who regularly ate cruciferous vegetables had a 35% reduced risk of lung cancer.[112] They also seem to be protective for prostate cancer.[113]

Cruciferous vegetables should be lightly cooked and chewed thoroughly when eaten if we are to fully benefit from their anti-cancer potential – for instance, the protective effects of broccoli are significantly diminished when it is cooked.[114]

Garlic and onions

Garlic is very well documented throughout history as a great medicinal food.[115] Current research suggests that it may play an important part in the prevention of prostate, stomach, colon and oesophageal cancers. French scientists have found evidence that eating garlic and onions is linked to a reduced incidence of breast cancer. Garlic and onions can slow the development of cancer and help to prevent cancer growth. The molecules responsible for these effects are released when garlic is crushed, chopped or chewed. Freshly crushed garlic is the best source of these molecules.

Citrus fruits

Citrus fruits such as oranges, grapefruits, mandarins and lemons are essential foods in cancer prevention. They can act directly on cancerous cells and have an anti-cancer effect.

Red grapes

Red grapes contain a compound in their skins called resveratrol which has an anti-cancer activity, so moderate consumption of red grapes or wine may be beneficial.

Tomatoes

Tomatoes have high amounts of lycopene, a pigment which gives tomatoes their bright red colour and their anti-cancer potential.

Lycopene's anti-cancer effect is increased by cooking tomatoes in the presence of vegetable fats such as olive oil. Eating at least two tomato-based meals a week may lower your risk of developing cancer.

Soy

There are great differences in the rates of hormone-dependent cancers – such as some forms of breast cancer and prostate cancer – between Eastern and Western countries.[116] This may be related to the higher consumption of soy-based foods in Asian countries, especially because consumption begins before puberty. Soy foods such as soybeans, soy flour, miso, tofu and soy milk contain isoflavones and phytooestrogens. Soy foods have also been found to be protective against colorectal cancer.[117]

To benefit from the anti-cancer effects of soy, studies have shown you need to consume about 50 grams per day of soy-based food. Only whole soy foods are considered cancer protective. Supplements containing isoflavones are not considered useful. For people with existing hormone-dependent cancers there is some concern regarding the safety of soy products although it is hard to delineate at the moment to what extent the risk is anticipated or real. Some studies have even suggested a protective role of genistein, a form of phytoestrogen, in reducing the risk of breast cancer recurrence.[118] To be cautious, at this stage of our knowledge those with hormone-dependent breast cancer should minimise soy food intake.

Green tea

Green tea contains large amounts of catechins which are compounds that have many anti-cancer properties. Try to have three cups of green tea per day.

Berries

Strawberries, raspberries, blueberries, goji berries and cranberries have high levels of antioxidants and anti-cancer compounds. They are a delicious part of an anti-cancer diet.

Omega-3 fatty acids

Omega-3 fatty acids, found in sardines, mackerel, salmon, flaxseed, soy and nuts, especially walnuts, can help to prevent cancer.[119] Studies have shown that consuming fish rich in omega-3s decreases the risk of developing breast, prostate and colon cancers.

Insoluble fibre

Insoluble fibre helps to prevent bowel cancer. If food, particularly red meat, stays in the gut too long because of constipation various chemicals are produced which can predispose us to cancer. Insoluble fibre is not absorbed from the gut and therefore it bulks up and loosens stools, which helps to reduce the time it takes for food to pass from one end of the gut to the other. Good food sources of insoluble fibre include wholegrain breads and cereals, brown rice, wholemeal pasta, and fruits and vegetables including skins and seeds where appropriate. It is advisable to include whole grains with every meal.

Herbs and spices

Season your dishes with turmeric, parsley, thyme, mint or capers as they contain extraordinary quantities of molecules that inhibit the growth of cancer cells and prevent the development of tumours.

Dark chocolate

Good-quality dark chocolate which contains 70% cocoa mass – that is, plenty of cocoa but not too much fat or sugar – contains polyphenols which can help to protect against cancer. Eating two 20 gm squares a day is enough.

More specific dietary advice follows at page 230 where we look at the Ornish program's cancer diet.

Connectedness

Connectedness can be important for different reasons at different times throughout the progression of cancer. People need support when they make the initial adjustment to a cancer diagnosis and face what it potentially entails. They need support in coping with cancer treatment. Cancer patients are often lonely as many people avoid contact with a friend or family member with cancer because they find it confronting or don't know how to deal with the potentially emotionally sensitive situation. A person with cancer may crave solitude, or conversely they may feel isolated. We will not know unless we ask.

Then there is the support required after treatment as they return to work and family life. Or if the cancer becomes advanced, then there is the important phase of palliative care and dealing with the prospect of death. The support a person receives makes a big difference to how they deal with it. There is potentially no more lonely time in a person's life and yet, with care and encouragement from others, this can be the most uplifting and inspiring. Ultimately, death is not optional for any of us, but how we confront death is. It is important for those caring for a dying loved one to help them find their way and not to project our assumptions and fears onto them.

Social isolation predisposes us to a whole range of illnesses, including cancer, and is associated with a higher mortality rate.[120] Population studies demonstrate that socially isolated men are two to three times more likely to die over the following nine to 12 years than those with good social networks, and socially isolated women are one and a half times more likely to die.[121] Our social support, or the lack of it, can also have a major effect on our ability to lead a healthy lifestyle. For example, having support to give up smoking makes it a lot easier, whereas a lack of support can make it all but impossible.

The most common sources of informal social support are family and friends, and it has been shown that cancer patients who are married or have a stable relationship survive for longer than would otherwise be expected. Women who have a better breast cancer prognosis are those who have social support and are married. Those who tend to minimise the importance of their cancer also have a better prognosis. Those with depression or who constrain their emotions have decreased breast cancer survival.[122]

In cancer management social support can be provided or enhanced by helpful and nurturing healthcare professionals, or formally, through cancer support programs. Such programs should really be a part of standard cancer care. The effect on survival of such programs has been discussed previously.

Environment

By and large, our environment is a safe place but there are a range of ways in which environment can increase the risk of cancer.[123] The list is extensive but following are the five most major risks.

POLLUTION AND PASSIVE SMOKING

Heavy air pollution makes a contribution to cancer risk, mostly lung cancer, and diesel fuel is the most problematic pollutant. The risk of heavy air pollution is nowhere near as great as smoking, though. Smoking increases the risk of lung cancer up to twenty-fold, as well as increasing the risk of mouth, throat and other cancers. Regular and long-standing exposure to passive smoking also increases the risk of some forms of lung and throat cancer; for those with heavy exposure the risk is nearly doubled.[124] Avoiding regular contact with passive smoking is advisable; fortunately, legislation that restricts smoking in public places has made this a lot easier.

ASBESTOS FIBRES

Asbestos was a common building and insulation material in the first half of last century. When asbestos materials become damaged and crumble the tiny fibres can be breathed in and cause cell damage that leads to a type of lung cancer (mesothelioma) and throat cancer. If having asbestos removed, it is important to have it done by persons qualified to do this work as there are a range of special procedures required to do this safely.

PESTICIDES, INSECTICIDES AND WEED-KILLERS

People who are exposed to agricultural chemicals are at a higher risk of a variety of cancers including lymphoma, leukaemia and prostate, skin and lung cancers. Farmers are at particular risk.

Only use pesticides, insecticides and weed-killers if really necessary. Natural methods such as companion planting and mulching should help to minimise their use.

The safe use and storage of these chemicals is important so use as little as possible, follow the safety precautions on the label, wear protective clothes, wash after use, and keep out of the reach of children and pets.

HOUSEHOLD CLEANERS, SOLVENTS AND OTHER CHEMICALS

There is not nearly enough research into the potentially harmful effects of household products. It is known, however, that products containing benzene and methylene chloride – found in some paint strippers and paints – can cause cancer. Use household cleaners, solvents, paints and other chemicals sparingly, and use environmentally friendly products wherever possible. Take the precautions recommended on the label, ventilate the area adequately, avoid contact with skin, wash after use, and store safely and securely away from children and pets.

ELECTROMAGNETIC FIELDS (EMF) AND RADIATION

Radiation and magnetic fields are a regular part of our environment. Low-level exposure from televisions, microwave ovens, electric blankets, mobile phones and computers probably does not increase cancer risk, according to the current balance of evidence.[125] Higher-level exposure, such as living within 200 to 300 metres of high-voltage powerlines or radio towers, probably does increase cancer risk, particularly for children.[126] Part of the reason may be because such fields upset melatonin secretion.

Having a simple procedure like a chest X-ray has been assumed to be safe, and this may be so for those with a low cancer risk, but the story may not be the same for those with a strong genetic predisposition to cancer. For example, women with genes that strongly predispose them to breast cancer (e.g. BRCA1 or 2) were found to have double the risk of getting breast cancer if they had a chest X-ray. If they had the chest X-ray before the age of 20 then their risk was fourfold.[127] This may be because it takes relatively less radiation exposure to cause DNA damage in genetically predisposed individuals. This should be taken into account before having radiological tests.

UV LIGHT

Sunburn increases the risk of malignant melanoma and high-level sun exposure increases the risk of less dangerous skin cancers such as SCC and BCC. Regular and moderate sun exposure, however, reduces the risk of a whole range of cancers, probably because of sunlight's beneficial effects on vitamin D, melatonin, immunity, mood and lifestyle.

The Ornish program for cancer

To date, Dean Ornish's program is the only comprehensive lifestyle program which has been trialled on any form of cancer. A study was done on 80 men with early prostate cancer [128] who had chosen to 'watch and wait' and monitor their disease rather than undergo treatment straightaway. Many prostate cancers are relatively dormant and not aggressive or life threatening, so it is a legitimate course of action with early prostate cancer to wait and see if the condition progresses rather than go through possibly unnecessary treatments which can have some very undesirable side effects. If monitoring reveals that the prostate cancer is aggressive then a man would certainly be advised to go on to have treatment.

Half the men were assigned to undertake the Ornish lifestyle program and the other half continued on with their usual lifestyle. The Ornish program, which is very similar to the Gawler Foundation cancer programs, comprised:

- Diet
  - Fruits, vegetables, whole grains, legumes and soy products such as tofu
  - Low fat (a total of 10% of calories from fat); particularly low in saturated fats and animal fats
  - Supplemented by fish oil (3 gm daily), vitamin E (400IU daily), selenium (200 mcg daily), vitamin C (2 gm daily)
- Exercise
  - Walking 30 minutes, six times weekly
- Stress management
  - Gentle yoga, meditation, breathing and PMR
- Support group for one hour, weekly

Over the following year, no men on the Ornish program went on to develop aggressive cancer, but six out of the 40 men in the non-Ornish group underwent conventional treatment because their cancer had progressed based on PSA levels, or MRI.

The researchers measured the men's PSA levels, which is a marker of prostate cancer activity. The graph opposite shows the average changes in PSA after one year. The Ornish group's PSA levels came down by an average of 4%, while the non-Ornish group's went up by an average of 6%. Furthermore, the greater their compliance with lifestyle changes – i.e. the better their adherence to the Ornish program – then the greater the improvement in their condition.

The belief that early cancer is an inevitably progressive condition may in fact be far from the truth, although more research is desperately needed into programs like Dean Ornish's to see:
- If a similar approach holds for cancers other than prostate;

PSA levels in Ornish prostate cancer study

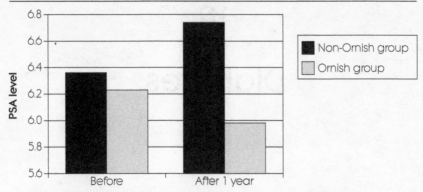

Relationship between degree of healthy lifestyle change and changes in PSA

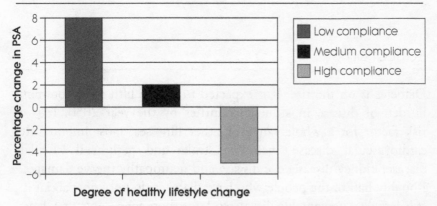

- If particular variations on the program are important for certain types of cancer;
- At what stage and to what extent such an approach can make a difference to cancer;
- To what extent it can minimise the need for invasive and expensive cancer treatments;
- How such programs affect cancer treatments and their side effects.

It is already well known that programs like Ornish's improve quality of life and mental health. If a patentable cancer drug had anywhere near this effect it would be widely publicised as a revolutionary cancer breakthrough and the discoverer would probably have a Nobel Prize for their efforts. But being undramatic, it is easy for the healthcare sector to fail to embrace such simple strategies. It is likely that times will change and some decades from now we will scratch our heads when we look back at the resistance to the simplest, safest and most effective strategies for fighting cancer.

12

Diabetes

Education

Diabetes is on the rise. It is expected to be the fifth most common burden of disease in affluent countries by the year 2030. It is a risk factor for a whole range of other illnesses, most importantly cardiovascular disease, including stroke and peripheral vascular disease, kidney disease, eye disease and neuropathy (nerve damage). Roughly half of the people who have diabetes do not know about it. It is largely a preventable disease and, for those who know they have it, readily treatable.

WHAT IS DIABETES?

Insulin is a hormone secreted by the pancreas largely in response to carbohydrate (sugar) intake. Insulin makes it possible for the sugar, in the form of glucose, to move from the bloodstream into the tissues so that it can be stored and used by the body's cells as fuel.

If the pancreas doesn't make enough insulin, or if our body becomes less sensitive to insulin, glucose stays in our blood rather than going to the tissues, and when it rises past a certain point it leads to tiredness. Then the glucose starts to get excreted in our urine. This requires that a lot of water be excreted in the urine along with the glucose, leading to dehydration. We also get acid and electrolyte imbalances in our blood. Furthermore, our tissues suffer from a lack of glucose, our cells' primary energy source, which leads to relative starvation known as ketosis. If our blood glucose level goes very high – mostly a risk in Type-1 diabetes – then these changes become acutely life-threatening.

There are two main types of diabetes which have different causes and treatments.

Type-1 diabetes

Type-1 diabetes – also known as juvenile-onset diabetes or insulin-dependent diabetes mellitus (IDDM) – accounts for about 5 to 10% of diabetes cases. Most commonly, Type-1 diabetes is an autoimmune condition which begins in childhood. In a genetically susceptible child an otherwise unremarkable viral infection can trigger the immune system to attack not only the virus but also the insulin-making cells of the pancreas; it is as if the immune cells mistake them for the virus. As a result, the pancreatic cells die and the body loses its ability to make insulin.

This profound and sudden insulin deficiency leads to a rapid rise in blood glucose and profound hyperglycaemia, ketoacidosis (high ketones with acid imbalance), electrolyte imbalance and dehydration. Before insulin was discovered this would have been rapidly fatal. Today, with regular insulin injections in conjunction with measured diet and physical activity, this is a readily treatable condition with a near normal life span. It does require a lot of discipline to maintain good control of Type-1 diabetes and ongoing monitoring for complications. Too high a dose of insulin or inadequate food intake can lead to a rapid drop in blood glucose called hypoglycaemia. In severe cases, hypoglycaemia can be fatal if glucose is not taken, by mouth if conscious, or intravenously if unconscious and not able to drink.

Type-2 diabetes

The more common form of diabetes is Type-2 diabetes, otherwise known as maturity-onset or non-insulin-dependent diabetes mellitus (NIDDM). It accounts for roughly 85% of diabetes cases and is largely a condition of affluent lifestyle: over-nutrition, high carbohydrate intake, overweight and obesity, physical inactivity and stress. A family history of Type-2 diabetes also predisposes us to developing it. Approximately half of Type-2 diabetics do not know they have it because, unlike Type-1 diabetes, it causes few if any symptoms until diabetic complications are well established.

The progression from non-diabetic to diabetic goes through an intermediate stage called 'impaired glucose tolerance'. In the early stages of Type-2 diabetes the pancreas still makes insulin, sometimes in high quantities, but because of poor lifestyle, the body has become less sensitive to insulin; this is sometimes known as 'insulin resistance'. The body gets less effect than it used to for the same amount of insulin, leading to high blood glucose and symptoms similar to but milder than Type-1 diabetes.

Type-2 diabetes is largely reversible if a person makes and maintains healthy lifestyle changes. Unfortunately many diabetics are unwilling to make such changes and so they take hypoglycaemic (blood-glucose-lowering) medications. If these medications are not enough to maintain a healthy blood glucose level, then insulin may need to be given by injection.

Today the old term 'maturity-onset diabetes' is no longer widely used. This is mainly because until recently Type-2 diabetes was a condition only seen in the elderly. It is now not uncommon to see Type-2 diabetes in pre-teens such is the level of inactivity and poor diet of many young people today. It is now estimated that over 4% of all adolescents have metabolic syndrome: high blood fats, blood pressure and blood sugar, and obesity around the trunk which predisposes them to Type-2 diabetes. Approximately 30% of overweight and obese adolescents have metabolic syndrome.[1] The long-term health implications are enormous and will be felt for generations to come.

Type-2 diabetes is easily diagnosed with a urine or blood glucose test.

There are other less common causes of diabetes. Any condition which injures or destroys the pancreas, such as cancer, severe pancreatitis or haemochromatosis (an inherited disorder where excessive amounts of iron are absorbed from food and retained in the body's organs), can secondarily lead to diabetes. Women can also develop insulin resistance during pregnancy in which case there is a higher likelihood of complications for mother and child during the pregnancy, and the mother is more likely to get Type-2 diabetes later in life.

Some medications can also aggravate diabetes by raising blood sugar levels.

THE IMPORTANCE OF MONITORING DIABETES

In the long term, monitoring diabetes on a daily basis is important for maintaining good control over the condition. Also important are regular checks with the GP, the care of a diabetic specialist – particularly for Type-1 diabetics – and education from allied health workers like dieticians and diabetes nurses. Effective management of diabetes is truly a team effort. Regular tests and consultations are required to help maintain control of blood glucose and complications, particularly the heart and blood vessels, kidneys, feet and eyes. Managing other cardiovascular risk factors is also central to the total management of diabetes. There are many websites which can provide more information on diabetes but try to source high-quality information such as that found through the International Diabetes Institute.

Type-2 diabetes, being far and away the most common form of diabetes and the one most amenable to lifestyle change, will be the focus of most of this chapter. There is clear evidence that adults who are physically active and maintain a normal BMI throughout adulthood are less likely to get diabetes.[2] Adults with impaired glucose tolerance who lose weight will reduce their risk. As important as lifestyle is for Type-2 diabetes, it is also important to emphasise that a healthy lifestyle is vital for reducing long-term complications in Type-1 diabetes.

Stress management

One of the effects of stress is to disrupt regulation of the immune system, so psychological stress can bring on a range of autoimmune conditions, including Type-1 diabetes.[3] Stress also increases sugar and fat levels in the blood. For this reason stress can also destabilise diabetes. Further, stress can multiply the chances of having diabetic complications like heart disease and can further destabilise diabetes by making us less likely to follow a healthy and disciplined lifestyle, maintain and monitor our blood glucose, and be more likely to get infections and other illnesses.

Research shows that stress management leads to a much better level of control over diabetes and lower rate of complications.[4] Good mental health makes for more stable diabetes control, a healthier lifestyle and better compliance with treatment and monitoring.

Spirituality

When we are diagnosed with a serious chronic condition it is commonly a time for an internal struggle and a review of our values. Spirituality is associated with better overall mental and physical health and a healthier lifestyle, all of which can be an important part of managing and coping with a chronic condition such as diabetes. Studies suggest that diabetic patients who have a spiritual dimension to their lives cope better with the condition and the complications that come with it.[5] Many diabetics have been found to be more diligent in lifestyle and self-management if they have a spiritual background.[6] Further, if a person is able to make meaning of the condition within their own cultural and religious background it can help to improve their ability to cope and their compliance with monitoring and treatment, particularly for indigenous groups that are especially prone to diabetes.[7]

Exercise

Physical activity is important for the whole population in the prevention of Type-2 diabetes. It is estimated that between a third and one-half of all new cases of diabetes could be prevented by regular physical exercise alone. If that was combined with healthy nutrition, the incidence of new cases of diabetes would plummet. Exercise is especially important for those who are at risk, in particular those who are overweight or who have a family history of diabetes.

There is strong and consistent evidence that physical activity is associated with a reduced incidence of Type-2 diabetes[8] and that it delays the onset of complications of all types of diabetes. Exercise also reduces the insulin requirements of people with well-controlled Type-1 diabetes. Type-2 diabetics who exercise vigorously and regularly are nearly 70% less likely to need medication[9] and have far better blood pressure and blood fat control.

Those who inject insulin need to carefully regulate exercise, food intake, insulin dose and timing in order to avoid highs and lows in blood sugar. As ever, those who are overweight or unfit should carefully choose the type, frequency, intensity and duration of exercise that suits them. Getting advice from a trained healthcare professional or sports instructor is advised.

Nutrition

The nutritional management of diabetes is about more than just reducing total calories; it is also about carefully selecting what types of foods make up those calories. Type-2 diabetics not only have problems with blood sugar levels, but also blood fat levels. This means that diet needs to look at saturated fat consumption (meat and dairy) as well as carbohydrate consumption. Trans-fatty acids may also increase diabetes risk. Complex carbohydrates, omega-3 fatty acids and low glycaemic index foods decrease the risk. Because of their immune-modulating effects, omega-3 fatty acids have also been found to reduce the chance of genetically at-risk children developing Type-1 diabetes.[10] Breastfeeding for the first six months of life may also protect against diabetes later in life. Milk containing the protein beta (β) 2 casein has also been implicated in causing Type-1 diabetes and should be avoided if possible.

The Finnish Diabetes Prevention Study[11] demonstrated that lifestyle changes reduce the risk of developing Type-2 diabetes. One group in the study received individualised counselling and had the following goals:

1. Weight reduction, optimally to a BMI of 20 to 23;
2. Total intake of fat less than 30% of overall calorie intake;
3. Intake of saturated fat less than 10% of overall calorie intake;
4. Increased fibre intake, at least 15 g per 1000 calories;
5. Moderate exercise for 30 minutes per day.

During the following few years of the trial their risk of diabetes was reduced by 58%. None of the people who reached four or five of the goals developed diabetes.

The dietary recommendations for the European Association for the Study of Diabetes and American Diabetes Association are as follows:[12]

- Carbohydrate and monounsaturated fatty acids: 60–70% of total calories
- Sucrose (sugar)   10% of total calories
- Fat (total)   less than 35% of total calories
  - Saturated fat   less than 8–7% of total calories
  - Polyunsaturated fat   less than 10% of total calories
- Protein   10–20% of total calories
- Fibre   intake encouraged
- Salt   less than 6 g per day

GLYCAEMIC INDEX

Adopting a low GI (glycaemic index) diet, in association with a high intake of dietary fibre, fruits and vegetables, is associated with far better diabetic control[13] as well as improvements in blood fat levels.

Low GI foods have been shown to reduce the blood glucose rise that occurs after eating a meal.[14][15] They also increase the sense of being satisfied after a meal, promote weight loss and improve insulin sensitivity. The European, Canadian and British nutritional guidelines for diabetes encourage the use of low GI foods. The glycaemic index ranks carbohydrates, according to their effect on our blood glucose level, on a scale of 0 to 100.

Low GI

If a food has a rating between 0 and 55 it is a low GI food. It is absorbed into the bloodstream slowly, which means there will be a consistent flow of glucose into the blood over a long period of time.

High GI

If a food is has a GI value of 70 or higher it is considered a high GI food. This food quickly raises our blood glucose level for a short period of time; it produces a greater surge of glucose and insulin that then drop rapidly.

GLYCAEMIC LOAD

Glycaemic index is only half of the story. The glycaemic load is actually a better indication of how good or bad a food is for control of blood glucose, and insulin. The high GI of some whole foods, like parsnip and dates, for example, is offset by their high fibre content. This gives them a low total glycaemic load. So, although many fruits and vegetables have a relatively high sucrose (sugar) content they are good for diabetics because of the fibre they contain.

Sucrose, a form of sugar made up of glucose and fructose, is listed as having a moderate GI. Many commercially produced foods contain high levels of refined sucrose (table sugar) but have very low fibre content and therefore have a very high glycaemic load. Hence, it is not sugar per se which is problematic for diabetics, but refined sugar. As a general rule, whole and high fibre foods are safer for diabetics. Many commercially produced fruit-juices and foods label themselves as having 'no added sugar' but actually have high levels of sucrose through the addition of things like fruit juice concentrate or corn syrup. Many 'low fat' foods also masquerade as being healthy for diabetics but they often have high levels of refined sucrose. It is important to develop the ability to understand food labels in order to get behind the appearances created by food marketing.

GI rating of major carbohydrates

Low GI (0–55)

All-Bran
All-Bran Fruit 'n Oats
All-Bran Soy 'n Fibre
Legumes: baked beans, soybeans, chick peas, etc.
Sweet potato, yam, taro
Bread: multi-grain, sourdough, rye or wheat pumpernickel, linseed rye, heavy fruit loaf
Barley
Semolina

Fruits: plum, peach, grapefruit, apple, banana, cherries, pear, orange, kiwifruit, grapes
Dried apricots
Yoghurt
Porridge
Pasta (except gnocchi)
Oat bran
Special K
Vita wheat biscuits
Rice bran

Moderate GI (56–69)

Breakfast cereals: e.g. Just right, Mini wheats, Sustain, Nutri-grain, Vita brits, Weet-bix, natural muesli
Breakfast cereal bars
Bread: light rye and rye bread, pita, wholemeal
Cornmeal
Cous cous

Honey
Basmati rice
Fruits: apricots, pineapple, paw paw, rockmelon, mango
Ryvita biscuits
Bagels
Gnocchi
Sucrose

High GI (70–100)

Watermelon
Parsnip
White potato
Baguette
Cornflakes
Rice bubbles
Rice (other than Basmati)
Lollies

Sports drinks
Dried dates
White bread
Crumpets
Bran flakes
Sultana bran
Rice cakes
Glucose

Source[16]

TIPS FOR MANAGING BLOOD SUGAR LEVELS

- Reduce the total GI of a meal by combining a small amount of high GI foods with a larger amount of low GI foods;
- Eat adequate protein at every meal to reduce blood sugar level fluctuations;
- Keep low GI snacks handy to eat when you feel hungry so you can eat these rather than high GI foods that reinforce the vicious cycle;
- Avoid regular consumption of sugar, cakes, sweets, soft drinks and drinks containing caffeine such as coffee, tea and cola;
- Enjoy a diet high in soluble fibre which helps stabilise blood sugar levels. Sources include legumes, apples, nuts, seeds, psyllium, pears, oat bran;
- Consume vinegar as it may help to improve control of diabetes.[17]

Connectedness

Psychological and social stress destabilises blood sugar levels, promotes an unhealthy lifestyle and increases the risk of children developing Type-1 diabetes and other autoimmune conditions. When a child develops diabetes there is not only the primary stress of the diagnosis to consider, but family and parental stressors too, because managing diabetes is not something that just affects the child.[18] The whole family feels the effects of having to care for the child, deal with complications, and experience limitations on their lifestyle.

Type-2 diabetes was almost unknown among indigenous cultures prior to their contact with the West. Changes in social structure, lifestyle and work all have their impact and now these groups have among the highest incidence of diabetes.

As with other chronic conditions, psychosocial support helps diabetics to cope and manage their illness.

Environment

Environment can play a role in diabetes in a number of ways.[19] Even the environment in the womb, before we are born, has a life-long effect on our risk of diabetes. Poor maternal health and poor growth within the womb increase the risk.

There is a relationship between inadequate sun exposure and autoimmune diseases including Type-1 diabetes which may partly explain the climate gradient and seasonal variation in the incidence,[20] i.e. Type-1 diabetes more commonly occurs in winter months and in countries further from the equator. Vitamin D also has effects on insulin production and activity.

Environment can be either more or less conducive to exercising and making good food choices, so it can contribute to our Type-2 diabetes risk. For example, moving to an area with better parks and recreational facilities might make us more likely to exercise, whereas moving somewhere with more fast-food outlets might increase our consumption of fast food. Nutrition tends to be poorer in lower socio-economic areas because these areas are heavily targeted by fast-food chains.

Different cultures have a significantly different incidence of Type-2 diabetes and this is only partially due to genetics. When we move from one culture or country to another, within a generation our risk for diabetes will largely match the average for our new environment.

13

Multiple sclerosis

Education

Multiple sclerosis is the commonest chronic neurological condition affecting young adults in developed countries and it is far more common in women than men. Despite decades of research, little is definitely known about its cause or the factors which trigger it, but it is thought to be an autoimmune condition in which the immune system attacks the myelin sheath around nerve fibres. Myelin is like insulation which helps the nerve impulses to pass along the axons – the connecting 'wires' – from one nerve cell to another. Without the myelin sheath the impulses are not transmitted properly and this leads to loss of function.

MS tends to have an up-and-down course, with exacerbations alternating with periods of partial recovery. During a period of exacerbation there will be a relatively sudden loss of function. The optic nerve – the nerve leading to the eye – is commonly the first affected, leading to blindness. Then, over the following weeks or months, there is a partial recovery of function – in the case of the optic nerve, there is a partial recovery of sight. Over the years, further episodes of exacerbation followed by only partial recovery lead to a steady loss of function and increasing disability, like difficulty walking or with coordination. There is a wide variation in how quickly the condition progresses. Some live a relatively unaffected life for many years; for some the condition almost halts its progress.

Some, however, have a rapidly progressive course leading to major disability.

There are few conventional treatments for MS which have a significant impact upon the course of the illness. The outcomes of medications like steroids and interferon – which try to lessen the immune activity attacking the nervous system – have been disappointing and overall they do not seem to significantly slow the progression of MS. Interferon is expensive and also has a number of very uncomfortable side effects including feeling like you have a viral infection. Glatiramer acetate is probably as effective as interferon but has fewer side effects. It is important for patients to have a full and frank conversation with their doctors about treatment options, expected outcomes, costs and side effects so that they can make an informed decision about which management plan to follow. The fact that there are no very effective drug treatments for MS does not, however, mean that there are no prospects for improving the outcome for MS.

A comprehensive and thoroughly researched book covering all the potential self-help and lifestyle strategies for MS is *Taking Control of MS* written by Professor George Jelinek. He is a professor of emergency medicine who got MS himself. His initial motivation for looking into self-help strategies was to improve his own outcome. He had an initially poor prognosis but after applying the information he found in the medical literature, his MS virtually stopped progressing at all and so he became interested in sharing it with other MS sufferers. Much of this chapter owes a debt to his work.

Unfortunately there is far less economic incentive to investigate the more natural approach to MS therapy than to research patentable drugs.

Stress management

Recent research shows that psychological health has a large impact upon a variety of autoimmune illnesses including MS.

Our mental and emotional state affects how we cope with MS. Having a condition such as MS is stressful in itself so it is not surprising that depression and anxiety are very common among MS patients. Managing mental health issues in MS is important in its own right but also because the influence of mental health on the progression of

MS has been underestimated. Life stress can activate MS or accelerate its progression. One trial showed that MS exacerbations were more likely after stressful life events.The MS patients most at risk of exacerbations were those with a high degree of SNS reactivity – high blood pressure, palpitations, raised adrenaline levels – to stressful events. [1] Those who have the greatest SNS reactivity to stress also have the greatest disturbance to immunity [2] when stressful events occur. Other studies have shown that for eight weeks after experiencing stress there was a 60% increased risk of an MS patient developing new lesions in the central nervous system. A more definitive review was undertaken by the BMJ as to whether stressful life events increased the risk of MS exacerbations. [3] It clearly showed a 'significant increase in risk of exacerbation after stressful life events.' Practising positive coping strategies has been associated with a reduced number of new brain lesions. [4] [5]

The aim of raising awareness of the impact of stress on MS is not so that MS patients might blame themselves for the progression of their condition – quite the opposite. To be informed is to understand and to be empowered about how to improve coping and mental health. As a side effect, this is likely to improve the prognosis.

The reason why stress worsens MS is being studied. [6] Stress is also known to affect particular hormones which are prognostic factors for MS. [7] Interferon, the principal medical treatment for MS, has a range of negative side effects when it is administered as a medication. Interestingly, interferon occurs naturally in the body and can be increased using self-hypnosis or mindfulness meditation. [8] [9] These strategies have good side effects, including better immunity and reduced inflammation, but the long-term clinical effects on MS are not proven as yet. Previously mentioned work on the role of mindfulness in neuroplasticity and neurogenesis may provide an enormous amount of optimism in the future. [10]

Spirituality

Finding meaning and deep sources of inspiration is vitally important when coping with a chronic, life-threatening and disabling disease like MS. This is borne out when MS patients are interviewed about what helps them to cope. 'Positive reinterpretation of disease' is of major importance. [11] This reinterpretation is really another way of patients finding meaning, of exploring themselves and their own values. A condition such as MS increasingly impacts upon virtually every aspect of patients' lives. Being able to adapt, redefine themselves, review their lifetime aspirations and eventually confront their mortality are all linked to the search for meaning which is at the core of being able to cope with an illness like MS.

Exercise

Exercise is of immense importance for MS patients in terms of maintaining strength, balance, function and general fitness as well as mental health, social interaction[12] and general health. The MS Society runs hydrotherapy programs – known as SWEAT – and these are associated with improved quality of life.[13] Studies have shown that exercise also helps MS patients to prevent or manage depression.[14] The role of exercise in reducing the frequency and severity of MS exacerbations has not been extensively studied, although a US study of MS patients showed that exercise slowed the progression of disability as well as improving quality of life.[15]

Fatigue and difficulties with mobility are common problems for MS patients, which can make exercising more difficult. Patients may need to seek advice from their doctor or other health practitioner about the most appropriate form of exercise, how vigorous it should be and how long they should do it. A carefully and gently graded exercise program is the safest, wisest and most enjoyable. Falling into a cycle of inactivity leading to greater immobility and then further inactivity will only worsen an MS patient's situation.

Nutrition

Almost at the same time as Dean Ornish was publishing his research on the holistic management of heart disease[16] in 1990 a study from Canada was also being published in the *Lancet* on a diet for MS patients.[17][18] The results were quite startling but received relatively little notice in the medical community, certainly much less than if a new MS drug had produced the same outcomes. Over a 34-year period only 31% of MS patients on a diet low in saturated and animal fats – less than 20 g per day – had died of MS complications. Meanwhile, approximately

80% of patients who weren't on the low-fat diet had died. Those on the low-fat diet also had slower disease progression and less disability. Other researchers have shown that MS patients who adopted a similar diet did not worsen significantly over a three-year period.[19]

Supplements of omega-3 fatty acids are associated with significant reductions in the frequency and severity of MS relapses.[20][21][22] The National Institute for Clinical Excellence in the UK currently recommends that 17 to 23 g per day of essential fatty acids such as the omega-3s may slow the progression of MS.[23] Fish and flaxseed oils, because of their omega-3 content, have significant anti-inflammatory properties. Supplementation with fish oil helps to regulate MS patients' immune systems to the same extent as drugs given to produce the same effect.[24] These studies reinforce other research suggesting strong links between high animal fat intake and an increased MS incidence. Studies have also found regular fish consumption and vegetable-based diets to protect against MS.[25][26][27][28] As with Type-1 diabetes it is likely that cow's milk consumption[29] plays a role in triggering MS, probably because a number of cow's milk proteins are targeted by the immune cells of people with MS.[30]

A low level of vitamin D, whether it be through poor diet or low sun exposure, is strongly associated with more aggressive MS.[31] Vitamin D supplements can reduce MS exacerbations.[32][33] A recent large study of over 7 million army personnel in the US showed that their risk of MS declined significantly as their vitamin D levels rose.[34] Vitamin D levels fluctuate throughout the year, being lower in winter and higher in summer, and more MS lesions develop in winter. Year-round supplements of 3000 to 4000 IU per day of vitamin D[35] are recommended, although in most places in Australia it should be easy to get the small amount of sunlight exposure required to keep vitamin D levels high. Even modest regular vitamin D intake and vitamin D supplements of only 400 IU per day were associated with a substantially lower risk of developing MS.[36]

Connectedness

One study showed that possible risk factors for MS exacerbations were 'interpersonal conflicts, loss and complicated bereavement, low perceived social support, anxiety and depressive episodes'.[37]

Unfortunately, the therapeutic potential for psychological and social support in MS has not been extensively explored, particularly in relation to long-term outcomes. What is clear is that coping with MS requires an enormous amount of support from family, friends, workplace and healthcare professionals. MS Societies and support groups provide an enormous amount of benefit in the form of social interaction, emotional support, education, resources and information for MS sufferers and their carers. As with other chronic illnesses, these should be considered as a standard part of management.

Environment

Stressful life events and unsupportive social environments are associated with the onset and progression of a variety of autoimmune diseases[38] but there may be an environmental factor as important if not more important: sunlight.

A consistent finding in studies is that countries with lower levels of sunshine have a significantly higher incidence of MS.[39][40] The incidence of MS in Australia per year is 13.5 cases per million women and 7.7 cases per million men, but the incidence varies, increasing the further south we go. It is roughly 6-7 times more common in cool Tasmania as it is in tropical Queensland. That is, MS becomes more common the further you get from the equator. In countries near the equator MS is nearly unknown whereas in countries such as Denmark the incidence can be as high as 48.6 cases per million for women and 43.0 for men.[41] This is likely to be due to the fact that exposure to sunlight increases the body's generation of vitamin D, a potent modulator of the immune system; sunlight also increases melatonin,[42] which plays an important role in immunity.

In one study, over an 11-year period the mortality rate from MS for people who already had the disease was nearly halved if they got regular sun exposure at home.[43] If they also had regular sun exposure in their work then their chance of dying was approximately one-quarter of those who didn't. Australian data has also shown that regular sunlight exposure reduces the chance of developing MS in the first place.[44] Tasmanian studies show that higher sunlight exposure between the ages of 6 and 15, particularly to winter sun, reduced the risk of having MS in adult life to approximately one third.[45][46][47]

Roughly 10 to 15 minutes daily of sunlight to most of the body

– for example wearing shorts or bathers – on a day with a moderate UV index of 7 produces 10,000 IU of vitamin D, which is plenty for a healthy immune system. If less of the body is exposed then we need to stay in the sun longer. Unfortunately, the message of avoiding sunburn has been heard by many in the community as avoiding sun altogether. The benefits of sunlight on MS are probably due to the direct effects of sunlight on immune function and melatonin as well as the indirect effects on vitamin D.[48] Many MS patients have poor heat tolerance and should go in the sun in the early morning or late afternoon, particularly in the warmer months.

14

Asthma

Education

Our understanding of asthma and its causes is changing. It used to be treated as one condition that was characterised by narrowing of the mid-size airways in the lungs, leading to wheezing and shortness of breath. But now we are coming to understand that there are a number of types of this airway narrowing, each with different causes. What this means in practice is that some treatments for asthma will work well for some people but not others. We know that three factors are involved in asthma:

1. Constriction of the muscle in the airway wall;
2. Inflammation and swelling of the airway lining;
3. Mucous secretion into the airway.

For some asthmatics the primary problem is muscle constriction; for others it is allergy and inflammation. For others there is much higher mucous secretion. Any of these make it difficult for air to pass through the airway, leading to shortness of breath and a wheezing sound because of air turbulence as it moves through the airway. A halving of the total diameter of an airway will reduce airflow 16-fold so even a slight narrowing of the airway can drastically cut our ability to breathe freely. Anything that makes the airway more likely to react by narrowing (this is called airway reactivity) can be a trigger for asthma. There are many things which can trigger episodes of this airway narrowing in asthmatics and different people have different triggers including:

- Upper respiratory infection such as a cold;
- Allergies to things like house dust mites, pollens, mould, fur, feathers;
- Inhaled irritants such as smoke;
- Weather changes;
- Occupational exposures to wood dust, chemicals, sprays, etc.;
- Certain medications;
- Some foods and additives such as colourings, monosodium glutamate, seafood, nuts;
- Exercise, particularly in cold weather;
- Emotional distress.

Asthma is a very common condition with between one in four and one in five children developing it. In most cases it is mild although some develop severe asthma. In rare cases severe attacks can be fatal. It generally begins between the ages of two and seven but it can come on even in adult years. Smokers in particular can develop it late in life, as a part of chronic obstructive pulmonary disease (COPD). Most children grow out of asthma by late adolescence but there is the potential for it to return. The incidence of asthma is increasing around the world which is likely to be due to a wide range of causes including changing diet, medication side effects, pollution, chemical exposures and sensitivities, smoking, lifestyle and psychological factors. The good news is that the number of deaths due to severe asthma attacks has dropped sharply over recent decades because of improved emergency care.

Asthma tends to be under-diagnosed, particularly among children. A common symptom like night-time cough often goes unrecognised as being associated with asthma. Once suspected, asthma is generally not difficult for a doctor to diagnose from the patient's history, examination and respiratory tests. There are many treatments available for asthma which are, by and large, safe and effective. These include:

- **Preventers:** These medications such as inhaled steroids help to reduce airway inflammation and prevent attacks. It takes hours for them to become effective and they tend to be used daily in people who have regular episodes of asthma.
- **Relievers:** These medications are designed to treat acute attacks and they act fast. They are generally used only as needed, but are sometimes also used to prevent an attack – for instance, an

asthmatic can inhale a dose prior to doing something they know is likely to trigger an asthma attack, like exercise. These medications are generally given via 'spacers' and 'puffers'.
- **Combinations:** Sometimes preventers and long-acting relievers are combined in the one medication.
- **Oral medications:** A number of oral medications such as steroids can be taken, particularly for acute, severe attacks. These will tend to be tapered off and then stopped once the worst of the episode is over.

Our doctor is best placed to advise on the optimal treatment regime. The aim is to take the lowest doses of medication required to produce good control so that the asthma does not negatively impact upon our life. It is advisable to regularly monitor asthma at home using a simple peak-flow meter and to discuss with our doctor and family an action plan in the case of a severe asthma attack. The important things for everyone to be clear about are when to use which medication, how to deliver it most effectively and when to seek emergency medical help. Because severe attacks can be fatal it is better to err on the side of caution when in doubt.

As important as conventional asthma therapies are, there is much that we can do for ourselves, not to mention a range of complementary therapies that can also help. Indeed, lifestyle and self-help strategies can often reduce the amount of medication required to maintain good asthma control. This helps to reduce the potential side effects of medication. It is important to mention that even though we might be using self-help strategies or complementary therapies to good effect, we still need to:

- Communicate with our doctor about what we are doing;
- Take necessary conventional treatments;
- Monitor our asthma control;
- Have an action plan in case of an emergency;
- Seek medical help immediately, when needed.

Stress management

That the mind has an impact upon asthma is not a new idea. Over a century ago it was observed that in people who were allergic to roses or cats an asthma attack could be brought on by the sight of a paper rose or the photo of a cat. This suggests that immune, allergic and inflammatory reactions can be brought on by thought as well as physical triggers. In those days not much was understood about how such a phenomenon could exist but now the science of psychoneuroimmunology (PNI) has gone a long way towards describing how such events take place.

The brain communicates with the airways and the airways communicate with the brain. A review indicated that in asthmatics, a suggestion that airways were narrowing or expanding can cause the airways to either narrow or expand, and that stress can also narrow the airways.[1] Panic and negative emotions affect asthma by causing hyperventilation, effects on the sympathetic nervous system (SNS), inflammation and poor healthcare behaviour. Panic and coping with stress by repressing feelings can increase the risk of dying from asthma.[2] Although the mind can have a negative effect on asthma it raises the potential that psychological factors can also play a part in the treatment of asthma.[3]

The fact that we have a genetic predisposition to a condition does not always mean that we are destined to develop that condition. Genes are often activated by environment and psychological factors. For example, children with a genetic predisposition to asthma are three times more likely to become asthmatic if the parents are coping poorly and they experience a high level of domestic stresses.[4][5] This does not mean that every child with asthma necessarily comes from an unsettled or dysfunctional family, or that every child from an unsettled background will necessarily get asthma. It simply means there is a greater risk. Negative emotional states are well known to be asthma triggers and can increase asthma severity and make acute attacks more severe.[6] One review of childhood asthma deaths found that there were 14 significant factors that predicted that a child was more likely to die of asthma. Seven of those 14 were psychological factors like depression, conflict and recent loss. The study concluded that 'psychological risk factors were prominent in severely asthmatic children who subsequently died of asthma'.[7][8]

Placebo, as with most other conditions, has a beneficial effect on acute episodes of asthma.[9] Although it could never be advocated as a treatment, the fact that the placebo effect holds for asthma does demonstrate the importance of the mind in asthma therapy. The patient's trust in their doctor or other health professional, good past treatment experiences leading to good expectations, and the health professional's enthusiasm and conviction all affect the outcome of therapy.

Reviews have also shown that relaxation and meditation have significant positive effects on subjective (the patient feels better) and objective (improved lung function tests) measures of asthma severity. Clinical trials examining the effect of relaxation showed benefits including less medication use, fewer hospital visits and less sick leave.[10] Biofeedback is also a promising strategy.[11] Feeling more able to self-manage and being provided with asthma education are beneficial,[12] cost-effective, improve adjustment, increase patients' compliance with their treatment, improve patients' feelings of competence and decrease their need for medical services. Family therapy is useful for asthmatics for whom family stress is a major trigger.[13][14] Hypnotherapy may also be helpful for asthma and allergy management.[15][16] A study on 16 severe asthmatics showed that after one year of hypnotherapy hospital admissions dropped sharply. Six of the asthmatics no longer needed to take steroids and eight were able to reduce their dose, and side effects were reduced.[17] Even keeping a journal about stressful life events has been found to improve long-term control of asthma.[18]

Current evidence suggests that most of the benefit of mind–body strategies for asthma are in helping reduce symptoms, improve outcomes for those with emotionally triggered asthma, and foster healthy lifestyle change. It is not clearly known to what extent the better outcome is attributable to reductions in inflammation.[19]

Breathing exercises are a very important adjunct to asthma management. Many such techniques, like yoga, are as much about focusing the mind as they are about breathing techniques. Their benefit is therefore likely to be a due to a combination of factors, including stress management.

In one study a two-week training program in yoga breathing resulted in fewer asthma attacks per week, better response to drug treatment and better lung function on tests.[20] It wasn't just that the patients felt better, their respiratory function had substantially improved. These improvements, as we would expect, depended upon the techniques being practised regularly. Similar results were demonstrated in a larger study.[21] The reasons for the improvement include that yoga breathing reduces reactions to allergens,[22] induces relaxation, relaxes muscles, reduces metabolic rate and settles panic associated with shortness of breath. Over the longer term such exercises improve respiratory function, and reduce reliever use, hospitalisations and sick leave.[23] In a 30-week study on breathing exercises for asthma, the participants were able to decrease their reliever use by an average of 86% and their preventer dose by 50%. A reduction in dose means reduced side effects and costs.[24]

One point to emphasise about the use of breathing exercises for asthma is to learn from an appropriately trained teacher such as a yoga therapist, one who is trained to use yoga for therapeutic reasons rather than just for flexibility or general wellbeing. Depending on your condition, some breathing exercises may be suitable and other not. The Buteyko method for retraining breathing is also coming up with some promising results.[25]

Spirituality

Faith or meaning is an important source of strength in our daily life and is associated with better mental health and therefore positive outcomes in chronic conditions such as asthma. Much of the benefit of faith for asthmatics is probably because of the social support of a religious community[26] but a significant part is related to our way of dealing with difficult emotions like anger, stress and depression which can trigger asthma. Spirituality can also play an important part in children managing a chronic condition like asthma.[27]

Exercise

Part of the explanation for the rise in asthma, particularly among children, may be lack of exercise.[28] Obesity also increases asthma incidence and symptoms. This is not only because of poor exercise tolerance but also because of inefficient breathing, airway constriction, hypoventilation, poor oxygen exchange and sleep apnoea due to the obesity itself.[29]

Exercise improves general fitness and wellbeing among asthmatics although these benefits may often be independent of a direct improvement on airway function due to exercise.[30] Exercise has been found to reduce airway hypersensitivity and thus reduce the need for medication in some asthmatics. (Exercise is also recommended for other chronic lung conditions; in cystic fibrosis it reduces coughing and sputum production, and improves the sense of wellbeing.)

When exercising it is important to keep well hydrated because dry airways are far more reactive in asthmatics. People with exercise-induced asthma do not need to avoid exercise but need to take steps to minimise its impact. This can include taking a reliever prior to playing sport and choosing a suitable sport and environment. Exercise is generally good for asthma and general wellbeing although swimming is often best for people with exercise-induced asthma;[31] the humidified air may be helpful. Avoiding outdoor sport on days with a high pollen count may also be beneficial. An asthmatic who has an attack while exercising or playing sport should stop and follow their asthma action plan.

Nutrition

Food can both help and hinder asthma. Some asthmatics have food allergies, intolerances[32][33] or sensitivities which can play a role. The typical foods that can be problematic are eggs, fish, shellfish, nuts and peanuts. Milk, chocolate, wheat, citrus and food colourings can also be a problem, however the onset of asthma is usually delayed with these foods and therefore it can be hard to link the symptoms with the particular food. Some people need to avoid foods containing monosodium glutamate (MSG), colourings (especially tartrazine which is used to give the yellow colour to some margarines) and other food additives.

In some cases foods containing salicylates may be a problem. Many fruits contain salicylates; this is ironic given that overall a diet high in fruit and vegetables has been shown to be protective against asthma. In this case one man's medicine can be another man's poison. Foods high in salicylates include chocolate, bananas, tomatoes, pineapples, strawberries, raisins, oranges, grapes, curry powder, hot paprika, rosemary, thyme, cordials and fruit flavoured drinks.[34] Aspirin is made of salicylic acid and possibly up to 20% of people have a low-level aspirin sensitivity. It is far less common to have a severe allergic reaction to foods containing salicylates. A high-salt diet appears to make exercise-induced asthma worse[35] and may increase airway reactivity.

Tryptophan in food is converted in the body to serotonin which can constrict the airways of some asthmatics, so limiting foods high in tryptophan may help some asthma sufferers. Tryptophan-rich foods include: milk, yoghurt, eggs, meat, nuts, beans, fish and cheese. Cheddar, Gruyere and Swiss cheese are particularly rich in tryptophan. As the body also uses tryptophan to make the important hormone melatonin, we should not totally exclude tryptophan from our diet.

Margarine is not a natural food. It is a manufactured food and is not quite as healthy as its public image would make out and it may be problematic for some asthmatics. Studies on children show that consumption of margarine increases wheezing.[36][37] Eating a diet high in polyunsaturated fats such as margarine, fried foods and omega-6 fatty acids (as distinct from healthy omega-3s) doubles the risk of asthma and may contribute to 17% of cases of asthma in three-to five-year-olds.[38]

To determine if we have food sensitivities which are contributing to asthma we can try an exclusion diet, in which certain foods or food groups are excluded and then reintroduced. It is important to seek advice from a suitably trained and experienced professional so that it is safe, effective and systematic.

Diet can also play a very therapeutic role in managing asthma. The following can be helpful as part of an asthma management program:

Fruit

Fruit is considered protective against asthma.[39][40] Communities with high-fruit diets have a lower incidence of asthma. Apples and pears[41] are considered especially effective.

Quercetin

Capers, apples, tea, onions, red grapes, citrus fruits, broccoli, cherries and raspberries are all high in quercetin which is a flavonoid with demonstrated anti-inflammatory action and is helpful in asthmatics.[42] Flavonoids are a variety of plant-based chemicals (phytochemicals) which have strong antioxidant properties. Quercetin has also been found in varieties of honey, including honey derived from eucalyptus and tea tree flowers.

Carotenes

Foods with high levels of carotenes are powerful antioxidants which can decrease inflammatory leukotrienes and hence help alleviate the inflammation of airways in asthma. Good sources are: carrots, pumpkin, broccoli, sweet potatoes, tomatoes, kale, collards, cantaloupe, peaches and apricots.

Vitamin E

Foods with high levels of vitamin E may be useful in asthma treatment and management because of vitamin E's effect on inflammatory chemicals in the body. Foods rich in Vitamin E include: wheat germ, nuts, seeds, whole grains, green leafy vegetables, vegetable oil and fish-liver oil.

Garlic and onions

Onions and garlic seem to also have an anti-inflammatory effect in the body.

Coffee and tea

Tea contains theophylline which is a mild bronchodilator – that is, it opens up the airways. Coffee has also a mildly beneficial effect on asthma.

Chilli

Surprisingly, chilli pepper[43] may actually desensitise airways to chemical irritants like cigarette smoke.

Omega-3 fatty acids

There have been mixed results from studies into omega-3 fatty acids and asthma, but given the anti-inflammatory effects of omega-3s (found in oily fish, flaxseed oil, walnuts and avocadoes) it is generally considered healthy to maintain good levels in your diet. Schoolchildren who ate fish more than once a week were found to have a third less chance of developing asthma than those who ate no fish.[44] Positive results have also been shown for taking supplements of fish oil[45] but some trials did not find a beneficial effect of dietary omega-3s on asthma.[46] On balance, the role of omega-3 fatty acids in preventing or managing asthma is still not completely resolved.[47] It may be beneficial for some forms of asthma but not others.

Vitamin and mineral supplements

There may be a role for antioxidant supplements such as vitamin C in asthma. One study showed that many adult asthmatics had a low intake of fruit, and the antioxidants vitamin C and manganese.[48] Although some reviews showed a big improvement in respiratory function in those who took 1 to 2 grams of vitamin C a day,[49] overall, the jury is still out.[50]

Asthmatics often have a low level of vitamin B6 and supplements may benefit asthma.[51] At a dose of 50 mg twice a day, vitamin B6 was able to reduce the frequency and severity of asthma attacks.[52]

Magnesium has muscle-relaxant properties and is used for acute asthma attacks.[53] Selenium may also be beneficial.

Connectedness

The impact of social connectedness and relationships on asthma can be direct or indirect.

The direct effect is when our emotions trigger changes in our airways. Unsettled social situations, emotions and relationships are all predictive of asthma attacks and deaths.[54] Conflict between an asthmatic child, his or her parents and therapists, in any combination, was particularly predictive. It is not only our psychological state and immune system that are linked – as we know from PNI – but our socio-economic background comes into play too. A study found that stress, especially in children from a low socio-economic background, put them at greater risk of dying of childhood asthma.

The indirect effects come from our social circumstances. How we live and the support we get can make us either more or less likely to catch infectious diseases that can trigger asthma attacks. It can influence whether we are likely to exercise or smoke, or be surrounded by smokers. Readily available support and supervision, especially for children, is also vital to asthma management, as is having access to support services. Depending on our social circumstances we are also more, or less, likely to receive education about asthma and its management, and be encouraged to monitor the condition.

Environment

Many of the triggers for asthma are environmental and therefore attention to environment can be an important part of reducing asthma's impact.

• **Upper respiratory infection:** an upper respiratory tract infection can trigger asthma so take simple hygiene measures like not coughing on others, thorough hand washing and where possible reduce exposure to viruses;

- **Allergies to house dust mites, pollens, mould, fur, feathers, etc.:** clean fresh air, a well-ventilated house, reducing dust and dusting regularly, avoiding exposure to particular plants, pollens or animals that may be problematic, low allergenic bedding and air filters.
- **Evaporative air conditioning:** This can be helpful for asthmatics because it filters the air as it cools it. It also humidifies the air, ensuring that our airways do not dry out, whereas refrigerative air conditioning dries the air.
- **Smoke:** Don't smoke and avoid passive smoking at home and work.
- **Weather changes:** Take care with sudden changes in temperature and breathe humidified air when possible.
- **Occupational exposure to wood dust, chemicals, sprays etc.:** Ensure adequate ventilation or protection such as using a mask if working in hazardous environments. Follow workplace safety regulations to create a safe work environment.
- **Some foods and additives such as colourings, monosodium glutamate, seafood, nuts:** For those with a serious food allergy it is vital to read all labels carefully and may even be necessary to ensure that the environment is completely free of the food, such as peanuts or sesame seeds.
- **Exercise:** dry air can be a problem as can temperature.
- **Emotional distress:** Establishing a safe and supportive emotional environment is important for everyone, and especially for people managing asthma.

15

Healthy ageing

Education

Jacques, the melancholic fool in Shakespeare's *Twelfth Night*, at one stage muses, 'and so from hour to hour we ripe and ripe, and then from hour to hour we rot and rot, and thereby hangs a tale'. Ageing is inevitable but how fast and how well we age is largely in our own hands.

We age for many reasons such as genetically coded 'inbuilt obsolescence', wear and tear, and oxidation. Oxidation is largely due to unstable molecules called 'free radicals' which can cause damage to other molecules including our genes.[1] Thus, antioxidants, which mop up these free radicals, have an important role in trying to neutralise these effects. Reductions in hormone levels are another part of ageing: there are declines in sex hormones – like oestrogen, leading to menopause and testosterone, leading to andropause – thyroid hormones, and others like growth hormone. This does not mean that taking these hormones artificially prolongs life. In the case of a pathologically low level of these hormones they can be useful but trials on taking them to slow normal ageing have been disappointing and they have many unwanted side effects. The rise and fall in the popularity of HRT has been a case in point.[2]

Obviously individuals vary enormously, but in general terms, the first third of our life is all about growth and strength, in the second third we largely hold our ground, and in the final third we start to reap what we have sown in the first two-thirds. Thus, old age can be a blessing or a curse.

Although there is much we can and should do to affect the rate at which the natural ageing process takes place, there has been an unfortunate tendency in our modern, youth-centred society to treat ageing as an illness. Natural stages of the life cycle, like menopause, have been treated as a disease. That approach not only helped to reinforce negative attitudes to healthy ageing but also did more damage than good to the health of a generation of women and consumed large amounts of health dollars in the process.

Life expectancy has steadily climbed since recorded history, but the most rapid increase in life expectancy has taken place in the last 150 years or so. The biggest reason for this has not been advances in medical science but something rather more down to earth: first and foremost is the introduction of sanitation, otherwise known as sewerage. Then come improvements to water, food and housing. It is the basics like clean water, better nutrition and living conditions that have made the biggest difference. It is easy to take these things for granted but how important they are becomes apparent during natural disasters, when these necessities are not available. In their absence a health system is hard pressed to make a difference. Medical advances, as important as they are, are largely dwarfed by the basic life essentials.

Japan currently has the longest life expectancy with the average Japanese man currently expecting to live for 78 years and woman for 84 years. Australia (77, 82) and Sweden (77, 82) are the world's next highest. In less affluent countries where the basics of sanitation, food and housing are far from optimal the life expectancy is like that before modern times in richer countries. Sierra Leone (33, 35), Niger (37, 40) and Malawi (37, 39), all in Africa, have the world's lowest life expectancy.[3]

Life expectancy in nearly all countries of the world has gone up significantly over the last century[4] and a commonly held belief is that it will continue to climb into the 21st century. Many government policies are based upon this premise. Healthcare, superannuation and pensions are just a few areas where policies assume an ageing population. Many experts predict that this current generation can expect to live into their 90s. 'Very long lives are the probable destiny of most people alive today. For everyone in his or her 30s and younger, especially children, a lifespan of 95 or 100 years will be common,'[5] according to expert J Vaupel from the US. If current trends are anything to go by, then this prediction seems to be reasonable.[6]

Greater longevity is no doubt much valued so this chapter looks at the factors which predict longer survival and the looming threats to continued extension of life expectancy.

Life expectancy is, of course, only part of the picture. Adding quality to life – living *well* in old age – is also a major aim. Ageing well means maintaining function and leading productive and active lives into old age. Defining old age is a topic for debate in itself. The 40 of yesteryear is now the new 60, and the 60 of yesteryear is now the new 80. The aim for a better life as well as a longer one can be summed up in the saying that we need to 'add life to years, not just more years to life.'[7]

THE COST OF LONGEVITY

Access to modern healthcare has to some extent reduced illness and death, but over and above providing the most basic healthcare there has always been a poor relationship between the amount of money spent on healthcare and longevity. More dollars do not necessarily mean greater health or a longer life, despite what many in the healthcare industry would have us believe. Healthcare expenditure now accounts for an average 9% of GDP among OECD countries, of which Australia is one. This is a steep rise from 5% in 1970. Different countries spend vastly different sums on healthcare. The US spends 15.3% of GDP, the UK 8.3% and Australia 9.2%.[8] Unfortunately, illness prevention and public health programs receive only about 3% at best of health expenditures in OECD countries.

It may appear that the big jump in healthcare spending over the last four decades is responsible for our increasing longevity, but what the data also shows is that income only determines life expectancy at the lowest end of the income spectrum. While the poorest countries have the lowest life expectancy, once a country has reached an income of only roughly one-eighth of an affluent country it has virtually the same life expectancy. High-expense healthcare, despite the public image, only makes a marginal rather than a major difference to longevity. The fact that people at the lower end of the socio-economic spectrum have poorer health than those at the upper end has less to do with access to expensive healthcare than it does with education, opportunity, employment, stress, lifestyle and empowerment.

Life expectancy by income

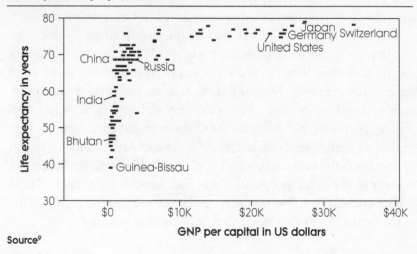

Source[9]

BURDEN OF DISEASE

In Westernised or affluent countries heart disease and cancer are the main causes of reduced longevity and disability for both men and women. For men, road accidents, HIV and substance abuse are the next top three. For women, they are depression, stroke and osteoarthritis. The global picture is somewhat different. Worldwide, the top five causes of reduced longevity and disability are malnutrition, poor water, unsafe sex (largely because of its role in spreading HIV), tobacco and alcohol abuse.

In Australia heart disease is the major fatal burden of disease while depression is the major non-fatal burden; overall, mental disorders account for 30% of the total burden of disease.[10] If current trends continue, in Australia it is predicted that depression will soon be the single biggest overall burden of disease (independent of its role in other illnesses, notably heart disease).[11]

WHICH WAY WILL LIFE EXPECTANCY GO?

There has been great optimism in the last century in regard to life expectancy. Every prediction assumes that we will be living longer in the future and this has led to considerable concern in most Western countries about how to fund an increasing number of retirees in what is expected to be an increasingly long retirement. But is this optimism well placed? As the saying goes, 'what goes up must come down' and this may be as true for life expectancy as it is for everything else.

We need to bear in mind that people living to an average age of 80 years today were born in the late 1920s under very different social, economic, lifestyle and environmental conditions to what we are experiencing now. Mental health, exercise patterns, obesity, over-nutrition and many other factors are very different now. What does a person born in the 1990s or 2000s have to navigate through that previous generations did not have to deal with? Any factors having an impact upon the health of young people now will not make themselves evident in life-expectancy data for at least another generation. There is the potential for life expectancy to plateau and then actually decline in the future. Signs that point to that possibility include:

- **Increasing levels of obesity, inactivity and a growing incidence of Type-2 diabetes in children:** This is associated with poor diet, high consumption of convenience food and sedentary pastimes like watching television and using computer.[12]
- **Climate change and other environmental factors:** Problems due to diminishing water and air quality will only accelerate as the population and pollution levels increase.
- **Increasing abuse of substances, illicit and prescribed:** The long-term effects of recreational drugs on mental and physical health will become an increasing problem within the next 20 years.
- **Increasing levels of stress, anxiety and depression, especially in our young:** These impact on growing suicide rates and also have effects on long-term physical health and the incidence of heart disease and cancer.
- **Overcrowding, poverty and inequity:** There is an increasing polarisation of wealth, resulting in problems especially for some urban population groups and children in single-parent families.
- **The increasing long-term impact of social isolation:** There are long-term effects on mental and physical health of increasing numbers of people living alone, increasing rates of marital break-up and a lack of community connectedness especially among the young.
- **The reduction in spirituality:** This affects resilience to stress, depression, physical health and longevity.
- **Increasing rates of illness due to medical treatment:** Due to the abundance of new medical technology and pharmaceuticals, illness

due to medical treatment is now a very common cause of death in most developed countries, particularly in the US.[13] There are also increasing concerns that bad side effects of drugs have been downplayed and benefits overstated.

- **The potentially negative impact of some forms of media, music and IT:** Apart from reducing physical activity, some forms of entertainment – television, aggressive music – may have other long-term effects on mental, social and physical health.
- **Trends in employment:** including the type and the amount. Under-employment is as much a detriment to health as over-employment.
- **Wild-cards:** Life expectancy could be reduced by potential self-inflicted disasters like genetically modified foods, war, terrorism, genetic engineering and xenografts (grafting animal organs and tissues into humans) leading to infections jumping across species.

If these problems are to be averted then individually and collectively we need to get back to basics by spending more resources and time on community building, relationships, education, health promotion, environment and lifestyle. Although it runs counter to currently accepted wisdom, the solutions may not be related to advances in technology but rather advances in common sense and collective action. The gains of the last century were hard won, but one suspects they can also be easily lost in this century.

WHAT AFFECTS HEALTHY AGEING?

The same factors commonly associated with chronic illnesses like heart disease and cancer have an impact on life expectancy and healthy ageing. For example, a study following people from 1981 to 2006 in the respected *Archives of Internal Medicine*[14] found that in men who were still alive at 70, smoking more than doubled their risk of dying before 90 years, diabetes nearly doubled it, obesity increased it by 40%, and high blood pressure by nearly 30%. Regular exercise, on the other hand, was associated with a nearly 30% lower risk of dying. It's not really surprising, but those with a healthy lifestyle not only lived longer but lived better, developed chronic illnesses later in life and had better mental health.

One series of studies, on people in Alameda County in the US, identified seven factors associated with poorer health and a shorter life.[15 16] It is pretty basic stuff, really:

- Excessive alcohol consumption;
- Smoking;
- Little physical activity;
- Being obese;
- Sleeping fewer or more than 7 to 8 hours per night;
- Eating between meals;
- Not eating breakfast.

Activities such as cognitive-behavioural therapy, meditation-based therapies, stress reduction, other strategies which reduce inflammation, calorie restriction and exercise may prolong the healthy life span in humans[17] due to their effects on DHEA (a steroid hormone), melatonin and inflammatory chemicals like interleukins, all of which influence ageing.

Some aspects of the anti-ageing industry will have an important role to play in the future but there are also some aspects of it which have more to do with market opportunities than with real improvements to wellbeing. It can be hard to distinguish between those products and therapies that are authentically useful and those that are market driven. Many products, operations, supplements and devices are promoted with greater claims than can be supported by reliable evidence, including beauty products, anti-wrinkle creams, plastic surgery procedures, injectables and hormones. For example, much has been made about the fact that testosterone levels fall in men and women when we age. Marketers have promoted the benefits of taking testosterone supplements in later life without strong evidence to back up their claims. We also have to weigh up the potential negative effects of administering hormones artificially. We should instead focus on healthy ageing strategies that are simpler, safer and better established, even though they require more effort and may be less glamorous and less heavily promoted.

Stress management

The mind is the main player in the drama of life. Over time, our state of mind can accelerate ageing by affecting our lifestyle decisions; by impacting upon genetics, physiology, immunity, oxidation and allostatic load; and increasing the incidence of a variety of chronic illnesses associated with ageing.

The more important thing to note is that the mind can work for us as much as it works against us. A recent paper identified a number of factors which could be identified at age 50 that were highly predictive of how long and healthy our life will be.[18] They included the seven factors highlighted in an earlier study – alcohol consumption, smoking, exercise, weight, sleep, eating between meals and eating breakfast – plus level of education, healthy coping mechanisms and whether or not we have depression. Depression is not only a risk factor for various illnesses but it also determines how we cope with those illnesses. If a person was happy, optimistic and had an attitude of wellness before the onset of a chronic illness, they had a longer and better life. It could be argued that the 'sad-sick' people in the study were unhappier because they were less well, but the data actually suggests that their unhappiness predated any illness or disability that could have caused it.

What is less clear from current evidence is to what extent one can change life-long negative attitudes and to what extent doing so can reverse the negative effects on health. But there is enough research on the beneficial effects of improving mental health for heart disease, cancer, immunity and other conditions to suggest that it can.

So, attitude is crucial for healthy ageing. Research has found that people who have more positive perceptions of ageing, lived seven and a half years longer than those with less positive perceptions.'[19] It could be that a negative attitude about ageing is a sign of poor coping or of a tendency to become inactive and withdrawn in later life. In any case, the seven and a half years gained by having a positive attitude to ageing compared well with the number of years of life we can gain through having lower blood pressure, cholesterol and BMI, exercising and not smoking. Such a finding challenges us to be careful about the attitudes we foster towards ageing. The way our culture views ageing and the elderly may affect how well we age.

Spirituality

A study following people over a nine-year period showed that the chance of dying from any cause was reduced and life expectancy increased for those with a regular spiritual dimension to their lives. Those without a spiritual dimension had an average life expectancy of 75 years, compared with 82 years for those with a spiritual dimension. Only a small amount of the difference could be explained by the commonly accepted lifestyle and social factors such as smoking and drinking patterns.[20] The study looked at churchgoing, but this is only a rough marker of meaning and spirituality generally. The finding is probably not isolated to those who attend church but would apply to people belong to any religion. In fact, it may not be related to religion per se, but rather that some people have a philosophical, psychological, cultural and community foundation which helps to sustain them.

Exercise

There is an old saying, 'if you don't use it you lose it' and never was this more true than in relation to ageing well. Much has already been said about the effects of inactivity and various illnesses associated with ageing including heart disease, diabetes and cancer.

As we age, we lose muscle mass, immune function, brain cells and bone density (our bones get thin). Our joints creak, our vitality diminishes and our hormone levels decline. We don't have to take this lying down. Age-related decline has been taken as inevitable, but just as medicine has had to reassess its belief that the brain cannot regenerate past adolescence, so too ideas about other aspects of ageing have had to change.

Many of us age before our time because our attitudes and practices accelerate the process. The assumed loss of muscle mass, for example, is not inevitable if we regularly exercise. To maintain muscle and bone mass we need to do weight or resistance training and not just aerobic training such as walking, jogging, swimming or cycling. We now know that muscle retains stem cells that can be stimulated to grow even late into life. Bone mass can be regained with the right approach to activity, diet, sun and mood. Regular physical exercise is important for healthy joints and cartilage. Physical exercise also stimulates brain cell growth and slows cell loss, which is discussed in more detail Chapter 18 on brain health and dementia.

The temptation is to avoid physical activity if our joints are sore, balance is poor and our vitality is low. This only gets us into a negative spiral of worsening pain, balance and vitality. Function lost late in life is hard to regain if we compound it through prolonged inactivity. This is one of the reasons that prolonged bed rest is not advocated in the way it once was. Conversely we can get into a positive spiral of increasing exercise and, gradually, increasing vitality and function.

If elderly it is important to start slow and build over time. Doing too much exercise too soon will be unpleasant, potentially harmful and off-putting. Extreme exercise when we are unused to it can bring on a heart attack and place our joints, tendons and muscles at risk. We should also consider that very gentle forms of exercise like tai chi and some forms of yoga can provide major benefits in function, vitality, balance and emotional wellbeing. For example, regular tai chi can significantly reduce falls in the elderly. At the same time involvement in physical activity within a group is a very important social outlet.

Nutrition

It would be hard to say that there is one diet which is 'the answer' to ageing long and well. Some dietary approaches may be very useful and some dietary supplements may also be useful. Overall, calorie restriction may be the single most important issue in healthy ageing, provided the calories we do get are from quality food sources.

One of the great successes of the developed world is to make food reliable, plentiful and of, generally speaking, good quality. Unfortunately, deprivation, which was once a threat in most countries, has now been overtaken by over-consumption as a health risk in affluent countries. The life expectancy of the whole globe could be improved by taking half the food from the developed countries and giving it to the developing countries. The contemporary Western diet, particularly if it contains large amounts of fast food and highly processed food, is often full of 'empty calories' in the form of carbohydrates and fat. Calorie restriction, which is largely a matter of not eating excess and empty calories, is well known in animal and human studies to be associated with significantly longer life expectancy and a lower rate of chronic illnesses.[21][22][23] Over-nutrition is a major factor in the onset and progression of many conditions including heart disease, cancer and diabetes.[24][25][26]

The Ornish and Mediterranean diets, discussed in chapters 10 and 11 on heart disease and cancer, may enhance the length and quality of life, as may the following dietary approaches.

LOW-CARBOHYDRATE DIET

This diet has attracted a lot of attention, some of it positive and some negative. It basically centres on reducing total carbohydrate intake which is not unreasonable considering the high-carb intake in most people's diet. According to this dietary philosophy, there is too much focus on fats and not enough focus on carbohydrate intake. At first the carbohydrate restriction in the low-carb diet is severe – severe enough to cause ketosis, a metabolic reaction similar to starvation – and the protein and fat intake are disproportionately high. Almost universally a person on this diet will see a significant weight loss in the early weeks. Slowly the carbohydrate intake is increased but not back to the original levels. It is clear that the low-carb diet reduces insulin resistance and improves glucose control. The long-term effects are not clear yet and many dietary experts say that the diet does not have the right balance of fats and plant-based products.

POLYMEAL

Evidence based on studies of the population living in Framingham in the UK suggests that some food items, including moderate wine intake, fish, dark chocolate, fruits, vegetables, garlic, and almonds, would have a significant effect on the incidence of heart disease and prolong life expectancy. Some experts call a diet which is rich in such foods the 'polymeal'. 'Combining the ingredients of the Polymeal would reduce CVD events by 76%. For men, taking the Polymeal daily represented an increase in total life expectancy of 6.6 years . . . The corresponding difference for women was 4.8 . . . years.'[27]

RISK REDUCTION DIETS

Risk reduction diets (RRDs) are the traditional diets of populations with the greatest human longevity and lowest illness rates, in particular the Okinawans in Japan, famed for their longevity, and some Mediterranean populations. In Crete and Okinawa the diet includes edible wild plants, culinary herb usage and traditional herbal medicines. These communities also enjoy a strong social network and have a high level of physical activity, especially at older ages. As a result these people enjoy a slower age-associated decline. There is good evidence that these diets reduce the risk of stroke, high blood pressure, CVD, Type-2 diabetes and death from cancer.

Nutritional features common to the RRD include:

- Nutrient intake from highly diverse sources;
- Calorie restriction;
- Omega-6 to omega-3 fatty acid ratio between 2:1 and 1:1;
- Soaked and fermented non-wheat grains: A recent report from the Insulin Resistance Atherosclerosis Study shows that consumption of whole grains decreases carotid artery atherosclerosis ('hardening of the arteries');
- Complex carbohydrates with low refined sugar;
- Protein predominantly from plant sources;
- Varied legume sources;
- Soured and fermented goat's and sheep's milk products;
- Plentiful intake of seeds, nuts and fish;
- Green tea: Consumption of green tea is associated with a lower prevalence of cognitive impairment and may slow progression of Parkinson's disease.[28] Two cups a day was shown to be markedly more protective than three to six cups a week. Studies have also shown that drinking green tea significantly reduced CVD, cancer and stroke deaths;[29]
- Moderate consumption of red wine;
- Highly diverse plant-based diet: Eating a range of fruit and vegetables results in a significant reduction in DNA ageing (oxidation);
- Bitter plant foods such as bitter endive, dandelion greens and artichokes: There is some evidence to sugget that these can slow the progression of illnesses associated with ageing;[30 31]
- Foods with high antioxidant concentrations (including the phytochemicals called polyphenols and flavonoids) such as goji berries, blackberries, walnuts, strawberries, artichokes, cranberries, raspberries, pecans, blueberries, ground cloves, grape juice and unsweetened baking chocolate: These have all been shown to slow the progression of illnesses associated with ageing;[32 33]
- Garlic and onion: Sulphur compounds in garlic and onion have anti-inflammatory, heart-protective, anticancer and blood-fat-lowering activity. Garlic decreases homocysteine (thought to be a risk factor for CVD) and blood pressure, and increases circulation in small blood vessels.[34] Garlic and onion also protect against prostate enlargement;[35]
- Carotenoids from pumpkin, squash, apricots and sweet potato;
- Lycopenes from cooked tomatoes;

- Lutein from apricots, broccoli, spinach, red peppers, spinach, beans and peas;
- Ferulic acid from cereal grains;
- Zeaxanthin from orange pepper, corn, spinach and tangerine;
- CoQ10 from mackerel, sardines and spinach;
- Lipoic acid from broccoli and spinach;
- Curcumin from turmeric: Researchers became interested in curcumin's potential to slow the progression of cancer and prevent or treat Alzheimer's disease after noting the low rate of dementia where curry is a staple part of the diet;[36]
- Mineral-rich seaweed products;
- Isoflavones from soy, tofu, tempeh and miso;
- Vegetable and grain-based dietary fibre;
- Abundant dietary sources of vitamins C and E.

DIETARY AND HORMONAL SUPPLEMENTS

Before considering the use of supplements for healthy ageing, it is best to seek advice from a suitably trained healthcare professional.

Many of the symptoms associated with ageing, including lack of vitality and strength, are due to a reduction in the capacity of our cells' energy factories, the mitochondria. Poor mitochondrial function is also implicated in a range of chronic diseases associated with ageing.[37] Antioxidants – including coenzyme Q-10 (CoQ10), which is available as a supplement – play an important role in protecting our mitochondria.[38][39] Supplements of sex hormones do not seem to have a safe and valid role in slowing normal ageing. A similar conclusion has been drawn about the long-term use of growth hormone.[40] Levels of DHEA (dehydroepiandrosterone), a hormone made by the adrenal gland, also decline with age. There is some evidence that DHEA supplements can help to reverse some of the symptoms of ageing[41] but more evidence is required and there are some potential risks such as prostate disease in men.

Connectedness

Again, much has been said in other chapters about the impact of connectedness on the progression of various illnesses. The researchers performing the Alameda studies also looked at the impact of social connectedness and personal relationships on longevity. They found that both were highly significant for living longer and living better.[42]

Even in affluent countries like Australia indigenous populations can have health statistics more representative of an undeveloped country, with life expectancy being at least 20 years less than the general population. This has much more to do with their cultural and community conditions than it does with access to basic healthcare. If a section of the community is alienated from the wider community, or if the healthcare provided is not culturally appropriate, then that section of the community is unlikely to avail themselves of it.

Environment

A vitally important aspect of service provision for the elderly is enhancing their environment and their opportunities for social interaction. Being in an unstimulating environment – such as in front of the television in a nursing home – will not help an elderly person to maintain their interest in life or their mental and physical capacities. Nor will being denied a useful role to play in daily life, or having their behaviour controlled through the overuse of sedative medication. These are sure ways to accelerate chronic degenerative diseases and cognitive decline, diminish mental health and lose functions needed for daily living. The environment for the elderly can be enriched with:

- **Social interaction:** Interaction with young people as well as peers helps to lift mood, slows cognitive decline and maintains social skills;
- **Music, art and other cultural activities:** These stimulate interest, engage attention and bring enjoyment;
- **Promotion of physical activity:** To whatever extent a person can safely maintain mobility, this should be seen as a goal.
- **Sunlight and fresh air:** This assists with mood and immunity, reduces the risk of infection, particularly in shared accommodation, and helps to improve vitality.
- **Interaction with nature:** This has similar effects to music and art. The appreciation of beauty, as a food for the mind, is a basic human need, not a luxury. Being able to care for a garden can give an elderly person a productive role, stimulate the mind and increase physical activity.

- **Contact with animals:** Pets, whether in individual or shared accommodation, have a profoundly positive effect on mood, emotions and stress.
- **Outings:** Variety in environment helps to maintain interest and stimulate responsiveness in elderly people. Regular outings are associated with better mental and physical health.
- **Hobbies and productive employment:** This does not have to be for pay but it helps to give a purpose and role in life as well as stimulate enjoyment.

16

Arthritis

Education

Arthritis simply means inflamed joints, 'arthro' meaning joint and 'itis' meaning inflamed. There are many different causes of joint pain and inflammation but the two commonest causes, which will be discussed in this chapter, are osteoarthritis and rheumatoid arthritis. There are other types, such as gout and arthritis secondary to viral and bacterial infections. Many of the comments in this chapter will be just as relevant for those other forms of arthritis not to mention musculoskeletal problems and osteoporosis.

It is important that if we have swollen and sore joints we see a doctor for a diagnosis.

OSTEOARTHRITIS

Osteoarthritis (OA) is the commonest cause of chronic joint pain. It significantly affects at least 10% of the adult population although a much higher percentage of people have OA but not severely enough to cause them major problems. OA is due to the long-term effects of wear and tear on the joints and therefore the incidence goes up with age. About 50% of people over the age of 60 have some level of OA.

In a healthy joint, cartilage forms a smooth surface over the ends of bones allowing them to move without friction over each other. In OA, over time the cartilage wears away and becomes pitted and inflamed. In severe cases eventually all the cartilage is worn away, leaving bone grinding on bone which can be very uncomfortable. The bone around the joint tries to compensate for this trauma and so can overgrow at the edges, leading to the deformities often associated with severe OA. Unlike in rheumatoid arthritis, in OA the joint tends not to be red or inflamed on the outside or very tender to touch.

OA mainly affects the large weight-bearing joints such as knees and hips but also ankles and other joints if they have been heavily used over a long period of time. OA can also be secondary to past joint injuries and is far more common in people who are overweight and inactive. Athletes, particularly those who play full-contact sports, are prone to OA later in life. A disposition to developing OA can also be inherited; and the pattern of joint involvement is a little different in these cases with the joints at the fingertips often being affected as well. The pain of OA tends to be at its lowest in the morning and increases with use of the joint throughout the day. OA is diagnosed with an X-ray, which will show narrowing of the joint – cartilage loss – and changes in the bone.

The best advice is to take steps to prevent OA before it occurs (which will be outlined over the following pages) but there are also many things that can be done to slow its progression, limit the pain and maintain mobility. The supplement glucosamine with chondroitin is as effective as any pharmaceutical, including anti-inflammatory medications, for pain relief for moderate to severe OA, although it works more slowly.[1] Glucosamine is safer and has far fewer side effects than pharmaceutical drugs and is cheaper although it is not subsidised. It also helps to preserve and possibly regenerate cartilage. The supplement SAMe (S-adeonsyl methionine) also shows potential for OA.[2]

Heat packs, physiotherapy, occupational therapy and a range of lifestyle changes are all helpful in the prevention and management of OA. When, however, OA progresses to a point where the pain and mobility problems are distressing and are impacting upon a person's life and functioning, and when more simple and conservative measures are not providing adequate relief, then surgery is the last option. Joint replacement can be effective in re-establishing function and reducing pain; they tend to last 10 to 15 years and then have to be repeated.

RHEUMATOID ARTHRITIS

Rheumatoid arthritis (RA) is an autoimmune condition in which, for reasons not entirely understood, the immune system has been sensitised to attack the joints as if they were foreign to the body. This causes inflammation, redness, swelling, tenderness and pain on movement. Sometimes RA is also associated with problems in other parts of the body such as the lungs, skin and blood vessels. RA affects women about three times as often as men and affects close to 2% of the population.

The joints commonly affected by RA are the hands – the finger joints, except for the joints at the fingertips – and ankles. Shoulders, elbows, knees, hips, neck and jaw can also be affected. The pain and stiffness associated with RA is often worse in the morning and settles somewhat when the person starts moving around. The progression of RA often waxes and wanes, with inflammation flaring up for days or weeks and then settling down. Over time the joint can become damaged, disfigured and less functional, leading to significant disability in severe cases.

RA is generally diagnosed based on the patient's medical history and a doctor's examination, and confirmed with X-rays and blood tests. As inflammation is the main problem in RA, anti-inflammatory medications are the mainstay of medical treatment. Steroids and a range of stronger drugs are used if the condition is severely disabling and progressive but, as ever, the benefits need to be balanced with the side effects.

Stress management

The psychological state is always important in any condition which involves chronic pain. Stress, frustration, anger or depression can all amplify the amount of impact that pain has. Negative emotional states:

* Increase inflammation;
* Increase muscle tension;
* Increase our perception of pain;
* Sensitise the nervous system to fire off pain messages more frequently;
* Reduce our ability to cope with pain.

Stress is pro-inflammatory. Stressful life events and unsupportive social environments are associated with the onset and exacerbation of a variety of autoimmune diseases, including RA.[34] Stress in the prior week is associated with increased arthritic inflammation and pain.[5] 'Irrational beliefs, the cause of much of our stress, are also associated with increased inflammation.'[6] How we learn to deal with stress early in life also affects the amount of inflammation we experience in response to stressors later in life. 'There is also a link between major depression and early life stress with poor health outcomes in inflammatory diseases such as RA.[7]

It is one thing to show that stress aggravates a medical condition but it is important to take the next step and show whether stress management helps to reverse or modify the condition. While there is ongoing damage associated with OA, the body is also attempting to heal itself. It has been shown that poor mental health slows healing. Conversely, better mental health is associated with quicker healing. Cognitive and mindfulness-based strategies that help a person to cope with, and be less reactive to, pain have been found to assist people with OA, RA and other chronic pain syndromes such as fibromyalgia.[8]

An innovative study tested whether stress reduction benefited two inflammatory diseases, RA and asthma.[9] Patients with moderate to severe asthma and RA were placed into two groups. Both groups received the usual medical care but one was given the exercise of writing in a journal for three consecutive days about the most stressful event in their lives. Follow-up four months later showed that the group that kept the journal had far fewer symptoms and their medical test results had improved. Interestingly, no psychotherapy was required to produce the benefit. Simply writing about and expressing what they had not expressed before helped these people come to terms with previously traumatic events, which in turn helped their medical condition. There is also considerable potential for CBT to alter the course of RA.[10]

Furthermore, when having to go through rehabilitation – say, after a joint replacement – a better mental state leads to quicker and better results.

Spirituality

Factors already discussed in previous chapters about coping, mental health and general wellbeing apply when dealing with a chronic condition like arthritis which is associated with ongoing pain and disability. In relation to arthritis specifically, a study showed that spirituality is one of the important coping mechanisms for women with a chronic, potentially debilitating and painful condition like OA or RA.[11]

Exercise

It has been accepted wisdom that exercise such as running damages cartilage but, like many things that are accepted wisdom, it may not be entirely true. Evidence suggests that regular exercise, including running,[12] helps to maintain cartilage whereas inactivity accelerates cartilage loss.[13] Sports that can more readily lead to cartilage damage, such as those involving a lot of turning at speed and full-contact sports, do increase the risk of later OA.[14] Carrying excess weight also puts weight-bearing joints like hips and knees at risk, but mainly if that excess weight is fat rather than muscle.[15] The reasons for this are not entirely clear but one important factor is that excess weight leads to a vicious circle of reduced exercise, poorer joint health, reduced muscle mass . . . and on it goes.[16] Weight control is imperative in patients with OA, especially those with OA in their legs or spine.

Exercise can interrupt the vicious circle of immobility and dependence triggered by OA. Furthermore, exercise increases mobility, increases strength and stability of joints, and diminishes pain, stiffness and swelling.[17] The extra muscle tone and strength actually help to protect joints and reduce the risk of falls. In the elderly, gains in strength, flexibility and balance can be more important than cardiovascular fitness.[18] Long-term benefits are largely dependent on maintaining exercise patterns over time therefore choosing a form of exercise we can and will maintain is important.

Exercise also becomes relevant for arthritis in rehabilitation after falls, fractures or operations. Physiotherapy helps here, by offering exercises specifically tailored to building flexibility, strength and stability.

It is tempting when joints are sore due to RA to get into a cycle of inactivity but this is not associated with good outcomes whereas regular physical activity is.[19] Convincing RA patients of this is a challenge. For RA patients also, physical activity improves strength, function and mobility, and can help to reduce pain.[20] Part of the reason may be due to effects on mood, joint stability and function, as well as an anti-inflammatory effect of moderate exercise. Tai chi is a gentle form of exercise which may suit many with RA. Early research has found that it reduces disability and depression, and enhances quality of life and mood for RA patients.[21] Hydrotherapy is another form of low-impact activity which suits many people with arthritis and many aquatic centres provide classes for the public.

Nutrition

Counselling on weight management and nutrition is a central aspect of maintaining healthy joints.[22] Foods can be both beneficial and, in a minority of cases, harmful for arthritis.[23] Glucosamine, chondroitin and SAMe supplements have already been mentioned and the following guidelines may also be useful to consider:

- Vegetarian diets are associated with lower weight and incidence of arthritis.[24] Over a decade ago, in a controlled trial RA patients fasted and then adopted a vegetarian diet for a year, resulting in a sustained improvement in their RA;[25 26] If considering fasting please consult a health professional.
- A diet high in fruit and vegetables and rich in antioxidants helps to slow the progression of chronic degenerative diseases;
- Some foods can help to reduce the pain of OA. High on the list are avocado and soybean but there is also some evidence for the Chinese herbal formula *Du Huo Ji Sheng Wan*, green-lipped mussels, and plant extracts from *Harpagophytum procumbens*;[27]
- Eat cold water fish (cod, tuna, mackerel, sardines or salmon) two to three times a week. Their omega-3 fatty acids have an anti-inflammatory effect beneficial for RA.[28] They also reduce pain[29] and help to slow the progression of OA. Ground flaxseed-meal and flaxseed oil, avocadoes and walnuts are also good sources of omega-3 fatty acids;
- Proteoglycans (found in oats, mussels, shark fin and tripe) are beneficial by providing the chemical building blocks for cartilage;
- Seafood contains high levels of chondroitin, beneficial for OA;
- Cooking with ginger and turmeric for their anti-inflammatory properties can be helpful;
- Increase intake of foods with high levels of flavonoids such as buckwheat, cherries and blueberries as these have anti-inflammatory properties;

- Probiotics – the 'good' gut bacteria found in yoghurt and some fermented milk drinks – can help to modulate immune function and reduce inflammation in a variety of autoimmune conditions such as RA;[30]
- Increase intake of nutrients that support bone.[31] These nutrients include calcium, magnesium, silica, zinc, manganese, bioflavonoids, copper and boron. A balance between all minerals is important. Adequate mineral intake throughout life also renders one less susceptible to osteoporosis. Foods rich in minerals such as calcium and magnesium include parmesan cheese, mozzarella, camembert, whitebait, sardines, salmon, canned fish with bones, almonds, brazil nuts, cashews, hazelnuts, unhulled sesame seeds, linseeds, pumpkin, sunflower, parsley, broccoli, green leafy vegetables, banana, avocado, dried figs, kelp, tofu.
- Enjoy good levels of vitamin C in foods such as blackberries, blueberries, cherries, raspberries, oranges, lemons, papayas, brussels sprouts, capsicum, tomatoes, asparagus, broccoli and strawberries.
- Vitamin D deficiency has been shown to increase the risk and progression of OA and osteoporosis. Foods rich in vitamin D include salmon, sardines, blue fin tuna and milk.
- Foods such as wheat germ, almonds, sunflower seeds, sunflower oil and hazelnuts have good levels of vitamin E[32] which appears to limit the breakdown of cartilage as well as stimulate cartilage synthesis.
- Including certain enzymes in the diet has been shown to be effective in reducing pain, inflammation and stiffness in RA.[33][34] Bromelain, which is found in pineapples, is one plant enzyme which may be useful.

Some patients with RA claim that their symptoms improve when they eliminate certain foods, but scientific support has been sparse.[35] No one food is believed to aggravate RA but food sensitivities can exacerbate joint inflammation. For example, foods in the nightshade family like tomatoes, potatoes, eggplant, capsicum and chilli can cause problems for some people. Identification of food sensitivities via an elimination diet can be helpful but before going on one it is best to receive guidance from an appropriately trained health professional, as restricted diets, if unbalanced, can lead to deficiencies and they need to be carefully managed.

Connectedness

A lack of social connectedness and unsettled relationships can trigger inflammatory diseases such as RA and are associated with greater levels of pain and disability. Isolation, and the lowered mood which often comes with it, significantly increase pain and disability. For example, women with stronger marriages were noted to deal with stress better and have lower levels of inflammatory hormones like interleukins.[36]

Arthritis and the disability or immobility associated with it can be a source of disconnectedness. It is hard to remain in touch with family, friends, the community and organisations we belong to, and difficult to go on outings, if we have mobility problems. The help of trained professionals like physiotherapists and occupational therapists, in conjunction with the use of mobility devices, can aid mobility enormously and have a major positive impact upon social engagement.

Environment

Environmental, socio-economic, occupational and personal factors impact upon the disability associated with arthritis in three main ways. They impact upon:

a. bodily function and structure;
b. the activities we undertake;
c. our level of participation.[37]

It is worthwhile being aware of these influences and, where possible, modifying them appropriately. Our environment can provide facilities to make it easy to undertake activities like exercise. The climate or perceived level of safety can make us more or less likely to participate in outdoor activities.

Our physical and social environment can be conducive to exercise and social interaction or antagonistic to it, and these can affect arthritis symptoms and progression. Regular moderate doses of sunlight are important for maintaining bone health (including preventing osteoporosis) by boosting vitamin D. By exercising outdoors, sunlight exposure and exercising can be combined as a part of our regular routine. Smoking, active and passive, is a well-established trigger for

RA.[38] Living in a smoke-free environment is important for this reason (and many others).

If arthritis is causing us a level of disability then fitting out our home and work environments with mobility aids can help us enormously to maintain function and independence. These can include ramps, rails and handles as well as things like cutlery specially suited for those with a poorer grip. Occupational therapists are best placed to advise about mobility aids.

17

Mental health

In keeping with the *illness* focus of our healthcare system, we have almost forgotten what mental *health* is. Mental health and happiness are natural, but just because they are natural does not mean that they are common. We could probably equate complete and total mental health with enlightenment, which is quite rare. For most of us there is a little bit of work to do to reach this lofty goal. One of the most unhelpful aspects of having a mental health problem is thinking, wrongly, that we are the only one. One of the most useful aspects of speaking with a health professional about it or being part of a support group is that we quickly discover that we are far from alone.

This chapter largely focuses on depression, anxiety and stress although many of the same principles and strategies will be equally applicable to other mental health problems like bipolar disorder, schizophrenia, phobias, obsessive-compulsive disorder (OCD), post-traumatic stress disorder (PTSD), attention deficit and hyperactivity disorder (ADHD) and personality disorders. Although the self-help strategies listed below are important for these conditions it is also important to seek advice, medication and supervision as appropriate from a suitably trained doctor, psychologist or counsellor. Those who seek help for a mental health issue have a significantly better long-term prognosis than those who don't. Depression, anxiety and other distressing mental states compounded by isolation are not a good recipe for mental health.

The causes or triggers for depression and anxiety are many and one rarely finds the one in the absence of the other, so the clinical picture is often a mixed one. We can inherit a genetic disposition to depression or anxiety but whether or not that disposition will be triggered depends on a wide variety of things, many of which are in our control. Major life stress can make a genetic predisposition more likely to express itself. Being overloaded or overly busy at home and work can create the conditions in which depression and anxiety can entrench themselves. Lifestyle factors such as smoking and physical inactivity can leave us more vulnerable. Substance abuse can trigger depression or anxiety, or exacerbate it if already present. Some medications can have side effects which impact upon mental health. Because the causes are so many, it also means that the potential solutions are many, and just as risk factors can build upon each other, so too can the solutions. To get the most benefit from this chapter, it is best to have first read Chapter 2, on stress management.

Education

DEPRESSION

Between 20 and 25% of people will experience a significant episode of depression during their lifetime. The incidence is slightly higher in women than men, but men with depression are less likely to see a healthcare professional.

The most extreme and concerning endpoint for severe depression is suicide. Suicide rates have increased notably in the years since World War II. Suicide is three to four times more common among men than women, suggesting that a lot of men in need of help are not willing to acknowledge or discuss their depression. The recent rise in suicide among males in late adolescence and early adulthood is of particular concern; in this age group it is the commonest cause of death. There is also a high incidence of male suicide after 65.

The biological view of depression is that it is largely a disruption of one particular neurotransmitter in the brain: serotonin. The view that this is the 'cause' of depression means that the 'cure' for depression is to take a medication to increase serotonin. Such a superficial view of the cause of depression ignores the important fact that many things influence the ways we think and live, and how we think and live affects the levels of serotonin in the brain. Serotonin is a secondary effect, not the cause. Although medications can help severe depression to a limited extent, if medication is used to the exclusion of dealing with broader psychological and social issues then the benefit is short-lived. Research suggests that the clinical effect of antidepressants for mild to moderate depression is largely a placebo effect and outcomes are largely independent of dosage.[12] This is not to say that there is nothing that can be done for depression, but medication by itself is at best a superficial answer.

Depression is primarily experienced as a persistently lowered mood. Everyone feels down from time to time but that's not depression. The persistently lowered mood of depression colours one's perception of oneself and the world leading to pessimism, chronic guilt, excessive rumination, an inability to take pleasure in normally enjoyable activities, irritability, lack of humour, lack of perspective, reduced focus, inability to cope and falling productivity. Depression also has other effects including poor appetite, lack of energy, poor sleep and reduced sex drive.

What makes depression hard to diagnose is that many people hide it and that many physical illnesses can masquerade as depression. These include things like cancer, anaemia and an underactive thyroid. Depression can also masquerade as many illnesses. It can therefore be important to exclude other health problems before settling on a diagnosis of depression. Because of the fact that many people are reluctant to be open about having depression there is often a delay in diagnosis and treatment.

Having depression is a risk factor for other illnesses – such as heart disease – but on the positive side, holistic management of depression substantially reverses the risk of such illness.

ANXIETY

We all have the propensity to get anxious about one thing or another from time to time but generally without a major impact upon our life, ability to cope or sense of wellbeing. When anxiety gets to that point we need to seek help. One definition of this kind of anxiety is a 'generalised and persistent anxiety or anxious mood, which cannot be associated with, or is disproportionately large in response to a specific psychological stressor, stimulus or event.'[3] In other words, we are anxious much of the time, or out of all proportion to the stresses we are facing.

There are many varieties of anxiety and sometimes the word 'stress' is used synonymously with it. 'Generalised anxiety disorder', as described above, is the most common form of anxiety. Panic attacks, which are sudden bursts of extreme anxiety, affect around 30% of the population at some stage, although for most people panic attacks do not become an ongoing problem. Phobias, OCD, and PTSD are also varieties of anxiety disorders. Often the picture is mixed and can fluctuate over time.

Anxiety generally expresses itself through restlessness, irritability, fatigue, poor concentration and performance, muscle tension and disturbed sleep. The mind can show a tendency to worry, particularly about future events. There are many physical effects of anxiety and stress, which are described in Chapter 2. As with depression, in the long term anxiety can predispose us to a range of illnesses like heart disease or poor immunity, but effective stress management can also reverse these risks.

DIAGNOSIS AND TREATMENT

A trained healthcare professional will ask a series of questions relating to the kinds of issues mentioned above and may also use a questionnaire to try and confirm depression or anxiety, and the severity of it. There is no simple blood test to diagnose depression or anxiety but it is possible that a doctor will perform blood or other tests, to exclude other illnesses.

The next step is to consider the most appropriate management plan. It is important that this is a cooperative process between the patient and the healthcare professional. Medication will often be a part of treatment but for best results it is important to include self-help strategies, such as those outlined below, counselling and group support where appropriate.

Stress management

Prolonged stress can bring on depression. Because it activates many of the same chemicals our body secreted during an infection or inflammatory illness, it can also trigger the 'sickness response' which may explain many of the symptoms experienced in depression like lack of appetite, energy and motivation.[4] A particular chemical pathways in the brain – the brain cytokine system – can become sensitised by stress early in life. If we learn to deal with stress and emotional challenges poorly at an early age this will leave us much more prone to depression in later life.

In terms of managing stress, anxiety and depression, mindfulness-based meditation and cognitive therapy are among a range of very beneficial strategies. Whatever approach we use, raising awareness and developing an ability to stand back from thoughts and feelings with a level of objectivity are crucial to improving mental health. These techniques are commonly more effective when we learn them as part of a support group. Chapter 2 describes this in more detail.

According to reviews of the available studies,[5] a range of other strategies can be helpful in the management of depression and increasing stress resilience. These include:

- Positive emotions and optimism;
- Humour;
- Being flexible in dealing with challenges;
- Being reflective;
- Acceptance;
- Religiosity/spirituality;
- Altruism;
- Social support;
- Having positive role-models;
- Positive coping styles;
- Exercise;
- Capacity to recover from negative events.

COGNITIVE BEHAVIOURAL THERAPY (CBT)

There is consistent evidence that Cognitive Behavioural Therapy (CBT) is an effective treatment for adults[6] and adolescents[7] with depression and anxiety.[8] It is also useful for the elderly[9] and can even help to prevent anxiety and depression in children.[10] It helps to improve physical health, immunity, reduce inflammation and aid recovery from illness and operations.[11] CBT can be delivered to individuals and groups.

CBT is aimed at examining, challenging and changing the way we think (cognitive) and behave (behavioural) and is based on the premise that anxiety and depression are the result of irrational and unexamined thoughts, beliefs, perceptions and attitudes. These thoughts affect our behaviour, which reinforces the irrational thoughts – but with insight we can change our thoughts and behaviour. The elements of CBT include:

- Education about depression, anxiety or any other mental health condition being treated;
- Identifying, examining and challenging irrational thoughts such as 'I always fail at everything I do' or 'Nobody loves me';
- Monitoring thoughts and reinforcing self-examination throughout the day;
- Discouraging behaviours which reinforce negative thought patterns – such as avoidance – and encouraging behaviours which reinforce new and positive thought patterns – such as confronting challenges.
- CBT will often be supplemented with other behavioural strategies like scheduling positive or enjoyable activities on a daily basis and learning relaxation techniques.

OTHER TYPES OF PSYCHOTHERAPY

Other forms of psychotherapy can also be helpful. These include Rational Emotive Therapy (RET), Acceptance-Commitment Therapy (ACT) and Dialectical-Behaviour Therapy (DBT) which use mindfulness, autogenetic training (using relaxation and hypnosis) and many others.

It is beyond the scope of this book to consider all these in depth, suffice to say that seeking help when we are dealing with significant mental health issues is the sensible thing to do.

OTHER APPROACHES

These approaches are generally used as adjuncts to psychotherapy. These therapies can be learned in courses or from appropriately trained counsellors, or other health practitioners:

- Meditation and relaxation techniques;
- Yoga or tai chi;
- Music therapy;
- Art therapy;
- Communication training;
- Assertiveness training;
- Keeping a journal;
- Bibliotherapy (books and other reading materials);
- Humour therapy.

Spirituality

The relationship between spirituality and mental health was discussed at length in Chapter 3, but let's remind ourselves of the key points and how they relate to depression and anxiety:

- Spirituality means different things to different people. One way of expressing it is the search for meaning.
- The search for meaning is a basic human need, not an option. Without it we fail to flourish and leave ourselves far more open to suffering, particularly in times of major adversity.
- There are many ways of searching for meaning, religion is one albeit an important one. We need to search for meaning in a way that suits our personal, cultural and philosophical outlook.
- Spirituality has a range of benefits for mental health. These include lower rates of depression and anxiety, and quicker recovery from depression and anxiety. Having a spiritual dimension to our life also helps us cope better with stressful life events.
- Spirituality protects us better from depression and anxiety (and other health problems) if it is instrinsic to our core beliefs rather than if we are just going through the motions, such as going to church out of convention.
- Spirituality, or the search for meaning, is an important part of any holistic approach to dealing with mental illness.
- A sense of meaning can help us to develop other helpful coping and lifestyle strategies.

Exercise

Exercise is a powerful, accessible and attractive but simple approach for depression that is effective at any age.[12] Exercise programs have been found to elevate mood, in both the healthy and the clinically depressed. Many studies have reported antidepressant and anxiety-relieving effects of exercise.[13] Higher-intensity exercise, such as running or team sports, seem to be more effective than low-intensity exercise, like walking. Exercise also helps combat a range of symptoms associated with depression including lack of vitality and concentration.[14] Exercise has also been useful in the management of alcohol and substance abuse, which commonly accompany anxiety, depression and other mental health problems.

Why exercise has this effect in depression and anxiety is not completely clear but some of the likely reasons include:

- Increased serotonin;[15]
- Improvement in sleep;[16]
- An increase in self-esteem by giving a sense of achievement and mastery;
- Acting as a distraction, stopping us from ruminating on our worries and concerns;
- Improvement in general health, vitality and physical fitness;
- Release of pent-up anger, frustration and hostility;
- Increase in social contact, particularly in team sports;
- Reduced need for medications that can aggravate depression such as sedatives or beta-blockers for high blood pressure.

In order for exercise to help mental health problems it needs to be done regularly, but one of the unfortunate aspects of depression and anxiety is that they often cause a lack of motivation. Although we may know that exercise is good for mood it is often hard to motivate ourselves while feeling emotionally down. This is why encouragement, structured programs, guidance and exercising with others are more likely to lead to success.

Nutrition

Nutrition has not generally been thought of as a core element in the management of mental health issues, but it should be. Dietary change in mental health needs to be very sensitively approached, though, because for many people food is a source of self-loathing and guilt, especially those who have eating disorders. Before considering making dietary changes that might be beneficial for mental health it is important to remember:

- Food is to be enjoyed. Take a look at the advice from healthy weight management expert Dr Kausman at the end of Chapter 5.
- The foods found beneficial for depression and anxiety are possibly helpful for other mental health problems including bipolar disorder and schizophrenia.
- Some foods have a therapeutic effect on depression and anxiety; others are just as important in offseting symptoms and physical health problems associated with poor mental health.

- Mental health is a complex area of health and diet is one piece of the jigsaw.
- For eating disorders, guilt or self-loathing, futher help and counselling from a health professional is advisable.

NUTRITION AND DEPRESSION

A review appeared in the *Medical Journal of Australia* regarding the evidence on the direct effects of food on mood and concluded the following:[17]

- Eating breakfast regularly leads to improved mood, better memory, more energy and feelings of calmness;
- Eating regular meals and nutritious afternoon snacks may improve cognitive performance;
- Slow weight reduction in overweight women can help to elevate mood.

Although we often eat sweet foods for comfort, a high level of refined sugar consumption is linked to a greater prevalence of depression. It is advisable to keep our intake of sugar as low as possible and read labels carefully as seemingly healthy foods can be deceptively packed with sugar. High levels of dairy consumption are also linked to a greater incidence of depression. If your intake is very high then limit consumption of milk and cheese and consider alternatives such as oat, soy or rice milk. By incorporating tahini, sardines and mackerel into the diet we can maintain our calcium intake.

There is a range of specific foods and nutrients which are beneficial for mood.

Omega-3 fatty acids

One key study[18] conclusively showed higher levels of depression in people with a low dietary intake of fish and seafood. Once again we see the importance of having a good level of omega-3 fatty acids in our diet, especially from fish. Taking omega-3 fatty acid supplements reduces symptoms of depression and bipolar mood disorder.[19] Regular omega-3 fatty acid consumption is associated with a 30% reduction in the risk of mental health problems.[20]

Chocolate

Happily, chocolate has now been confirmed as a food which improves mood,[21] although that does seem to be stating the obvious. It does not seem to be so useful when it is consumed in excess as a comfort food rather than in moderation. Dark chocolate (high cocoa mass) is best, because it has plenty of the nutrient value of chocolate and not as much of the fat and sugar.

Starchy root vegetables

A higher intake of starchy root vegetables may be beneficial for depression. Potatoes, yams, Jerusalem artichokes and sweet potatoes are examples.

Low GI

A low GI (glycaemic index) diet can help protect against metabolic disorders such as insulin resistance and in so doing, can provide some protection against depression. For more information on the glycaemic index, see Chapter 12, 'Diabetes'.

Folate

Folate is well known for preventing birth defects and is taken by most pregnant women. Studies have also shown it to be useful in the treatment of major depressive disorders.[22][23][24] You will find it in foods such as tomato juice, green beans, broccoli, spinach, asparagus, okra, black-eyed peas, lentils, navy and pinto beans, and chick peas.

SAMe

SAMe is a chemical occurring naturally in our bodies. Supplementation has been shown to be effective for some people with mild to moderate depression.[25] Our body usually manufactures all the SAMe it needs from the amino acid methionine, which is found in meats, soybeans, eggs, seeds and lentils.

B vitamins

Foods high in B vitamins, particularly B6, have long been thought to help with prevention of depression. [26][27] We need a constant daily supply of B vitamins in our diet as they are water soluble and not stored in our body. Foods rich in a range of B vitamins include potatoes, bananas, lentils, chilli, tempeh, liver, turkey, spinach, broccoli, mushrooms and tuna.

5-HTP

5-HTP is an amino acid which is used to make serotonin in the brain and can enhance mood and sleep.[28] Foods that contain the amino acid tryptophan can help raise levels of 5-HTP. Such foods include red meats (beef, pork, lamb and wild game), poultry (chicken and turkey) and seafood (tuna, salmon, halibut and shrimp), as well as cottage cheese, Swiss cheese, peanuts, cashews and avocadoes.

Vitamin C

Vitamin C assists in the production of 5-HTP and is a fabulous antioxidant. It is always useful to include vitamin C-rich foods in your diet. These foods include citrus fruits, like oranges, cantaloupe, strawberries, tomatoes, broccoli, cabbage, kiwifruit and capsicum.

Iron

Iron levels can have an effect on cognition, depression and memory.[29] Good food sources of iron are wholegrain cereals, meat, poultry and fish. Liver is an especially rich source of iron, but pregnant women should avoid this source due to its high level of vitamin A which can cause birth defects. Because iron absorption can vary for different foods, vegetarians who exclude all animal products from their diet may need almost twice as much dietary iron each day as non-vegetarians. Sources include dark green leafy vegetables such as spinach, raisins, nuts, seeds, beans, peas, and iron-fortified cereals, breads and pastas. Vitamin C increases iron absorption. Cut back on tea and coffee around mealtimes, since the tannins in tea and coffee bind to iron and interfere with absorption.

NUTRITION AND ANXIETY

Much of the nutritional information above for depression applies for anxiety also.

It is also worth considering removing stimulants from the diet as these can add to anxiety. Typically stimulants include coffee, tea, excessive chocolate, caffeine-based energy drinks, and Coke or Pepsi. Coffee and other foods containing caffeine make us more alert but can increase heart rate and aggravate agitation and depression. This is particularly important for the increasing numbers of adolescents attempting to use caffeine as a mood-enhancing drug.[30] To make decaffeinated tea simply soak the teabag for 45 seconds, discard the tea and then add fresh hot water. Nearly all the caffeine is leached out in the first 45 seconds.

During times of anxiety and increased stress there are greater demands for our body's nutrients. They are used more rapidly to meet the increased biochemical needs of metabolism, so we require increased amounts of nutrients. You may like to consider including some of the following foods in your diet.

Antioxidants
One effect of stress on the body is an increase in oxidation and free radical production, so antioxidants are an especially important part of the diet. There is more detail on antioxidants in Chapter 5, 'Nutrition'. The herbal supplement licorice provides adrenal support – valuable for anxiety due to the increased secretion of adrenaline by the adrenal glands – and can help as an antioxidant.[31]

Essential fatty acids
There is some evidence that omega-3 fatty acids may reduce symptoms of anxiety.[32]

Amino acids
Amino acids such as tyrosine, phenylalanine, glutamine and choline provide our body with the building blocks to make essential brain chemicals (neurotransmitters) such as dopamine, GABA and acetyl-choline. Providing your body with adequate amounts of these amino acids helps to ensure there are adequate levels of these useful brain chemicals. Good sources of these amino acids include oats, cabbage, beets, beef, chicken, fish, beans, dairy products, cauliflower, tofu and eggs.

Low GI foods
Avoid low blood sugar (hypoglycaemia) as this can make you feel more anxious. If you are prone to hypoglycaemia then ensure you eat regularly – every three hours if possible – and snack on healthy low GI foods. Have your blood sugar checked by your doctor before assuming you have hypoglycaemia.

Starchy foods
Oats and other starchy foods can have a calming effect.

Fluid intake

Ensure you have adequate fluid intake. Use an electrolyte-based drink if you have sweated a lot after exercise or on a very hot day.

Inositol

Inositol[33] has been shown in studies to be useful in panic disorder conditions.[34] Inositol can be found in wheat germ, brewer's yeast, bananas, liver, brown rice, oat flakes, nuts, unrefined molasses, raisins and vegetables.

Chamomile tea

Chamomile tea has been found to have some antioxidant effects. Many people find it has a relaxing and calming effect although there is not much evidence on this.[35]

Magnesium

Magnesium is a mineral with many uses in the body including relaxing tense or cramping muscles, maintaining normal nerve function and heartbeat, and helping to maintain stable blood sugar levels and immune function.[36][37] You can find magnesium in green vegetables such as spinach, some legumes, nuts and seeds, and whole, unrefined grains.

B vitamins

As in depression, the B vitamins[38] are considered helpful in general, but B6 seems to be particularly important. Vitamin B6 can be found in potatoes, bananas, chicken breast, sunflower seeds, trout, spinach and avocadoes. Some of the symptoms of B5 deficiency are fatigue, headache, sleep disturbances, nausea and abdominal discomfort, so you can start to see the value of foods rich in B vitamins for managing anxiety. Mushrooms are an excellent source of vitamin B5, along with broccoli, cauliflower, turnip greens and sunflower seeds.

Connectedness

Upbringing and social circumstances profoundly influence the way we think and cope, and hence affect whether we are vulnerable to developing depression or an anxiety disorder later in life. Social isolation, a relationship break-up, a poor education, socio-economic disadvantage and unemployment can all predispose us.

The sub-cultures we identify with in society and the music we listen to can create an atmosphere which reinforces depression and anxiety. It is hard and almost impossible to make substantial and sustainable progress with mental health issues without attention to our mental and emotional environment. The importance of supportive and stable relationships – for example, partner, family and friends – cannot be over-emphasised. Consciously seeking and nurturing such relationships has a flipside in that we may need to be prepared to leave behind relationships which consistently undermine our efforts for growth.

Connectedness is also nurtured through engaging with our community and being involved with clubs and interest groups. Attending these can be therapeutic in itself. Connectedness and support can be fostered in other ways too, including via healthcare professionals, support groups, group therapy and over the Internet. There are increasing numbers of Internet-based mental health services which are useful in providing information for self-help techniques and links to healthcare programs.

Connectedness and support has a beneficial effect on mood and self-esteem and also, depending on the group, can help us to make other healthy changes such as improving diet or exercise.

Environment

Our environment can have a range of good or bad effects on our emotional state. It is not hard to observe the effect of a sports crowd on our mood, or the effect of a beautiful garden or park. It is hard to feel good about ourselves or the world if we live in a war zone. Our environment can also affect our behaviour for better or worse, whether it be a casino, shop, or a doctor's surgery.

Environment influences us at every stage of our life cycle. Our mother's womb can influence us. A mother who is smoking during pregnancy increases the risk of mental health problems in her child later in life.[39] Extreme stress for a pregnant woman, particularly in the first trimester, can substantially increase her child's risk of schizophrenia. At the other extreme of the life cycle, elderly people who are living in a non-stimulating environment have declining mental health as a result. Environment can foster and support social interaction, opportunities and learning.

Environment can impact mental health in other ways. Air

pollution, for example, may exacerbate depression.[40] Climate change and drought impact upon economies and communities and these can have secondary effects on the mental health of the people involved.

Sunlight is an important modulator of mood. There is a natural rise and fall in mood with the seasons but for some, winter is enough to lead to depression. Regular, moderate sun exposure has been found to be beneficial for mental health, particularly in those with Seasonal Affective Disorder (SAD) which is a type of depression.[41] Light stimulates brain chemicals and mood (this is probably a hangover from earlier days in our evolution when we would have gone into a relative hibernation when food was scarce). Sunlight may also have a beneficial effect on schizophrenia.[42]

18

Brain health
and dementia

Education

Dementia is the name given to a cluster of conditions which lead
to progressive memory loss and disability. To some extent, cognitive
decline and loss of brain cells is a normal part of the ageing process,
but for some the rate of loss is so great that it has a major impact upon
their life.

In dementia, short-term memory is affected first, until in the late
stages even long-term memories are lost. The progression of the
condition can be insidious, beginning with forgetfulness but the
presence of forgetfulness does not necessarily mean dementia; it might
mean things such as depression, being overly busy or inattentive.
Dementia is often present for some years before it becomes obvious
enough – usually to others – that there is something wrong. The
course of the disease can be long, with a slow decline in functioning,
increasing dependence on others and behavioural problems such as
wandering or aggression. Institutionalisation is a common outcome in
the latter stages as the burden of care becomes too great or dangerous
for the carer, most often an elderly spouse. The varieties of dementia
include:

- **Alzheimer's disease (AD)** which accounts for nearly two-thirds
  of dementia cases. It is associated with plaques, protein (amyloid)
  deposition and 'tangles' between brain cells followed by cell

loss. The triggers for this progression of events are not entirely understood but factors mentioned in this chapter obviously play an important part.

- **Frontal lobe dementia** accounts for about one in 10 cases; personality changes are early and prominent.
- **Vascular dementia** accounts for about one in 7 cases and is typically associated with long-standing CVD.
- **Alcohol abuse** accounts for about one in 20 cases of dementia. In the future there may be other variations of dementia seen increasingly in in association with abuse of recreational drugs.
- **Other types** of dementia can occur in association with conditions such as Parkinson's disease, AIDS, brain tumours and syphilis.

Dementia is common and becoming more common in the community due to an ageing population. It is one of the major burdens of disease in affluent countries. It is not only a burden for the person who has it but also for family, carers and the community, and this is why supporting patients and their carers is such an important part of the management of dementia. Currently approximately 10% of people over 65 years old are affected with dementia, although many only mildly, and 20% of people over 80 have the condition. Recent figures in the US showed that nearly 14% of the population had dementia at the age of 70 and over 37% by the age of 90.[1] If lifestyle and mental health patterns deteriorate further, the future incidence of dementia may rise more than we expect.

Risk factors for dementia include a family history, chronic depression and other mental health problems, CVD, social isolation, substance abuse, inactivity (passive leisure activities) and other life-style factors that will be discussed. The fact that many of the risk factors for dementia are reversible means there is a lot we can do to prevent its onset or to intervene early, before the condition is well established. There are things which accelerate brain cell loss and things that slow it.

Education is important in preventing dementia because education and mental stimulation, whether early or even late in life, helps to protect the brain from age-related decline.[2] Exercising the brain preserves the brain cells we have and may even stimulate new cell growth. For example, one review of research in the field showed that, compared to those with five years or less of formal education, those with nine or more years' formal education had approximately one-seventh the chance of developing dementia later in life.[3] This was not explainable by other risk factors.

If concerned about the possibility of early dementia in ourselves or others, proper assessment, confirmation of the diagnosis and testing to look for any underlying illnesses is required. For example, sometimes dementia is difficult to distinguish from severe depression.

The management of dementia includes treating any underlying illnesses, modifying risk factors, particularly cardiovascular risk factors, supervision and attending to basic care and hygiene. Undiagnosed illnesses like urinary tract infections or an underactive thyroid can often compound the severity of dementia in the elderly and when treated will often lead to a significant improvement in wellbeing. The drug treatments for dementia – such as cholinesterase inhibitors – have shown only very limited and short-term benefits despite the fact that they have created a lot of interest and been widely promoted. The conclusion from one review was, 'Because of flawed methods and small clinical benefits, the scientific basis for recommendations of cholinesterase inhibitors for the treatment of Alzheimer's disease is questionable.'[4]

This does not mean there is nothing we can do to prevent or manage dementia, but if any of the following strategies are to be helpful then they need to be implemented early and over the longer term. According to a review in the *Postgraduate Medical Journal*, 'A healthy life both physically and mentally may be the best defence against the changes of an ageing brain.'[5]

Stress management

Probably the most obvious mind–body link of all is between mind and brain. In short, stress, via many stress hormones, can accelerate age-related brain cell loss. This is described in Chapter 2.

The central nervous system has many mechanisms to allow it to adapt to the environment, repair damage and slow the ageing process. These mechanisms include reduction of stress and inflammatory chemicals, proteins that promote cell survival, enzymes that repair our DNA, and the mobilisation of stem cells to replace damaged brain cells.[6] [7] These protective mechanisms can be impaired by some toxic chemicals and processes that lead to more oxidation, including psychological stress. Stress is implicated in disorders like AD and

Parkinson's disease. Studies showed that middle-aged to elderly people who were prone to becoming distressed had twice the risk of developing AD than those who weren't.[8] Major psychiatric illness such as major depression and psychosis is three to four times more common in people who develop dementia.[9][10] It has also been found that levels of amyloid – the protein implicated in AD – are much higher in the brains of people with depression.[11] Default states of brain – including going over the past and rumination – also involve areas of the brain affected by AD.

Stress, emotion, memory of past experience, how focused we are, and the way we use our leisure and work time all influence our risk for developing AD.[12] Therefore, they have implications for the prevention and management of AD.

Leisure activities occupy a significant part of our day. Whether we are aware of it or not, we are practising a state of attention for hours of the day depending on what kind of leisure activities we engage in. Passive leisure activities that lull us into a state of inattentiveness, non-engagement and lack of tactile experience look to be the most unhelpful for maintaining cognitive function. Number one among passive leisure activities is television watching.[13] Simple observation and common sense might suggest that if we don't use some capacity then nature withdraws it, just as not using our muscles leads to their wasting away whereas exercise builds them up. The evidence is becoming strong now that this is also the case with the brain. It has been shown that in middle adulthood, each additional daily hour of television viewing increases the risk of developing AD by 1.3 times (i.e. a 30% increase). The researchers noted that 'participation in intellectually stimulating activities and social activities reduced the associated risk of developing AD'.[14] We do not know whether more intellectually stimulating forms of television content have a less harmful, or possibly protective, effect. In another study, people who had the least diverse leisure activities, spent the least time on them and practised more passive activities (principally watching television) were nearly four times as likely to develop dementia over a 40-year period than people with more active leisure pursuits.[15] What protects against cognitive decline are having diverse leisure activities, intellectually engaging activities such as playing music or games, or reading, or physical exercise.[16] Music, art, looking after pets and other stimulating activities can all help to increase enjoyment and bring back memories even in those with quite advanced dementia.

A range of lifestyle factors have been implicated as causes of dementia. A major 16-year study[17] undertaken in Dubbo, NSW, found that moderate intake of alcohol was associated with a 34% lower risk (although high alcohol intake increases the risk), daily gardening with a 36% lower risk and daily walking with a 38% lower risk. Poor respiratory function was associated with an 84% higher risk and depression with a 50% higher risk. Obviously we should do our best to do more of the things that protect us against dementia and minimise the risk factors.

Psychological and social factors affecting dementia risk

Risk factors	Protective factors
• Major psychiatric illness	• Physical exercise
• High stress	• Diverse leisure activities
• Television watching and other passive leisure activities	• Intellectually stimulating leisure activities
• Living alone or living with a dominant spouse and having no close social ties	• Marriage and social contact
• Unproductive working style	• Stimulating work

Sources[18] [19]

All of the data about risk factors for dementia needs to be contrasted with the increasing number of studies showing that practices that help us to improve our mental health, reduce stress and improve our focus – such as mindfulness-based practices and CBT – also help to slow age-related brain cell loss, particularly in important parts of the brain like the memory centre (hippocampus) and frontal lobes. Brain cell loss may even be a reversible process to some extent. Mindfulness-based practices and CBT can be successfully integrated into care even for those who already have a mild level of dementia.[20] It is long overdue that the attention in dementia research became more focused on outcomes from psychological and lifestyle improvements.

Spirituality

A spiritual perspective can help a person and their carers[21] to cope with a condition as debilitating as dementia. To maintain dignity and to see this adversity in a larger context will help to buffer some of the mental and emotional impact of the illness. Considering the psychosocial factors which are risk-factors for dementia it would not be surprising if spirituality or an active religious life were protective. Indeed, this may be part of the reason why 'a slower rate of cognitive decline was associated with higher levels of spirituality and private religious practices', according to a review in the journal *Neurology*.[22]

How spirituality or the search for meaning is integrated into care is certainly going to be influenced by the patient's and carer's outlooks as well as the skill of the health practitioner. As E Mackinley wrote in the *Medical Journal of Australia*:

> *Providing spiritual care is about tapping into the concept of spirituality: core meaning, deepest life meaning, hope and connectedness. The search for meaning, connectedness and hope becomes more significant as older people are faced with the possibilities of frailty, disability and dementia. Spirituality, ageing and meaning in life can be discussed in the context of an alternative view of 'successful ageing'.*[23]

Exercise

Physical exercise, even if moderate, protects against cognitive decline and dementia later in life and directly stimulates the growth of new nerve cells at any age.[24] [25] [26] [27] [28] To quote one review, 'physical activity reduces the risk of cognitive decline and dementia in later life.'[29] In a study[30] of over 10,000 people aged 35 to 55 participants' exercise levels were measured and categorised as low, medium or high. When their cognitive function was tested 12 years later, a low level of physical activity doubled the chance for poor cognitive performance. Persistent low exercise was particularly harmful, more than doubling the risk of cognitive decline and dementia.

Exercise at any time of life can help to preserve brain function and concentration. It improves academic performance by increasing blood flow to the brain; increasing the levels of hormones which help to stimulate growth of brain cells; increasing alertness, focus and awareness; reducing depression and stress; and increasing self-esteem.

Care needs to be taken when starting exercise later in life. Start slowly and gently build up exercise duration and intensity, within reasonable comfort levels. Gentle forms of exercise such as walking or water aerobics may be the safest first options. The benefits are even greater if the exercise increases social interaction at the same time.

Nutrition

As ever, nutrition plays an important role. Many of the guidelines for heart disease and stroke (Chapter 10) apply in the case of dementia. Below are some key points to consider.

- Calorie restriction, folate and antioxidant supplements, especially when combined with regular intellectual and physical activities, are helpful for dementia prevention and management.[31] Large population studies convincingly show that a plant-based, low-calorie, high-nutrient diet reduces the risk of developing AD by 40%.
- Antioxidants have an anti-inflammatory effect which protects brain cells. Thus, fruits and vegetables lower the risk of developing age-related neurodegenerative diseases such as Parkinson's disease and AD. Vary the colour of the vegetables you eat to get the best balance. The polyphenolic compounds found in fruits such as blueberries seem to have a beneficial effect.[32]
- Eat fish regularly.[33] Omega-3 fatty acids in fish may be particularly useful, possibly because of their anti-inflammatory effects. 'There is a growing body of evidence . . . that suggests a protective effect of omega-3 fatty acids against dementia,'[34] according to a Cochrane review. DHA (one type of omega-3 fatty acid), best obtained from fish, walnuts and flaxseeds, reduces stress hormone levels, and hence dementia risk.
- Whole, unprocessed grains increase the B vitamins in your diet.
- Olive oil is emerging as an important food for reducing our risk of chronic disease. Olive oil is rich in fatty acids and antioxidants, vitamin E and other trace plant nutrients. There is extensive evidence supporting olive oil as beneficial to cognitive health.
- There is a high prevalence of vitamin B12 deficiency in elderly people and this has been associated with brain diseases.[35] Food sources include egg, fish, chicken, turkey, lamb and yoghurt, but depending on the blood level sometimes a supplement is needed.
- Egg yolks are packed with the amino acid choline which is used to make acetylcholine, a crucial molecule in the brain responsible for memory.
- Managing blood sugar levels and proper control of diabetes is important. This helps to ensure optimal circulation to all parts of the body, including the brain. When diabetes is not properly controlled, you increase your chances for dementia.

- Maintain good fluid intake as dehydration and electrolyte imbalances can aggravate poor cognitive function.

Connectedness

The table on page 303 listed some of the psychological and social factors which can impact upon the incidence and progression of dementia. To expand on this a little, working in a job one finds interesting and stimulating is protective against cognitive decline[36] but a daily occupation which creates little interest or intellectual stimulation is associated with greatly increased risk.

Although some might find it hard to believe, marriage is also protective against dementia. It is nearly two and a half times more common in the never-married.[37] Long-term cohabiting relationships are also protective. It is unknown exactly why marriage protects against dementia, but it could be because it protects against mental illness, increases our communication and diversifies our leisure activities.

With dementia looming as such a major problem in an ageing population more attention needs to go towards prevention. The abovementioned research has many implications for structuring work, leisure and social life in such a way that the risk of dementia is reduced, although any benefits might take generations to be felt. If current trends in work, leisure and social life are anything to go by we could have a dementia epidemic far greater than we ever imagined. The responsibility lies as much with legislators and policy makers as it does with individuals.

One of the hardest things for dementia patients and their carers to achieve is to remain socially engaged. Dementia not only makes it difficult to converse with people but can also cause behaviour which is potentially embarrassing and confronting. The impact of the illness on a person's ability to interact often makes social outings a difficult proposition, but it is a vital aspect of the management plan.

One last point on connectedness is that carers for dementia patients need social support as much as the patients do.

Environment

It is already clearly established that family, social, school and occupational environments can impact upon our cognitive abilities throughout life. Creating enriching and stimulating environments at home and in aged-care facilities[38] is one of the most valuable things that can be done for dementia sufferers. It is a vital pillar supporting all the other strategies to minimise the incidence of dementia and slow its progression. Improving the environment for people with dementia can be achieved with music, interaction with people and animals, interaction with nature, dance and many other things. The worst possible environment, although convenient in staff- and resource-strapped aged-care facilities, is being put in front of the television or left in bed alone.

For dementia sufferers a consistent and familiar environment is also crucial because any change in environment can feel threatening. Going to a new place provokes fear in a person with dementia because they are unable to assimilate the new environment into memory. Even relatively late into the illness, if they remain in a familiar environment like home, people with AD can often maintain a limited range of independence that they could not if they were moved somewhere else.

From a different perspective on 'environment', chemical exposures, such as to fumigants and defoliants, are associated with a substantially increased risk of AD.[39] Heavy air pollution has also been implicated.[40] Exposure to mercury and lead are also risk factors.[41] The assessment of some AD patients may need to include these chemicals and metals and if their levels are found to be high then steps should be taken to limit exposure. Once again, the importance of a clean and healthy environment cannot be denied.

19

Healthy immunity

Education

Our environment is full of micro-organisms: viruses, bacteria, fungi and yeasts among others. Some are friendly and helpful, others are a nuisance and others – some germs or pathogens – are potentially life-threatening. We are exposed to germs all the time but rarely do they cause a clinical infection and symptoms. This is because our body has defences to keep them out or, if they get in, to immobilise or kill them. After a germ gets past the physical barriers such as skin or stomach lining, our immune system is our front-line defence against infection. The war between potentially harmful pathogens and the body's defences is finely balanced. Things that put the balance in favour of the pathogen or reduce our body's defences can shift the balance, making it more likely that we will come down with an infection.

The cells of the immune system are called white blood cells (WBC) and there are a variety of them. There are lymphocytes, which have two main families: T-cells and B-cells. There are a variety of different T-cells, such as Natural Killer T-cells, which are like combat troops. They attack and destroy foreign cells, viruses or bacteria by injecting them with toxic chemicals. The B-cells are largely involved with producing immunoglobulins or antibodies which can attach to viruses and bacteria, either immobilising them or making them easier for T-cells to recognise and attack. Other varieties – known as helpers

– give off chemical messages which help to inform, mobilise and clone other WBCs. Other cells turn off the immune response. There are WBCs responsible for the allergic response, and WBCs called macrophages which are like scavengers mopping up dead bacteria and cells; macrophages also play a role in our body's cancer defences.

WBCs collect in large numbers in certain tissues like lymph glands, the gut wall, the bone marrow and the spleen. They also circulate around the body in the bloodstream and can move into tissues when directed to by chemical messages. Many of the inflammatory chemicals such as cytokines and interleukins are the chemical messengers used by the immune system. The immune cells talk to each other and they also talk to the brain, particularly the limbic system (associated with emotions) and the frontal lobes (responsible for reasoning and emotional regulation among other things). The brain also talks to the immune system and has a key role in regulating its function.

The immune system largely works on the ability to distinguish between 'self' and 'not-self'. Self denotes our own cells and tissues. They have our own personal 'name' written all over them in the form of antigens, so our WBCs don't attack them. A micro-organism such as a virus or bacteria wears its own antigens on the surface. Because its antigens are different to ours, the virus or bacteria looks foreign to our immune system which will therefore attack it. Some cancer cells, as they mutate, can start to look more and more foreign to our immune system which will then attack the cancer cells.

There are basically two forms of immune system dysfunction: immuno-suppression, and inflammation and autoimmunity.

IMMUNO-SUPPRESSION

Immuno-suppression is when the immune system doesn't do what it is meant to do, that is, defend the body against pathogens. Immuno-suppression can be caused by psychosocial factors (e.g. stress, depression and social isolation), drugs (e.g. steroids and chemotherapy), unhealthy lifestyle (e.g. poor nutrition, inactivity, over-activity, poor sleep), cancer (e.g. those that infiltrate the immune system and bone marrow like leukaemia, lymphoma and multiple myeloma) and infections (e.g. HIV-AIDS).

Immuno-suppression occurs when the number of WBCs becomes too low or when they function poorly. Either way, it leaves the body far more open to infection. Our immune function tends to decline with age and babies have immature immune function, so both the elderly and very young are more prone to life-threatening infections.

INFLAMMATION AND AUTOIMMUNITY

The second form of immune system dysfunction is when it does things it is not meant to do: over-reacting, which is called inflammation, and attacking the self as if it were foreign, which is called autoimmunity. Inflammation does have a role to play in healthy immunity, as it is needed to defend and repair tissues when they have been injured such as with physical trauma, chemical exposure, infection or radiation. When inflammation is activated inappropriately or becomes excessive it becomes a disease in itself. Our genetic makeup can predispose us to inflammatory diseases and they can be aggravated by psychological and social stress and poor lifestyle.

Autoimmune conditions include diseases as diverse as Type-1 diabetes, rheumatoid arthritis, inflammatory bowel disease and MS. They can be triggered by an infection, psychological or social stress, vaccinations[1] and other factors, some of which remain a mystery, in a person who is genetically predisposed. For reasons not entirely understood, there has been a steep rise in the incidence of autoimmune conditions in recent decades.

The immune response is so complex that we really don't understand that much about it, what activates it, over-activates it, switches it off. That we don't understand the full complexity of what the immune system does, and how it does it, does not prevent us from understanding simple principles about what helps it to work better. These principles follow below.

Stress management

Stress, depression, social isolation and other things which negatively affect our psychological wellbeing result in:

- **Lowered immune defences:** The number and/or function of our WBCs are reduced. Immunoglobulins are also lowered.
- **Increased susceptibility to infections:** We are therefore more likely to get an infection when exposed to a virus or germ.
- **Increased severity and progression of infections:** If we get an infection it is more likely to be severe and prolonged.

- **Increased relapse of chronic and latent infections:** Chronic infections as diverse as glandular fever, herpes, cold sores and HIV are far more likely to relapse.
- **Increased activity of inflammatory illnesses:** Stress is pro-inflammatory and this aggravates inflammatory conditions as diverse as asthma, dermatitis, psoriasis and arthritis.
- **Increased activity of autoimmune conditions:** Autoimmune conditions are more likely to be triggered and to progress.
- **Poor response to immunisation:** Our immune system's response to immunisations is slower and less vigorous.
- **Increased activity of allergic conditions:** Allergic conditions can be conditioned and aggravated by psychological factors.
- **Lowered defences against some cancers:** Immune cells are an important defence against some cancers. Increased inflammation also has a detrimental effect in cancer.

For an extensive discussion about psychoneuroimmunology – PNI, the effect of mind on immunity – see Chapter 2, 'Stress management'.

Spirituality

The positive effects of spirituality on our mental and emotional state suggest that it should also have a beneficial effect on immunity. What little work that has been done to examine the relationship between spirituality and immune system health has suggested such a link.[2] For example, studies found that women with breast cancer who rated spiritual expression as more important than other women had higher numbers of WBCs, including more helper and NK cells;[3] and that spirituality impacted upon the immune function of carers of HIV patients.[4] None of this is surprising because anything which helps us to foster positive emotions, transcend negative emotions, experience compassion, or express our emotions in a better way, would be expected to positively impact upon immune function.

Exercise

Regular physical exercise helps to stimulate immunity at either end of the age spectrum. It protects children from infectious diseases[5] and in the elderly helps to reverse the age-related decline in immunity.[67] Further, exercise also has an anti-inflammatory effect[8] which may partly explain why exercise slows the progress of age-related and chronic illnesses which involve inflammation. Put the other way, inactivity is associated with poor immune function and an increased susceptibility to infections. Exercise stimulates WBCs to be more responsive (that is, it increases healthy lymphocyte activity and the number of circulating T-helper cells). The immune-enhancing effect of exercise is important for the management of various conditions involving the immune system such as HIV/AIDS and cancer. For example, patients with HIV/AIDS who do aerobic or resistance training for around 20 minutes, four times per week, have better mood and coping ability, and a slowing of the progression of the illness.[9]

Extreme exercise, on the other hand, places a strain (allostatic load) on the body and can potentially suppress immune function. The immuno-suppression is greatest 'when exercise is continuous, prolonged, of moderate to high intensity and performed without food intake'[10] and the disruption can be greater still in extreme weather conditions. This may explain why elite athletes often have relatively poor immune function, take longer to get over infections and are prone to chronic fatigue syndrome.

Nutrition

INFECTIONS

Nutrition can have a very positive effect in boosting our immunity and therefore limiting our susceptibility to infections. Various antioxidants and trace elements have important roles to play and we need to have the right balance of these compounds in our diet.

Nutrient deficiency is generally regarded as a major contributor to immune system deficiency. We tend to think of nutrient deficiencies as a third-world problem – however the typical teenage diet can be very deficient and a lot of food consumed in the Western world is of little or no nutritional value. The elderly may also struggle to extract enough nutrients from food because their digestive systems do not function as well and they may have difficulty buying and preparing healthy, fresh foods. This is a particular problem for elderly people living alone.

General tips for boosting and balancing immunity and therefore preventing infections include:

- Adequate protein is essential for optimal immune function. Intake of amino acids in protein-rich foods, such as arginine and glutamine, are particularly important.[11][12]
- Too much refined sugar may lower immune function and reduce the ability of your body to destroy bacteria.[13]
- Healthy body weight is associated with good immune function. Conversely, obesity is associated with decreased immunity, and sickness and death from infections.
- Garlic contains glutathione and allicin which can assist in boosting immunity.[14]
- Pomegranates score highly on the antioxidant scale and have powerful anti-inflammatory substances (punicalagin and ellagic acid) which help to protect against cell damage.
- A healthy vitamin intake is important for effective immune response in terms of antioxidant value [15] and because they enable our body to make important chemical messengers and they support cellular function.[16] See pages 114–117 for foods rich in important vitamins.
  - The B vitamins are essential for the production of antibodies. Vitamin B6 and folic acid have important influences on immune responses, especially T-cells.
  - Vitamin D is vital for healthy immunity.[17] Dairy, eggs, oily fish and shitake mushrooms are all good sources of vitamin D.
  - Vitamins A, C and E are also important for healthy immunity.
- Of the micronutrients zinc, selenium, iron and copper are important for immunity.[18][19]
  - Foods rich in zinc include lean meats (beef, other red meats and shellfish), nuts, beans, whole grains and fortified breakfast cereals are good sources.
  - Foods rich in selenium are Brazil nuts, tuna, beef, turkey and chicken breast.
  - Adequate iron intake helps prevent infections and studies show that populations that are iron deficient get fewer infections when their diet is supplemented with iron.[20]
  - Copper is found in barley, beef, crabmeat, lobster, oysters, almonds and cashews.
- Probiotics help restore and maintain good gut bacteria which not only help to prevent gastrointestinal infections but also

benefit health in other ways. Eating good-quality natural yoghurt containing live bacteria has been found to boost immunity.[21][22] This may be particularly helpful for people who have just taken a course of antibiotics which are known for depleting good gut bacteria.

- Seaweeds such as spirulina and chlorella are packed with vitamins and minerals and considered beneficial to immunity.

AUTOIMMUNE CONDITIONS

The principles of nutrition for autoimmune conditions have been covered to some extent in the chapters on the autoimmune diseases multiple sclerosis (Chapter 13) and rheumatoid arthritis (Chapter 16). The same principles apply to most autoimmune conditions but there are some specific dietary guidelines related to other particular autoimmune conditions.

Coeliac disease

In coeliac disease, an autoimmune condition triggered by gluten sensitivity, the immune system attacks the lining of the gut. Gluten is found in grains such as wheat, oats, rye, barley and spelt. There is some evidence that the onset of coeliac disease may be delayed or moderated if babies are breastfed for longer, particularly at the time grains are introduced into their diet.[23] In coeliac disease gluten needs to be removed from the diet. Longer breastfeeding time may also be associated with a reduced risk of Type-1 diabetes.[24]

Inflammatory bowel disease

Like other autoimmune conditions, inflammatory bowel disease (the most common types being ulcerative colitis and Crohn's disease) has been on the increase. Nutrition has a major role to play in the management of IBD and possibly the prevention of it. As the bowel's ability to absorb nutrition is poor due to inflammation in this disease, the diet should aim to help prevent and treat malnutrition, promote growth and development in children, optimise bone health and prevent osteoporosis. There are a number of dietary factors worth considering in inflammatory bowel disease (IBD).

- Pre- and probiotics help maintain healthy bowel flora and may be valuable in the management of IBD[25] and possibly other autoimmune conditions.[26] Friendly gut bacteria, such as lactobacillus,[27] as found in good-quality natural unsweetened yoghurt, appear to be helpful in the treatment and prevention of IBD.

- Omega-3 fatty acids (in oily fish, avocadoes walnuts and flaxseed) and polyphenols (found in green tea) may reduce the symptoms of gut inflammation.[28] The ratio of omega-6 to omega-3 is very important. Omega-3 from fish oil[29] appears to protect the bowel lining against damage from inflammation.

- A low-fibre, high-sugar, high-animal fat Westernised diet has been proposed as a risk factor for developing IBD.[30] The increasing incidence of Crohn's disease in Japan, for example, is probably related to an increasingly Westernised diet.[31] The foods implicated include refined sugar,[32] fast food,[33] margarine[34] and dairy products.[35]

- Germinated barley foodstuff (GBF),[36] a by-product from breweries has been shown to improve ulcerative colitis. GBF is high in glutamine-rich protein and dietary fibre. Its benefits for ulcerative colitis may be due to the glutamine and other antioxidants such as B vitamins. It can be found in some health food stores.

- Oat bran has been shown to help reduce abdominal pain.[37] You can increase your intake of oat bran by including it in your breakfast cereal.

- Vitamin D[38] is frequently low in patients with IBD.

- Various minerals are important for IBD. Low bone density occurs in approximately half of all IBD patients; maintaining a good calcium intake and possibly using calcium supplements may be helpful. Anaemia, iron deficiency and folate deficiency are also common among patients with IBD.[39] Magnesium can be lost due to reduced absorption and diarrhoea and may need to be supplemented.

- Vitamin B12 can be low in an IBD patient either because of poor absorption due to gut inflammation or because they have had an operation to remove part of the bowel which absorbs B12 vitamin. B12 is easily given as supplements or injections.

- Antioxidants are important to help reduce inflammation in IBD.[40]

ALLERGIES

We have also experienced a large increase in the incidence of allergies in Westernised countries and part of the reason may be diet and lifestyle.[41] The following nutritional information may help:

- Breastfeeding babies helps to reduce the incidence of allergies in the early years of life.[42] Adverse reactions to foods, mainly cow's milk protein and eggs, are most common in the first two to three years of life.[43] Goat's milk is often a better tolerated alternative to cow's milk. Children often outgrow their food allergy.
- There is some evidence that a diet low in fresh fish, omega-3 fatty acids or antioxidants, or high in sodium (salt), may influence respiratory symptoms and aggravate asthma in some asthmatics. [44] [45] [46]
- The probiotic lactobacillus has been shown to provide protection against allergy-based eczema or dermatitis.[47]
- Some people are allergic to foods such as peanuts, sesame seeds, wheat, eggs, cow's milk or seafood.[48] If we suspect a food allergy it is important to be assessed by a trained health professional. Food reactions may also occur due to dyes (e.g. tartrazine), flavourings and preservatives (e.g. nitrates, nitrites, MSG) and toxins in food. Read labels carefully. For food allergies the best form of management is avoidance of the food or additive.

Connectedness

The quality and extent of our relationships with each other and the wider community has a profound effect on our emotional health and thereby our immunity. Studies have shown that factors like social isolation, bereavement and marital separation put us at risk of developing or worsening a range of illnesses related to immune system disruption such as the common cold, pneumonia, progression to AIDS in people who have HIV, asthma, rheumatoid arthritis and multiple sclerosis. [49] [50] [51] If we want our immune system to thrive then we need to feel happy with the quality and amount of our social interaction.

One aspect of social interaction that can be problematic is living in shared accommodation, particularly if it is overcrowded and has poor ventilation. Many infectious diseases spread easily in such conditions.

Environment

The general principles of healthy environment apply to healthy immunity. They include:

- Ensuring a good social environment;
- Getting adequate sun exposure (to boost vitamin D);
- Avoiding exposure to:
  - Environmental toxins such as air pollution, and the heavy metals lead and mercury which can suppress immunity or increase inflammation;
  - Chemical additives, antibiotics and hormones now commonly used in food production and processing;
  - Powerful electromagnetic fields (EMFs). Avoid living within 200 to 300 metres of high-voltage powerlines as it can affect melatonin and thereby immune function;
  - Known allergens. For those with severe allergies, such as to nuts, total avoidance of those allergens, even in minute quantities, is strongly advised;
- Infectious diseases such as malaria or dengue fever. Protection from mosquitoes will be important.
- Avoiding outdoor activities on days when pollen counts are high as this can help prevent hay fever and asthma episodes;
- Ensuring that you have a pleasant environment to exercise in, as exercise can benefit immunity;
- There is a theory which is gathering momentum that a lack of exposure to normal pathogens in childhood may predispose people to the later development of allergies and asthma.[52]

20

Chronic fatigue
syndrome

Education

Chronic fatigue is a common symptom in the community and affects
between 10 and 25% of people. It can be due to a number of physical
illnesses or poor mental health. Chronic fatigue *syndrome* (CFS), on
the other hand, is less common, probably affecting between 0.2 and
0.7% of the community. CFS can affect people of any socio-economic
group or age, although it is most common in young adults. Women
are affected roughly three times as often as men.

CFS is a diagnosis that is made when other causes of severe and
chronic fatigue have been excluded. There is a recognisable pattern
of symptoms which may be the result of disturbed brain function or
immune dysregulation although the cause is still not clear. Contributing factors may be psychological upset, the aftermath of a viral
infection, an impairment in the body's regulation of the autonomic
nervous system, sleep disturbance, food intolerances, exposure to
toxins and metabolic disturbances. There also looks to be an inherited
component to CFS[1] but as we come to understand it better, CFS will
probably prove to encompass a range of conditions rather than just
one specific 'disease'.

Experts in Australia suggest that it is important to distinguish
between 'disease', 'illness' and 'disability'.[2] A disease is an entity we
can identify, diagnose and understand. The term 'illness' describes the
subjective experience of the patient – their suffering and symptoms –

318

regardless of whether doctors can understand and define it. Disability is the physical, psychological and social impairment related to the disease or illness. Even though CFS is not well defined as a disease the illness and disability of CFS are obvious. The levels of illness and disability associated with CFS are often comparable to multiple sclerosis or severe rheumatoid arthritis.

CFS is diagnosed on the patient's clinical picture which means that the doctor looks for characteristic symptoms. The following table shows the symptoms of CFS according to the current Australian guidelines published in the *Medical Journal of Australia*.[3]

CFS symptoms

1. Fatigue

Clinically evaluated, unexplained, persistent or relapsing fatigue persistent for six months or more, that:

- is of new or definite onset;
- is not the result of ongoing exertion;
- is not substantially alleviated by rest;
- results in substantial reduction in previous levels of occupational, educational, social or personal activities;

and

2. Other symptoms

Four or more of the following symptoms that are concurrent, persistent for six months or more and which did not predate the fatigue:

- Impaired short term memory or concentration
- Sore throat
- Tender cervical or axillary (armpit) lymph nodes
- Muscle pain
- Multi-joint pain without arthritis
- Headaches of a new type, pattern, or severity
- Unrefreshing sleep
- Post-exertional malaise lasting more than 24 hours

It is important for a doctor to exclude other causes of chronic fatigue such as thyroid problems, diabetes, anaemia and depression. CFS can exist alongside other health problems, which makes the diagnosis more difficult; it often coexists with other syndromes such as fibromyalgia and irritable bowel syndrome. CFS commonly causes depression, so it is important to try and determine which came first, the chronic fatigue or the depression.

The fatigue associated with CFS typically comes on with relatively minor exertion and may last for hours or days afterwards. The fatigue is different to symptoms such as weakness, shortness of breath, excess sleepiness or low motivation – all of which are likely to be related to other causes. Physical signs like unexpected weight loss or a rash, which are not typically associated with CFS, may indicate other illnesses. There are generally few physical signs of CFS.

There are no simple tests to confirm a diagnosis of CFS or to monitor its progress but tests like a blood count or thyroid function tests may be useful to exclude other health problems. A self-diagnosis of CFS should not be made. A GP is generally well placed to diagnose and manage CFS but a range of other healthcare practitioners can also make valuable contributions. These can include a psychologist or counsellor, lifestyle adviser or health coach, complementary health practitioners, occupational therapist, physiotherapist and others. It all depends upon a person's needs. Referral to specialists may be helpful if the diagnosis is not clear or there are other complex physical or mental health concerns.

There are no successful drug treatments for CFS although medications to treat concurrent medical problems or symptoms may be useful. The mainstays of treatment, which are mostly backed up by solid evidence, are cognitive behavioural therapy (CBT) and graded exercise programs.[4]

Stress management

Prolonged psychological stress can make it much more likely for someone to come down with CFS.[5] Once triggered, CFS can be a difficult thing to turn off again using stress management alone, but enhancing the coping skills and mental health of a CFS sufferer is vital to improving their outcome. Finding the support of a concerned and empathic healthcare professional is the first step in being able to manage the often considerable stress of having CFS. Other people often disbelieve that someone with CFS has a real illness, which compounds the CFS sufferer's stress.

CBT has been found to help people with CFS cope better, improve their functioning, reduce their symptoms and improve their outcomes.[6,7] It is important in CFS to take a measured and gradual approach to resuming activities, whether physical, intellectual or social. This is called 'pacing'. The person slowly increases their activity according to their response and capacities. CBT helps a person to do this, by overcoming their negative attitudes and beliefs about the illness, treatments and outcomes. Beliefs such as 'It is all futile' or 'I can't do any activity' do not aid wellbeing or recovery and need to be gently challenged. Interestingly, the placebo response in CFS patients is very low which is perhaps linked to the low expectations that many patients have[8] and also indicates that there are major disease processes going on in their bodies.

Stress management is far less effective in the absence of a graded exercise program and other strategies. Mindfulness-based CBT has not been extensively trialled for CFS but is likely to be of use.

Sleep disruption is a common problem in CFS particularly when the patient also has fibromyalgia. The temptation for people with CFS to take long naps in the daytime can disrupt normal sleep patterns at night, compounding the issue. Key tips to help people with CFS get a good night's sleep include:

- Have a regular sleep routine and go to bed when *sleepy* rather than *tired*. There is a difference – you can be tired physically but not sleepy.
- Avoid watching television in bed;
- Try and rise at the same time each day, using an alarm clock if necessary;
- Avoid sleeping tablets or use them sparingly;
- If taking a daytime nap then limit it to no more than 20 minutes;
- Maintain gentle daily exercise.

Meditation and relaxation exercises can be helpful adjuncts to counselling. They improve people's coping ability and help them deal with any mental health problems they might have as well as CFS, but they do not seem to have a major impact upon fatigue. This is not surprising as CFS is a problem where the sympathetic nervous system is commonly under-activated rather than over-activated.

Spirituality

Dealing with a chronic and undefined illness like CFS can be enormously taxing on resilience and resources. Fears about our future prognosis, concerns about having our life aspirations undermined, watching our family and career roles potentially be eroded, and being unable to participate in previously enjoyable pastimes can all make life seem like it has little meaning or direction. For this reason finding new meaning, direction, roles and fulfilment are a part of managing CFS that should not be ignored. A diagnosis of CFS is commonly a stimulus to examine our values and come to a deeper understanding of ourselves.

Exercise

Exercise is one of the mainstays in the management of CFS. Many people with CFS understandably adopt a strategy of prolonged rest but this is unhelpful in the long term. Exercise programs have consistently been shown to increase the activity levels of people suffering CFS.

It is important to take a measured approach to increasing exercise. A person with CFS might have more vitality one day and feel tempted to 'make hay while the sun shines' but this often leads to a big drop in energy for days afterwards. That is why experts recommend graded exercise. Graded exercise, if undertaken sensibly, brings improvements in people's capacity to do physical work as well as improvements in psychological wellbeing and cognitive functioning.

Graded exercise also helps a person with CFS reduce the tendency to avoid activity[9] and social engagement. Waiting only for 'good days' can lead to a negative spiral of lowering activity, mood and falling exercise tolerance.

According to Royal Australian College of General Practitioners (RACGP) Working Party, people with CFS should be encouraged to exercise body and mind regularly. We begin at a level of exertion that we can tolerate without significantly worsening our symptoms. Short sessions are preferable to longer ones at first. The duration and intensity of physical and mental activity can be gently increased as tolerance improves.

CFS sufferers should be involved in negotiating their own individual management and exercise plan with their doctors and this program should also be reviewed on a regular basis.

Nutrition

To date there are no proven nutritional approaches for CFS although there are a number of promising initial findings. This reflects a lack of research funding in the field, or the possibility that CFS comprises a range of conditions that might respond to different nutritional approaches. While the evidence builds there are nevertheless a few things to note about the role of nutrition for CFS patients:

- Maintaining a balanced and healthy diet is important. Help the immune system with a wholesome diet high in unprocessed, unrefined foods, especially fruit and vegetables;
- Oxidative stress is observed in many patients with CFS so a diet rich in antioxidants may be of benefit;[10]
- Food sensitivities are problematic for many CFS sufferers so an elimination diet may be useful to rule out food sensitivities. Consult with your doctor or other trained health professional before going on an elimination diet;
- A nutrient-dense diet is helpful and including 'super foods' such as blueberries, quinoa, seaweeds, garlic and shiitake mushrooms may help. Carefully selected supplementation may be required to ensure adequate levels of vitamins and minerals.[11] Folinic acid, which the body converts into folic acid, shows some promise in the treatment of CFS.[12] Sources include those for folic acid;
- Avoid pro-inflammatory foods like excessive sugar, coffee, excessive red meat and processed foods;
- Eating oily fish regularly[13] may help because of the antioxidant omega-3 fatty acids they contain;
- D-ribose, a carbohydrate found in many foods including brewer's yeast, has been shown to substantially reduce symptoms in people with CFS.[14]

Connectedness

CFS sufferers should be encouraged to adopt a broad approach to managing the illness. It used to be advocated to take prolonged rest which led to social withdrawal but it is now clear that this is not a good strategy for CFS. Although continuing full-time work may be difficult, there may be other practical options such as part-time or flexible working hours. Those of school or university age need to consult with their healthcare professionals and family so they can make decisions about how much workload they can safely take on and how to retain contact with friends and family. CFS has a big impact on a person's family and so involving family in consultations and management of the illness is crucial. This is not just a consideration for the person with CFS; the family may also need considerable support.

Many people can make a contribution to the management of CFS. The assistance of supportive healthcare practitioners makes a major difference. Joining one of the CFS support groups can be of enormous benefit as it is easy to feel alone.

Environment

Environmental factors such as lack of sunlight, or lead exposure, can cause or exacerbate chronic fatigue, but have not been linked to CFS itself. Exposure to a range of viruses may be a trigger for many CFS cases. Some environmental toxins may trigger CFS or make symptoms worse in some people with CFS. These toxins include:

- Chlorinated hydrocarbons; and other insecticides and pesticides;
- Industrial solvents;
- Silicone breast implants;
- Ciguatera poisoning through eating fish infected by certain algae.

Environmental factors are key in helping to optimise energy levels for people with CFS. An environment conducive to exercise will help CFS sufferers to maintain a graded exercise program. A stimulating social and academic environment will help to maintain social and cognitive functioning.

21

Genetics

The human mind is not capable of grasping the Universe. We are like a little child entering a huge library . . . The child knows that someone must have written those books. It does not know who or how.
  Albert Einstein, quoted in *The Next Thousand Years*, by A. Berry

The genetic code is like a vast and mysterious book. Crick and Watson described the alphabet making up our DNA in the 1950s and since then the human genome has been mapped or 'spelled out'. We have cracked the genetic code but this does not mean that we understand the intricacies of the book we have opened. Nor does it mean that we are necessarily qualified to be editors of it. The rush into the genetic age has certainly hailed in a brave new world; one of much potential but one that is also potentially dangerous.

Education

Our DNA determines many of our physical and psychological characteristics; it is the blueprint for our body and every chemical or function within it. DNA is made up of four different components – like a four-letter 'alphabet' – that link together in a particular sequence. It forms a 'double helix' strand, like two intertwined strings. There are 46 (23 pairs) pairs of these strands – known as chromosomes – in our body's cells. Each chromosome is divided up into segments called genes. According to a gene's specific four-letter DNA sequence, it gives the body's cells instructions to make proteins that influence everything

325

from what colour eyes we have to our chances of developing certain diseases. Each of us has 99.9% of our genetic makeup in common with other humans, meaning that the other 0.1% determines all the differences between individual humans and races.

We inherit one half of a chromosome pair from our father and one half from our mother, and therefore inherit our characteristics from both of them. There are some characteristics – including illnesses – that we develop if just one of the chromosomes in a pair has the gene that codes for it. This type of inheritance is called 'autosomal dominant'; Huntington's disease is an example of an illness inherited this way. There are some characteristics and illnesses where the gene must appear on both chromosomes in a pair in order for us to have the characteristic or disease. This type of inheritance is called 'autosomal recessive'. If only one of our chromosomes has the gene then we won't have the condition ourselves but we will be a carrier, potentially handing it on to our offspring. Cystic fibrosis is an example of an illness inherited this way.

There are other characteristics and illnesses that are not inherited in such a mathematically simple way and whether or not we have them will be the result of the interaction of many genes. Such inheritance shows up in our family history as an increased risk of coming down with an illness such as cancer or heart disease.

Our 'genotype' is the name for what is in our genes – our DNA code. Our 'pheonotype' is the name for what our genes are expressing, for instance how tall we are or the colour of our hair. Just because we have a gene in our genotype does not mean that it will express itself, just as having a program loaded onto a computer's hard-drive does not mean that the program is necessarily active. At any given time, not all genes are expressing themselves; many are lying dormant. The activation and deactivation of certain genes can trigger the onset, progression and halting of many diseases. The study of this process is called epigenetics. Genetic dispositions to illnesses can be triggered and cause illness by a range of psychological and lifestyle factors. As with every other aspect of human health, in genetics there is no one factor that affects our wellbeing independently from the rest.

For a long time the view was that genes didn't change much unless they were damaged by chemicals or radiation. But, it seems, genes are far more malleable than we previously imagined. When our cells multiply each new cell is meant to be a genetic replica of the cell it came from but sometimes 'spelling errors' are made in our DNA when our cells divide. These are called genetic mutations. Most genetic mutations are insignificant and do not change cell function; in other words, they do not change the meaning of the text. Some mutations do change genes in a significant way, and thereby change cell function, sometimes with beneficial effects but sometimes with disastrous effects. These 'spelling errors' certainly do change the meaning of the text. Our body does have a 'spell-check' function: cells have the ability to repair genetic damage. This is called DNA repair capacity (DRC). Some of the factors affecting DNA damage and repair will be discussed in more detail, following.

DNA damage is particularly important in the genesis of cancer[1] as well as other diseases. For example, some inherited genetic mutations only slightly increase the risk of breast cancer compared to the rest of the community but some mutations can very substantially increase the risk. It has already been mentioned, in discussing breast cancer genes and X-rays, that it may take relatively little radiation damage to cause cancer in people who have inherited one of the high-risk genes.

Although we may have a genetic or family inherited predisposition to cancer, the cancer can be switched off by the action of cancer suppressor genes. Damage to these suppressor genes can also lead to cancer.

The discovery of the genetic code has led to a rather mechanistic view of the human being. As Francis Collins, the head of the Human Genome Project, said, 'We will not understand important things like "love" by knowing the DNA sequence of homo sapiens . . . If humanity begins to view itself as a machine, programmed by this DNA sequence, we've lost something really important.'[2]

Stress management

Our mental state is a major but possibly under-recognised factor in determining the development, expression and repair of our genes. To what extent thought, emotion, motivation and the search for meaning can affect genes is not completely known, but it is clear that genes affect mind and mind affects genes.

Psychological stress increases DNA damage.[3] Initial research came from animal studies[4][5] but more recently studies on humans have shown increases in DNA damage in humans under stress. A study on healthy medical students showed that during the exam period, there was an increase in DNA repair capacity (DRC) in nearly all of them.[6] Stress was damaging their DNA and thereby stimulating the body's DNA repair mechanisms. However, there were some students who actually had no increase in DRC or a *fall* in DRC. These were the students with the highest and most consistent levels of emotional stress and mood disturbance at exam time. This suggests that high levels of emotional stress, apart from increasing DNA damage, can also impair our DNA repair mechanisms. This has big implications for some kinds of cancers. For example, a study showed that women with breast cancer have a lower DRC than women who don't.[7]

Stress increases the incidence of genetic mutations, probably impairs the body's ability to repair them[8] and increases oxidation. Coping with emotional trauma also increases damage of DNA.[9] To some extent stress-related DNA damage may be reduced through techniques like yoga,[10] but there is relatively little research in this field at the moment.

Our psychological state also affects genetic expression – that is, our state of mind and our emotions influence our chances that our genetic predispositions to certain illnesses (our genotype) will be expressed and that we will get sick (our phenotype). This link has been shown with conditions as varied as addictions,[11] cardiovascular disease,[12] depression,[13] schizophrenia[14] and asthma.[15] This begins to explain why stress is such a common trigger for so many diseases. This variation in gene expression comes about partly because our genes are programmed by the 'epigenome' which are chemicals and proteins laid down over the genes and which alter their expression. Epigenetic patterns are sculpted during our development, right from the time we were a foetus and are affected by what our mother eats, our exposure to environmental toxins and psychological stress.[16]

To illustrate how our psychological state can activate the expression of genes, chronic pain is well known to be associated with depression. A study has suggested that how much we react emotionally and physiologically to chronic pain sensitises the brain to pain messages, and it also increases the likelihood that if we have genes that predispose us to depression, those genes will be activated and we will go on to develop depression. Further, chronic pain associated with depression impairs the ability of the brain to activate the genes make new brain cells (neurogenesis).[17]

Not only is DNA function, damage and repair affected by our

psychological state, but our mind also affects genetic ageing. At the end of each chromosome is a segment of DNA called a telomere; it stops the DNA from unravelling, which causes cells to die. A way to gauge the rate at which our DNA is ageing is to measure the length of our telomeres – shorter telomeres indicate ageing – and our telomerase activity. Telomerase is the enzyme that repairs telomeres; a low level suggests rapid ageing.

A study on healthy pre-menopausal women under psychological stress (because they were caring for someone with a major disability) found that the women who were coping less well had higher oxidative stress, lower telomerase activity and shorter telomere length – that is, their genes were ageing rapidly. The genes of the women who felt the most stressed showed the equivalent of between 9 and 17 years of additional ageing than those who felt the least stressed.[18] A similar finding has been demonstrated for people with depression.[19]

These landmark studies help us to understand how our mental state may promote or slow the onset of age-related diseases. For example, poor mental health is a major risk factor for CVD, and this may be partly because of rapid genetic ageing. Low telomerase activity is associated with high allostatic load (physiological wear and tear), and other risk factors for heart disease and stroke such as smoking, high blood fats, high blood pressure, high blood glucose and metabolic syndrome.[20]

What does it all mean? The science is complex. The message is simple: looking after your mind is an investment in looking after your genes. This may be a previously unrecognised reason why a healthy mind leads to a healthy body.

Spirituality

The relationship between spirituality, genetics and health can be looked at from a number of points of view.

- Spiritual beliefs and philosophies can impact upon how one looks at genetic engineering, gene therapy, cloning and stem-cell research. People with a religious view are more likely than others to look upon such new technologies in a negative light.
- It can affect attitudes and practices in relation to contraception or abortion. The latter is often offered as a solution to genetic abnormalities in a foetus.

- The benefits of spirituality, a sense of meaning and religiosity on mental and physical health may partly be due to their effect on immunity and genetics. The only study of its type looked at Falun Gong practitioners and found they had enhanced immunity and genetic function.[21] (Of course, the physical exercise practices and meditation of Falun Gong may be responsible for these benefits, aside from any influence of spirituality.)
- Spirituality and religion have been shown to have a beneficial effect upon lifestyle, including lowering rates of substance abuse in those genetically at risk of addiction.[22] This may be due in part to the reduced risk of expressing a genetic disposition to smoking and other addictive behaviours in those with a high level of religiosity.[23]

Exercise

There is no part of our bodily makeup which is not affected by physical activity, and that includes our genes.[24] Exercise helps our healthy genes to express themselves and reduces the activity of unhealthy genes, due to an infinitely complex interaction of chemicals. It is not necessary to understand how it works in order to enjoy the benefits, just like one doesn't need to know how a car works in order to enjoy the benefits of driving.

Regular moderate exercise helps to reduce oxidative damage and is associated with improved DNA repair which may help explain why exercise is associated with slower ageing and cell death.[25] Part of the reason exercise protects our genes may be because, just like a calorie-restricted diet, it changes the balance of calories coming into the body and calories being used up. The anti-inflammatory effect of exercise may also be a factor.

Extreme physical training, on the other hand, is associated with more oxidative damage[26] – although it does stimulate DNA repair as a part of the body's attempt to compensate.[27] These effects can be seen for a week after extreme exertion such as a marathon.[28]

Exercise also has beneficial effects on mental health and as we know from the preceding section, there is a link between our psychological state and the health of our genes. All in all, healthy genes are just another reason to exercise regularly.

Nutrition

Nutrition, as we would expect, has an pivotal role in the function, repair, expression and ageing of DNA.[29][30][31] In relation to the genetics of cancer and other illnesses, nutritional supplements seem to be far less protective than a nutrient-rich diet. There is strong evidence that several vitamins and minerals are required for DNA synthesis (which happens constantly, as our cells die and are replaced), prevention of oxidative damage to DNA and the maintenance of DNA. To help protect and care for your DNA:

- Calorie restriction is associated with less DNA damage and better DNA repair which is part of the reason calorie restriction helps protect against cancer.[32] A 40% reduction may decrease the incidence to near zero.[33][34] On the other hand, malnutrition in children, which is different to calorie restriction, is associated with higher DNA damage.[35]
- The amino acid arginine is required for DNA production. Arginine is found in cashew nuts, brown rice, watermelon seeds, garlic, green and root vegetables, and walnuts.
- Low levels of folate are associated with poor DRC and increasing the intake of folate is associated with better DNA repair.[36]
- The minerals selenium, manganese and zinc are proven to be necessary for the activity of DNA repair enzymes.[37]
- Calcium and magnesium may have stabilisation effects on DNA.
- Coenzyme Q-10 supplement was found to improve DNA repair significantly.[38]
- Carotenoids in foods such as carrots and pumpkins, rather than carotenoid supplements, have been shown to decrease DNA damage.[39]
- Cruciferous vegetables such as broccoli, brussels sprouts and cabbage decrease DNA damage in humans.
- The Mediterranean diet, rich in olive oil and vegetables, is associated with a reduced incidence of cancer partly because it protects our DNA from damage and helps it to repair itself.[40]
- Reductions in DNA damage have been reported for green tea drinkers.
- Red wine contains resveratrol (found in the skins of red grapes) which has been shown to reduce DNA damage.
- Soy milk reduces DNA damage.

- Various omega-3 fatty acids affect DNA replication pathways.[41] DHA can be obtained from wild salmon, scallops, shrimp, halibut, tuna, navy beans, soy beans, tofu, flaxseed oil, walnuts, cabbage, kale and broccoli.

Connectedness

Genetic predispositions often lie dormant and can be triggered by events and social circumstances. This activation of genes is rather like clicking onto an icon on a computer to start up a program. For instance, we can have a genetic tendency towards addictive behaviour. The kinds of things that can 'click' this addictive tendency on and send us seeking drugs are the experience of injecting, being exposed to a drug culture and emotional stress.[42] We can have a genetic predisposition towards psychosis, and this may be activated by drug use and social adversity in adolescence and early adulthood.[43]

We can inherit a predisposition to a mental health problem like depression but it is the interaction between heredity and our upbringing which is crucial for our risk of actually developing depression later in life. Childhood trauma and genetic factors are known to contribute to the development and effects of depression. In fact, 80% of adults with depression experienced at least one type of childhood trauma. The common childhood traumas include physical neglect, emotional abuse and emotional neglect. The greater the childhood trauma, the earlier the onset of depression.[44]

To what extent these genetic dispositions and damage can be switched off we do not know but it may be one of the ways in which social support is so helpful therapeutically.

Environment

Environment has an enormous influence on genetic function and expression through a variety of different pathways.

SOCIAL ENVIRONMENT

Children raised in deprived environments can have severe cognitive and behavioural difficulties and poor response to stress, lasting into adulthood. 'These changes reflect permanently altered gene expression, so-called "environmental programming"', according to the journal *Trends in Neurosciences*.[45]

It is not entirely known how malleable genetic expression is but some long-held beliefs are being challenged. The psychological and social environment may even influence the speed and timing of strongly inherited illnesses. Huntington's disease being an autosomal dominant disorder (we need the gene on only one chromosome in a pair to inherit it), it is assumed that if a person has the gene then they will come down with this condition. It is a severely debilitating, progressive disorder which affects the brain's ability to control movement and leads to early death. There is no known cure. Animal studies, however, show that a socially, intellectually and physically enriching environment delays the onset of Huntington's disease. One in seven mice genetically predisposed to Huntington's who were placed in an enriched environment came down with symptoms. All seven mice who were not placed in an enriched environment developed symptoms.[46] The therapeutic potential of these findings has not been explored in humans but the findings do suggest the possibility of a new approach using mind–body-based gene therapies.

CHEMICAL ENVIRONMENT

Exposure to many toxic chemical and trace metals can lead to genetic damage. This has implications for cancer among other illnesses. The number of cancer-causing substances is enormous with over 400 found in cigarette smoke alone, therefore it is not surprising that passive smoking contributes to DNA damage. Heavy air pollution is also problematic. So ubiquitous are chemicals in our homes and workplaces that it is all but impossible to avoid them. There are some chemicals we are exposed to whose risks we are not certain of yet. If you have concerns about chemical and heavy metal exposure it is advisable to be assessed by a doctor trained in environmental medicine or a toxicologist. A range of tests can be performed to identify problems.

RADIATION EXPOSURE

A little radiation is normal and even healthy; a lot can be life-threatening. The main way that radiation kills cells is through DNA damage. Common household exposures are probably nothing to be concerned about. What is of more concern is living within close proximity to high-voltage powerlines; multiple X-rays, particularly in cancer-prone people; and exposure to radioactive elements from nuclear reactors. These are of concern not just for the generation exposed but many generations afterwards.

Appendix 1

Lifestyle assessment

The questionnaire on the following page will help you monitor your progress with regard to lifestyle change by comparing your responses before and after the program. First, photocopy the chart, then based on the *last month* give yourself a rating in each of the following areas. Add your scores for your total out of 40 and keep the completed questionnaire so that you can compare your results after finishing the program.

		2 points	1 points	0 points	Your score
Family and Friends	My communication with others is open, honest and clear	almost always	some of the time	hardly ever	
	I get the emotional support that I need	almost always	some of the time	hardly ever	
Activity	I do 30 minutes exercise, e.g. running, cycling, fast walking	4 or more times a week	2–3 times a week	hardly ever or never	
	I relax and enjoy leisure time	almost daily	some of the time	hardly ever	
	Maintenance of my exercise program	has been consistent for more than 2 years	has not been consistent	never exercised regularly	
Nutrition	I eat 5 or more serves of fruit and vegetables daily	almost always	some of the time	hardly ever	
	My diet includes excess sugar, salt, animal fats or junk foods	rarely	some of the time	frequently	
	My BMI (body mass index – see page 94)	20–25	25–30 / 18–19	over 30 / less than 18	
Tobacco and toxins	In the past year I have used tobacco	never	socially	on a daily basis	
	I abuse drugs (prescribed or un-prescribed)	hardly ever or never	some of the time	frequently	
	I drink the following amount of coffee, tea or cola daily	less than 3 cups per day	3–6 cups per day	6 or more cups per day	
Alcohol	I drink the following amount of alcohol daily	Males: 2 or less drinks / Females: 1 or less	Males: 3–4 drinks / Females: 2 drinks	Males: more than 4 drinks / Females: more than 2 drinks	
Sleep	I get 7–9 hours' sound sleep per night	almost always	some of the time	hardly ever	
Stress	I tend to cope well with stress	almost always	most of the time	some of the time	
	I have had the following number of major stressful events in past year	none	1–2	3 or more	
Personality	I am a positive thinker	almost always	some of the time	hardly ever	
	I get anxious and worried	hardly ever	some of the time	almost always	
	I have depression	hardly ever	some of the time	almost always	
	I have a sense of time pressure, urgency, impatience, anger or hostility	hardly ever	some of the time	almost always	
Career	I am satisfied in my job or role	almost always	some of the time	hardly ever	
				TOTAL/40	

Adapted from the 'Fantastic Lifestyle Assessment'[1]

Appendix 2

Eight-week course outline

The following course structure is given as a guide. It could be used by a healthcare practitioner running the Essence program in his or her practice; it could be used to train healthcare practitioners or as a foundation for a school curriculum. The program can be tailored to the audience, and time and resources available. To fully implement the program, two hours per week should be useful.

WEEK 1

Introduction
In the first week introduce yourself and the program with its aims, principles (see Chapter 9) and structure. Invite the participants to introduce themselves to the rest of the group and say why they are there. This puts you and the group in the picture. Also establish some group rules for the course such as:

1. A person is listened to by the whole group when they are speaking. This is part of participants having respect for each other.
2. Participants need to confirm that they will keep the confidentiality of other group members. Although participants might discuss principles and general issues covered in the course with family or friends, what individuals say about their own situation and lives should stay within the group.
3. Self-criticism is not one of the course aims or practices. Emphasise the unhelpful causes and effects of self-criticism.

4. The course is educative and the leader is there to encourage, facilitate discussion and draw out insights – not to sit out the front and deliver a series of weekly lectures on the given topic. Experience, reflection and questions are the catalysts for change.

If wishing to compare lifestyle pre- and post-course it would be useful to ask the participants to complete the lifestyle assessment.

Behavioural strategies

Explore and discuss the behaviour change strategies outlined in Chapter 8, 'Changing behaviour'. These include understanding motivation, SMART goals and the cycle of change. Help people to provide examples relating them to their experience and also to acknowledge how difficult it can be to implement change. Understanding the strategies will deepen with application over the weeks but it is important to become acquainted with them. Good homework to set in the first week is:

1. Set a SMART goal related to one of the elements of the Essence program and be prepared to report back in week 2 on the experience of trying to apply it.
2. Complete the table on page 168 outlining the costs and benefits of change for that SMART goal.

Education

Introduce the first element of the Essence model, Education. The whole program is an educational intervention in itself. Emphasise that education includes more than just information; it is a 'drawing out'. It includes raising awareness, understanding ourselves and learning skills. If they haven't already, encourage the participants over the following week to read:

1. Chapter 1, 'Education';
2. Pre-read Chapter 2, 'Stress management' for next week's class.

Mindfulness

Take some time to introduce the basic principles of mindfulness and then take everyone through the mindfulness exercise for approximately five minutes. Be sure to practise it yourself while you are taking others through it. Suggest that participants practice at home for five minutes twice a day as a 'starting dose', preferably before breakfast and dinner. Also invite the participants to reflect on mindfulness, or the absence of it, in day-to-day life. What is the effect of being more mindful (e.g. on stress, work, communication, study, performance, sport, eating) and what is the effect of being unmindful?

Introduce the **perception task** (see page 63) and see if some participants can give brief examples of the relationship between perception and stress in their day-to-day life. Don't spend too long and avoid too much theory or the attempt to explain it too much or to convince anyone of anything. This introduction of the mindfulness-based cognitive task each week is to open up the inquiry, not to close it down. Set 'perception' as a homework task for the week (see Chapter 2) and invite them to relate their discoveries to the group in week 2. Even if they report that they were in a day-dream all week, or that they realised how stressed they get, that is a useful discovery.

The mindfulness practices are an important foundation to help participants be more self-aware and objective. Direct them to the section on mindfulness beginning on page 53.

Journal
Encourage the participants to begin a journal and to use it to help facilitate questions and insights for discussion the following week.

WEEK 2

Debrief of behaviour change
See how the participants got on with the homework from the previous week.

1. **Motivation:** What insights did they have into their motivation arising from the cost-benefit exercise?
2. **The SMART goal:** How did they go? Was the goal achieved? What were the challenges? If the goal was not achieved then what got in the way?
3. **The cycle of change:** Are there any insights into the cycle? What stage are they at with regard to important Essence elements they would like to work on? What stands in the way of moving on to the next stage?
4. **The readings:** Were there any questions or discussion points?

Stress management

Practise the mindfulness exercise for at least five minutes with the group, guiding them through it.

Facilitate a discussion on the principles of the mind-body relationship and the effects of stress on health. There may be some questions arising or clarifications required. Try to avoid losing important principles among the complexity.

Debrief the mindfulness homework from the previous week.

1. **Mindfulness exercise:** Was it practised and if so what was noticed? What did it show up? What was the effect at the time of practice and after re-engaging with daily activities? Anything, so long as it is drawn from experience, will be useful, even if the mindfulness has revealed how distractible the mind is, or how reactive we get to daily events. If it wasn't practised, why not and what got in the way? Are there any questions or difficulties?
2. **Mindfulness in day-to-day life:** What was found from reflecting on mindfulness, or the absence of it, in day-to-day life? What was the effect of being more mindful (e.g. on stress, work, communication, study, performance, sport, eating) and what was the effect of being unmindful? How much of the time do we tend to be mindful?
3. **Perception and stress:** Debrief the task set last week. What did the participants discover about this in their day-to-day life?

Mindfulness

Introduce the mindfulness homework for the following week:

1. **Mindfulness practice:** Continue with the 'starting dose' of five minutes' practice twice a day.
2. **Introduce the 'comma' or short mindfulness practice:** Encourage participants to practise this during the week as often as they remember. Natural times are in the space between activities. (For more on the 'comma' see page 59.)
3. **Introduce the letting go/acceptance task:** See page 65. Ask if some participants can give brief examples of the relationship between letting go/acceptance and stress in their day-to-day life. Don't spend too long and avoid too much theory or the attempt to explain it too much or to convince anyone of anything. Set this task as homework for the week and invite them to relate their discoveries to the group in week 3.

4. **A SMART goal for stress management:** Is there a goal they would like to set themselves for the coming week with regard to stress management?

Reading

Encourage the participants to pre-read Chapter 3, 'Spirituality' and be prepared to discuss any questions or reflections the following week.

In closing

See if there are any final questions before finishing. Finish with a comma.

WEEK 3

Start with a comma if possible.

Debrief

See how the participants got on with the homework from the previous week.

1. **The SMART goal:** Are there any insights and reflections on the SMART goal for stress management? Was the goal achieved? What were the challenges? If the goal was not achieved then what got in the way?
2. **Motivation:** What further insights have they had into their motivation?
3. **The cycle of change:** What stage are they at with regard to stress management? What assists or stands in the way of their moving on to the next stage?
4. **The readings:** Were there any questions or discussion points?

Stress management

Practise the mindfulness exercise together for six to seven minutes and debrief their experience and deal with any questions. Keep it practical and based on experience.

Debrief the mindfulness homework from the previous week.

1. **Mindfulness exercise:** Was it practised and if so what was noticed? What did it show up? What was the effect at the time of practice and after re-engaging with daily activities? Anything, so long as it is drawn from experience, will be useful, even if the mindfulness has revealed how distractible the mind is, or how reactive we get

to daily events. If it wasn't practised, why not and what got in the way? Are there any questions or difficulties?

2. **Commas:** Were they practised and if so what did it show us about our state of mind and body? If it wasn't practised, why not? What gets in the way?

3. **Letting go/acceptance:** Debrief the task set last week.

Introduce the homework for the following week.

1. **Mindfulness practice:** Continue with the 'starting dose' of five minutes' practice twice a day. If some feel ready and motivated, they may wish to do 10 minutes twice a day.

2. **Continue with the 'comma' or short mindfulness practice:** Encourage participants to practise this during the week as often as they remember.

3. **Introduce the limitations task:** See page 68. Again, in introducing it, see if some participants can give brief examples of the relationship between limitations and stress in their day-to-day life. Set this task as homework for the week and invite them to relate their discoveries to the group in week 4.

Spirituality and meaning

This discussion should be facilitated around spirituality and meaning related to wellbeing rather than moving towards more religious, political or social issues. The discussion is not designed to indoctrinate any ideology, nor impose a belief in God; it is more about opening minds to the question of spirituality and meaning and how it fits into their own lives. Sensitivity to, and respect for, the diverse cultural and religious backgrounds of the participants is paramount. Although humour may help to facilitate discussion at times, please take care that participants do not ridicule others' beliefs. The following questions may be helpful in facilitating discussion.

1. **Spirituality and religion – definition:** Ask whether spirituality and religion are the same; and if they are different, what are the differences? Spirituality may be seen as a more internal process, whereas religion provides an external framework that may or may not lead to an internal process.

2. **Relationship between spirituality and health/wellbeing:** Respond to any questions or responses to the reading and elicit participants' understanding of the relationship between spirituality

and wellbeing. Wellbeing can also be broken down into physical, emotional and social wellbeing.

3. **Spirituality and resilience:** Ask how spirituality or meaning help people cope with very difficult circumstances and cultivate resilience. Discuss whether people can find meaning in suffering, and/or ask whether they have had such experiences in their lives. Opportunities to illustrate this with personal experiences may arise, but please don't create an impression of prying into areas that participants are uncomfortable to talk about.

4. **Individuals' meaning or the search for meaning in life:** Ask how they find meaning in their lives. How do they cope in difficult circumstances? Do they believe there is a purpose in their lives and how does this guide their life?

Reading
Encourage the participants to pre-read the Chapter 4, 'Exercise' and be prepared to discuss any questions or reflections the following week.

Closing
See if there are any final questions before finishing. Finish with a comma.

WEEK 4
Start with a comma.

Debrief
See how the participants got on with the homework from the previous week.

1. **Spirituality:** Are there any further insights and reflections about the role of spirituality and meaning in their lives?
2. **The readings:** Were there any questions or discussion points?

Stress management
Practise the mindfulness exercise together for six to seven minutes and debrief their experience and deal with any questions. Keep it practical and based on experience.

Debrief the mindfulness homework from the previous week.

1. **Mindfulness exercise.**

2. **Commas.**
3. **Limitations.** Debrief the task set last week.

Introduce the homework for the following week.

1. **Mindfulness practice:** Encourage the group to practise for 10 minutes twice a day, although if some do not feel ready and motivated, do not force the issue.
2. **Continue with the 'comma' or short mindfulness practice:** Encourage participants to continue practising this during the week as often as they remember.
3. **Introduce the 'presence of mind' task:** See page 67. In introducing it, see if some participants can give brief examples of the relationship between presence of mind and stress in their day-to-day life. Set this task as homework for the week and invite them to relate their discoveries to the group in week 5.

Exercise
Inquire as to what the group believe the health benefits of exercise are and inquire which are most relevant for individuals in the group. Be sure to include physical and psychological wellbeing gained from exercise. Discuss the basic level of exercise needed for health benefits. Ask participants about their personal practice of exercise and whether they are happy with the amount they do and what benefits they get from it. Ask participants what motivates them or inhibits them to do exercise. Discuss possible ways to overcome these barriers.

Exercise homework for the week:

1. Ask participants to set a SMART exercise goal for themselves.

Reading
Invite the participants to pre-read Chapter 5, 'Nutrition' over the following week and to pay particular attention to Rick Kausman's strategies for healthy eating on page 127.

Closing
See if there are any final questions before finishing. Finish with a comma.

WEEK 5

Start with a comma.

Debrief
See how the participants got on with the homework from the previous week.

1. **The SMART goal:** Are there any insights and reflections on the SMART goal for exercise? Was the goal achieved? What were the challenges? If the goal was not achieved then what got in the way?
2. **Motivation:** What further insights have they had into their motivation, particularly in relation to exercise?
3. **The readings:** Were there any questions or discussion points?

Stress management
Practise the mindfulness exercise together for 10 minutes and debrief their experience and deal with any questions.

Debrief the mindfulness homework from the previous week.

1. **Mindfulness exercise.**
2. **Commas.**
3. **'Presence of Mind':** Debrief the task from last week.

Introduce the homework for the following week.

1. **Mindfulness practice:** Encourage the group to practise for 10 minutes twice a day, although if some do not feel ready and motivated, do not press the issue. It is important that people are encouraged to practise but at the same time to be comfortable to move at their own pace.
2. **Continue with the 'comma' or short mindfulness practice:** Encourage participants to continue practising this during the week as often as they remember.
3. **Introduce the listening task:** See page 70. In introducing it, see if some participants can give brief examples of the relationship between listening and stress in their day-to-day life. How often do we listen to the mental chatter and rumination? What is its content and effect? Set this task as homework for the week and invite them to relate their discoveries to the group in week 6.

Nutrition

Inquire as to what the group believe the health benefits of healthy nutrition are and inquire which are most relevant for individuals in the group. Ask participants to share something about their personal nutrition and whether they are happy with the current situation. Inquire as to their attitudes towards food and eating. Ask participants what motivates them or inhibits them to eat a more healthy diet. Discuss possible ways to overcome these barriers. Inquire as to the participants' attitudes and practices with relation to weight management.

Nutrition homework for the week:

1. Ask participants to set a SMART nutrition goal for themselves.
2. Invite them to reflect on their own motivations and attitudes around food.

Reading

Invite the participants to pre-read Chapter 6, 'Connectedness' over the following week.

Closing

See if there are any final questions before finishing with a comma.

WEEK 6

Start with a comma.

Debrief

See how the participants got on with the homework from the previous week.

1. **The SMART goal:** Are there any insights and reflections on the SMART goal for nutrition? Was the goal achieved? What were the challenges? If the goal was not achieved then what got in the way?
2. **Motivation:** What further insights have they had into their motivation, particularly in relation to eating and healthy nutrition?
3. **The readings:** Were there any questions or discussion points?

Stress management

Practise the mindfulness exercise together for 10 minutes and debrief their experience and deal with any questions. Keep it practical and based on experience.

Debrief the mindfulness homework from the previous week.

1. **Mindfulness exercise.**
2. **Day-to-day mindfulness.**
3. **Commas.**
4. **Listening.** Debrief the task from last week.

Introduce the homework for the following week.

1. **Mindfulness practice:** Encourage the group to practise for 10 minutes twice a day.
2. **Continue with the 'comma' or short mindfulness practice:** Encourage participants to continue practising this during the week as often as they remember.
3. **Introduce the self-discipline task:** See page 72. In introducing it, see if some participants can give brief examples of the relationship between self-discipline and stress in their day-to-day life. Set this task as homework for the week and invite them to relate their discoveries to the group in week 7.

Connectedness
Open up a discussion about connectedness and the role of relationships in wellbeing. The following topics and questions may be useful in facilitating that discussion.

1. **The connection between social support and wellbeing:** What are the advantages and disadvantages of social support or the lack of it? Ask for their understanding of social support in relation to health and wellbeing and whether there are any questions or comments in relation to the previous readings. Ask for personal examples of how connected the participants feel and how this helps their wellbeing.

   Has their social support changed with new phases in their personal or work life? Have they had to create or recreate new social networks?
2. **The support of the group:** In what way has the support of the participants in the Essence program been helpful? This is an

important question which helps to bring home the point that the Essence program is an exercise in fostering social support.

Connectedness homework for the week:

1. Ask participants to set a SMART goal for themselves in relation to connectedness or relationships.
2. Invite them to reflect on their own motivations and attitudes around relationships and social engagement.

Reading
Invite the participants to pre-read Chapter 7, 'Environment' over the following week.

Closing
See if there are any final questions before finishing with a comma.

WEEK 7

Start with a comma.

Debrief
See how the participants got on with the homework from the previous week.

1. **The SMART goal:** Are there any insights and reflections on the SMART goal for connectedness? Was the goal achieved? What were the challenges? If the goal was not achieved then what got in the way?
2. **Motivation:** What further insights have they had into their motivation, particularly in relation to connectedness and relationships?
3. **The readings:** Were there any questions or discussion points?

Stress management
Practise the mindfulness exercise together for 15 minutes and debrief their experience and deal with any questions. Keep it practical and based on experience.

Debrief the mindfulness homework from the previous week.

1. **Mindfulness exercise.**
2. **Day-to-day mindfulness.**

3. **Commas.**
4. **Self-discipline:** Debrief the task from last week.

Introduce the homework for the following week.

1. **Mindfulness practice:** Encourage the group to practise for 15 minutes twice a day, although if some do not feel ready and motivated, do not press the issue. It is important that people are encouraged to practise but at the same time to be comfortable to move at their own pace.
2. **Continue with the 'comma' or short mindfulness practice:** Encourage participants to continue practising this during the week as often as they remember.
3. **Introduce the emotions task:** See page 74. In introducing it, see if some participants can give brief examples of the relationship between emotions and stress in their day-to-day life. Can we be aware of but non-attached to emotions? Set this task as homework for the week and invite them to relate their discoveries to the group in week 8.

Environment

Open up a discussion about the role of environment in wellbeing. The following topics and questions may be useful in facilitating that discussion.

1. **What constitutes the environment:** Brainstorm their understanding of what an environment is. It is more than air, water and soil; does it include the mental, emotional and social environment? What of their living/home environment? What do the environments we live in communicate to us and what effects do they have? Does environment have effects on work, study, personality, health or other behaviours?
2. **Seeking different environments:** Ask what sort of environment participants seek. Discuss what effects (both positive and negative) their current environment has on their health and wellbeing.
3. **The level of control over our environment:** Discuss the amount of control that they have in the environment in which they live. Ask them how they deal with things in the environment that they cannot control and the effect this has on their wellbeing. Inquire as to whether they have taken any conscious steps to modify their environment.

4. **Creating a healthy environment:** Ask participants to discuss the compromises they had to make when choosing their environment and possible changes they could bring about to their immediate environment to make it conducive to their own wellbeing.

Environment homework for the week:

1. Ask participants to set a SMART goal for themselves in relation to environment.

Closing
See if there are any final questions before finishing with a comma.

WEEK 8
Start with a comma.

Debrief
See how the participants got on with the homework from the previous week.

1. **The SMART goal:** Are there any insights and reflections on the SMART goal for environment? Was the goal achieved? What were the challenges? If the goal was not achieved then what got in the way?
2. **Motivation:** What further insights have they had into their motivation, particularly in relation to enhancing their environment?

Stress management
Practise the mindfulness exercise together for 15 minutes and debrief their experience and deal with any questions. Keep it practical and based on experience.

Debrief the mindfulness homework from the previous week. Are there any final reflections or insights in relation to the following?

1. **Mindfulness exercise.**
2. **Day-to-day mindfulness.**
3. **Commas.**
4. **Emotions:** Debrief the task set last week.

Introduce the nature of ongoing homework now that the course is drawing to a close. It is important to see the end of the course as a beginning. What we have been considering over these eight weeks is a way of life which will be sustainable in the long term.

1. **Mindfulness practice:** Encourage the group to continue to practise for 15 minutes twice a day or, if not for 15 minutes, for whatever amount of time they feel is sustainable.
2. **Continue with the 'comma' or short mindfulness practice:** Encourage participants to continue practising this as often as they remember.
3. **Introduce the expanding self-interest task:** See page 75. See what discussion arises around the relationship between expanding self-interest and stress in their day-to-day life.

Final debrief

Take some time to discuss the following:

1. What insights have been gained throughout the course in relation to:
   a. Changing behaviour;
   b. Mindfulness: meditation, day-to-day mindfulness, the cognitive tasks?
2. What benefits have been derived? Were there any challenges?
3. What were the one or two main insights we learned from our experiences?
4. How have we progressed in relation to the goals we set for ourselves?
5. What challenges have we met and how did we respond to them?
6. How do we intend to consolidate in an ongoing way what we have learned during the course?

If the lifestyle assesment was completed in Week 1 then you might like to invite the group to complete the assessment again now. Then compare the pre- and post- course assessments. What changes were noticed?

Closing

See if there are any final questions before finishing with a comma.

Followup gatherings can be useful to help reinforce the course content and practices.

Appendix 3

Useful health websites

The Quit Program: www.quit.org.au

The Cancer Council of Victoria: www.accv.org.au

Australian Health Promotion Association:
www.healthpromotion.org.au.

Public Health Association of Australia: www.phaa.net.au

VicHealth: www.vichealth.vic.gov.au

International Union Health Promotion and Education:
www.iuhpe.org

The Centre for Mindfulness: www.umassmed.edu/cfm

Nutrition: www.nutrition.gov

MedlinePlus (nutrition/exercise): www.nlm.nih.gov/medlineplus

PubMed: www.ncbi.nlm.nih.gov/pubmed/

References

Introduction

1 www.vichealth.vic.gov.au

2 Mathers CD, Loncar D. Projections of global mortality and burden of disease from 2002 to 2030. PLoS Med. 2006 Nov;3(11):e442.

3 Campbell SM, et al. Identifying predictors of high quality of care in English general practice: an observational study. BMJ 2001 Oct 6; 323(7316): 784–7.

4 Astin J. Why patients use alternative medicine: results of a national study. JAMA 1998;279(19):1548–53.

5 Hassed C, de Lisle S, Sullivan G, Pier C. Enhancing the health of medical students: outcomes of an integrated mindfulness and lifestyle program. Adv Health Sci Educ Theory Pract. 2008 May 31. [Epub ahead of print]

6 Friedman LS, Richter ED. Relationship between conflict of interest and research results. J Gen Intern Med 2004;19:51–56.

7 Turner EH, Matthews AM, Linardatos E, et al. Selective publication of antidepressant trials and its influence on apparent efficacy. N Engl J Med. 2008 Jan 17;358(3):252-60.

8 Linthorst G, Daniels J, Van Westerloo D. The majority of bold statements expressed during grand rounds lack scientific merit. Medical Education 2007;41(10):965–967.

PART 1 – THE SEVEN PILLARS OF WELLBEING

Chapter 2: Stress Management

1 Murray C, Lopez A. The global burden of disease. 1996, World Health Organisation.

2 Rey J. The epidemiological catchment area study: implications for Australia. MJA 1992;156:200–3.

3 Rutz W. Rethinking mental health: a European WHO perspective. World Psychiatry. 2003;2(2):125–7.

4 Miller M, Rahe R. Life changes scaling for the 1990's. J Psychosom Res 1997;43(3):279–92.

5 Cantor C, Neulinger K, De Leo D. Australian suicide trends 1964–1997: youth and beyond? MJA 1999;171:137–41.

6 Ustun TB, Ayuso-Mateos JL, Chatterji S, et al. Global burden of depressive disorders in the year 2000. Br J Psychiatry. 2004;184:386–92.

7 Mathers CD, Vos ET, Stevenson CE, Begg SJ. The Australian Burden of Disease Study: measuring the loss of health from diseases, injuries and risk factors. Med J Aust. 2000;172(12):592–6.

8 Muller N. Ackenheil M. Psychoneuroimmunology and the cytokine action in the CNS: implications for psychiatric disorders. Progress in Neuro-Psychopharmacology & Biological Psychiatry. 1998;22(1):1–33.

9 Porter RJ, Gallagher P, Watson S, Young AH. Coritcosteroid-serotonin interactions in depression: a review of the human evidence. Psychopharmacology (Berl). 2004 Apr;173(1-2):1-17.

10 McKelvey R, Pfaff J, Acres J. The relationship between chief complaints, psychological distress, and suicidal ideation in 15–24 year-old patients presenting to general practitioners. MJA 2001;175:550–2.

11 Jureidini JN, Doecke CJ, Mansfield PR, Haby MM, Menkes DB, Tonkin AL. Efficacy and safety of antidepressants for children and adolescents. BMJ. 2004;328(7444):879–83.

12 Vitiello B, Swedo S. Antidepressant medications in children. N Engl J Med. 2004;350(15):1489–91.

13 Resnick MD, Bearman P, Blum R, et al. Protecting adolescents from harm; findings from the National Longitudinal Study on Adolescent Health. JAMA 1997;278(10):823–32.

14 Hallfors DD, Waller MW, Bauer D, et al. Which comes first in adolescence-sex and drugs or depression? Am J Prev Med. 2005;29(3):163–70.

15 Bressan RA, Crippa JA. The role of dopamine in reward and pleasure behaviour – review of data from preclinical research. Acta Psychiatr Scand Suppl. 2005;(427):14–21.

16 Covey LS, Glassman AH, Stetner F. Depression and depressive symptoms in smoking cessation. Compr Psychiatry 1990;31:350–4.

17 Hall SM, Muñoz RF, Reus VI. Cognitive behavioural intervention increases abstinence rates for depressive-history smokers. J Consult Clin Psychol. 1994 Feb;62(1):141–6.

18 Brake WG, Zhang TY, Diorio J, Meaney MJ, Gratton A. Influence of early postnatal rearing conditions on mesocorticolimbic dopamine and behavioural responses to psychostimulants and stressors in adult rats. Eur J Neurosci. 2004;19(7):1863–74.

19 Kjaer TW, Bertelsen C, Piccini P, et al. Increased dopamine tone during meditation-induced change of consciousness. Brain Res Cogn Brain Res. 2002 Apr;13(2):255–9.

20 Girdler SS, Jamner LD, Shapiro D. Hostility, testosterone and vascular reactivity to stress: effects of sex. Int Jour Behav Med 1997;4:242–63.

21 Taylor SE, Klein LC, Lewis BP, et al. Biobehavioural responses to stress in females: tend-and-befriend, not fight-or-flight. Psychological Review 2000;107(3):411–29.

22 Uvans-Moberg K. Oxytocin-linked antistress effects – the relaxation and growth response. Acta Psychologica Scandinavica 1997;640(suppl.):38–42.

23 Altemus M, Deuster A, Galliven E et al. Suppression of hypothalamic-pituitary-adrenal axis response to stress in lactating women. Journ Clin Endocrin Metab 1995;80:2954–9.

24 Holstrom R. Female aggression among the great apes: a psychoanalytic perspective. In K Bjorkqvist & P Niemela (eds.) *Of Mice and Women: aspects of female aggression* (pp. 295–306). San Diego, CA: Academic Press.

25 Brown MA, Buddle ML, Martin A. Is resistant hypertension really resistant? Am Journ Hypertens 2001;14(12):1263–9.

26 McEwen BS. Protection and damage from acute and chronic stress: allostasis and allostatic overload and relevance to the pathophysiology of psychiatric disorders. Ann NY Acad Sci. 2004;1032:1–7.

27 Lazar SW, Kerr CE, Wasserman RH, et al. Meditation experience is associated with increased cortical thickness. Neuroreport. 2005;16(17): 1893–1897.

28 Dunn AJ, Swiergiel AH, de Beaurepaire R. Cytokines as mediators of depression: what can we learn from animal studies? Neurosci Biobehav Rev. 2005;29(4–5):891–909.

29 Novack DH, Cameron O, Epel E, et al. Psychosomatic medicine: the scientific foundation of the biopsychosocial model. Acad Psychiatry. 2007 Sep–Oct;31(5):388–401.

30 Astin J. Why patients use alternative medicine: results of a national study. JAMA 1998;280(9):784–7.

31 Shorter E. *A History of Psychiatry: from the era of the asylum to the age of Prozac.* (John Wiley, New York, 1997).

32 Mayberg HS, et al. The functional neuroanatomy of the placebo effect. Am J Psychiatry. 2002;159(5): 728–37.

33 Kirsch I, Deacon BJ, Huedo-Medina TB, Scoboria A, Moore TJ, et al. Initial Severity and Antidepressant Benefits: A Meta-Analysis of Data Submitted to the Food and Drug Administration PLoS Medicine 2008 Feb;5(2):e45 doi:10.1371/journal. pmed.0050045

34 Goldapple K, et al. Modulation of cortical-limbic pathways in major depression: treatment-specific effects of cognitive behaviour therapy. Arch Gen Psychiatry. 2004;61(1):34–41.

35 Wager TD, et al. Placebo-induced changes in FMRI in the anticipation and experience of pain. Science. 2004;303(5661):1162–7.

36 Singer T, et al. Empathy for pain involves the affective but not sensory components of pain. Science. 2004 Feb 20;303(5661):1157–62.

37 Moseley JB, O'Malley K, Petersen NJ, et al. A controlled trial of arthroscopic surgery for osteoarthritis of the knee. N Engl J Med. 2002;347(2):81-8.

38 Page SJ, Levine P, Leonard A. Mental practice in chronic stroke: results of a randomized, placebo-controlled trial. Stroke. 2007 Apr;38(4):1293–7. Epub 2007 Mar 1.

39 Ursin H, Eriksen HR. Sensitization, subjective health complaints, and sustained arousal. Ann N Y Acad Sci. 2001 Mar;933:119–29.

40 Siegel DJ. *The Mindful Brain.* Norton, New York: 2007.

41 Pawlak R, Margarinos AM, Melchor J, et al. Tissue plasminogen activator in the amygdala is critical for stress-induced anxiety-like behaviour. Nat Neurosci 2003;6(2):168–74.

42 Wang J, Rao H, Wetmore GS, et al. Perfusion functional MRI reveals cerebral blood flow pattern under psychological stress. Proc Natl Acad Sci USA. 2005;102(49):17804–9.

43 Small DM, Zatorre RJ, Dagher A, et al. Changes in brain activity related to eating chocolate: from pleasure to aversion. Brain 2001;124(Pt 9):1720–33.

44 Plassmann H, O'Doherty J, Shiv B, Rangel A. Marketing actions can modulate neural representations of experienced pleasantness. Proc Natl Acad Sci U S A. 2008 Jan 22;105(3):1050–4. Epub 2008 Jan 14.

45 Davidson RJ, Kabat-Zinn J, Schumacher J, et al. Alterations in brain and immune function produced by mindfulness meditation. Psychosom Med. 2003;65(4):564–70.

46 Matsunaga M, Isowa T, Kimura K, et al. Associations among central nervous, endocrine, and immune activities when positive emotions are elicited by looking at a favorite person. Brain Behav Immun. 2007 Oct 29; [Epub ahead of print]

47 Lazar SW, Bush G, Gollub RL, et al. Functional brain mapping of the relaxation response and meditation. Neuroreport. 2000;11(7):1581–5.

48 Lazar SW, Kerr CE, Wasserman RH, et al. Neuroreport. 2005;16(17):1893–1897.

49 Gross CG. Neurogenesis in the adult brain: death of a dogma. Nature Reviews Neuroscience. 2000;1(1):67-73.

50 Arias-Carrion O, Olivares-Bunuelos T, Drucker-Colin R. Neurogenesis in the adult brain. Revista de Neurologia. 2007;44(9):541–50.

51 Yang Y, Raine A, Lencz T, et al. Prefrontal white matter in pathological liars. Br J Psychiatry. 2005;187:320–5.

52 Irwin MR. Human psychoneuroimmunology: 20 Years of discovery. Brain Behav Immun. 2007 Sep 30; [Epub ahead of print]

53 Watkins A. *Mind-body Medicine: a clinician's guide to psychoneuroimmunology.* Churchill Livingston, London, 1997.

54 Glaser R, Kiecolt-Glaser JK. Stress-induced immune dysfunction: implications for health. Nat Rev Immunol. 2005;5(3):243–51.

55 Cohen S, Herbert T. Health Psychology: psychological factors and physical disease from the perspective of human psychoneuroimmunology. 1996;47:113–42.

56 Knapp P, Levy E, Giorgi R, et al. Short-term immunological effects of induced emotion. Psychosom Med 1992;54:133–48.

57 Jemmott J, Hellman C, McClelland D, et al. Motivational syndromes associated with natural killer cell activity. J Behav Med 1990;13:53–73.

58 Jandorf L, Deblinger E, Neale J, Stone A. Daily vs. major life events as predictors of symptom frequency:

a replication study. J General Psychol 1986;113:205–18.

59 Herbert T, Cohen S, Marsland, et al. Cardiovascular reactivity and the course of immune response to an acute psychological stressor. Psychosom Med 1994;56:337–44.

60 Sieber W, Rodin J, Larson L, et al. Modulation of human natural killer cell activity by exposure to uncontrollable stress. Brain, Behaviour and Immunity 1992;6:141–56.

61 Marsland A, et al. Stress, immune reactivity and susceptibility to infectious disease. Physiology and Behaviour 2002;77(4–5):711–6.

62 Cohen S et al. Reactivity and vulnerability to stress-associated risk for upper respiratory illness. Psychosom Med. 2002;64(2):302–10.

63 Tendulkar AP, Victorino GP, Chong TJ, et al. Quantification of surgical resident stress 'on call'. J Am Coll Surg. 2005;201(4):560–4.

64 Gouin JP, Kiecolt-Glaser JK, Malarkey WB, Glaser R. The influence of anger expression on wound healing. Brain Behav Immun. 2007 Dec 8; [Epub ahead of print]

65 Kiecolt-Glaser JK, Loving TJ, Stowell JR, et al. Hostile marital interactions, proinflammatory cytokine production, and wound healing. Arch Gen Psychiatry. 2005 Dec;62(12):1377–84.

66 Bosch JA, Engeland CG, Cacioppo JT, Marucha PT. Depressive symptoms predict mucosal wound healing. Psychosom Med. 2007 Sep–Oct;69(7):597–605.

67 Cohen S, Tyrrell DA, Smith AP. Psychological stress and susceptibility to the common cold. N Engl J Med. 1991 Aug 29;325(9):606–12.

68 Cohen S, Doyle WJ, Skoner DP. Psychological stress, cytokine production, and severity of upper respiratory illness. Psychosom Med. 1999;61(2):175–80.

69 Glaser R, Kiecolt-Glaser J, Speicher C, et al. Stress, loneliness and changes in herpes virus latency. J Behav Med 1985;8(3):249–60.

70 Van Rood Y, et al. The effects of stress and relaxation on the in vitro immune response in man: a meta-analytic study. J Behav Med 1993;16(2):163–81.

71 Leserman J, Jackson E, Petitto J et al. Progression to AIDS: the effects of stress, depressive symptoms and social support. Psychosom Med 1999;61(3):397–406.

72 Cohen M, Arad S, Lorber M, Pollack S. Psychological distress, life stressors, and social support in new immigrants with HIV. Behav Med. 2007 Summer;33(2):45–54.

73 Evans D, Leserman J, Perkins D, et al. Severe life stress as a predictor of early disease progression in HIV infection. Am J Psych 1997; 154:630–34.

74 Antoni MH, Cruess DG, Cruess S, et al. Cognitive-behavioural stress management intervention effects on anxiety, 24-hr urinary norepinephrine output, and T-cytotoxic/ suppressor cells over time among symptomatic HIV-infected gay men. J Consult Clin Psych. 2000;68(1):31–45.

75 Cruess DG, Antoni MH, Kumar M, et al. Cognitive-behavioural stress management buffers decreases in dehydroepiandrosterone sulfate

(DHEA-S) and increases in the cortisol/DHEA-S ratio and reduces mood disturbance and perceived stress among HIV-seropositive men. Psychoneuroendocrin. 1999;24(5):537–49.

76 Kiecolt-Glaser J, Glaser R. Psychoneuroimmunology: can psychological interventions modulate immunity? J Consult Clin Psych 1992;60:569–75.

77 Kiecolt-Glaser J, Glaser R. Stress and the immune system: human studies. In Tasman A. and Riba M. (eds.) Annual Review of Psychiatry 1991;11:169–80.

78 Rossen R, Butler W, Wladman R. The protein in nasal secretion. JAMA 1970;211:1157–61.

79 Jemmot J, McClelland D. Secretory IgA as a measure of resistance to infectious disease. Behav Med 1989;15:63–71.

80 Ring C, Carroll D, Hoving J, et al. Effects of competition, exercise, and mental stress on secretory immunity. J Sports Sci. 2005 May;23(5):501–8.

81 Jemmott J, Magloire K. Academic stress, social support and S-IgA. J Pers Soc Psychol 1988;55:803–10.

82 He M. A prospective controlled study of psychosomatic and immunologic changes in recently bereaved people. Chinese J Neurol Psychiatry 1993;24:90–93.

83 Annie C, Groer M. Childbirth stress – an immunology study. J Obst Gynecol & Neonat Nursing 1991;20:391–7.

84 McClelland D, Floor E, Davidson R et al. Stressed power motivation, sympathetic activation, immune function and illness. J Human Stress 1980;6:11–19.

85 Pawlow LA, Jones GE. The impact of abbreviated progressive muscle relaxation on salivary cortisol and salivary immunoglobulin A (sIgA). Appl Psychophysiol Biofeedback. 2005 Dec;30(4):375–87.

86 Labott S, Ahleman S, Wolever M. et al. The physiological and psychological effects of the expression and inhibition of emotion. Behav Med 1990;16:182–9.

87 Dillon K, Minchoff B, Baker K. Positive emotional states and enhancement of the immune system. Inter J Psychiat Med 1986;15(1):13–6.

88 Rein G, Atkinson M, McCraty M. The physiological and psychological effects of compassion and anger. J Advance Med 1995; 8(2):87–105.

89 Jemmott J, Borysenko J, Borysenko M, et al. Academic stress, power motivation, and decrease in secretion rate of salivary secretory immunoglobulin A. Lancet 1983;1(8339):1400–2.

90 Marsland A, Manuck S, Fazzari T, et al. Stability of individual differences in cellular immune response to stress. Psychosom Med 1995;57:295–8.

91 Boyce WT, Chesney M, Alkon A, et al. Psychobiologic reactivity to stress and childhood respiratory illnesses: results of two prospective studies. Psychosom Med 1995;57(5):411–22.

92 Kiecolt-Glaser J, Dura J, Speicher C, et al. Spousal caregivers of dementia victims: longitudinal changes in immunity and health. Psychosom Med 1991; 53:345–62.

93 Eriksen HR, Ursin H. Subjective health complaints, sensitization, and sustained cognitive activation (stress). J Psychosom Res. 2004;56(4):445–8.

94 Ursin H, Eriksen HR. Sensitization, subjective health complaints, and sustained arousal. Ann N Y Acad Sci. 2001 Mar;933:119–29.

95 Kabat-Zinn J, Lipworth L, Burney R. The clinical use of mindfulness meditation for the self-regulation of chronic pain. J Behav Med. 1985;8(2):163–90.

96 Carmody J, Baer RA. Relationships between mindfulness practice and levels of mindfulness, medical and psychological symptoms and well-being in a mindfulness-based stress reduction program. J Behav Med. 2007 Sep 25; [Epub ahead of print]

97 Gonsalkorale WM, Miller V, Afzal A, Whorwell PJ. Long term benefits of hypnotherapy for irritable bowel syndrome. Gut. 2003;52(11):1623–9.

98 Elias AN, Wilson AF. Serum hormonal concentrations following transcendental meditation – potential role of gamma aminobutyric acid. Med Hypoth. 1995 Apr;44(4):287–91.

99 Harte JL, Eifert GH, Smith R. The effects of running and meditation on beta-endorphin, corticotropin-releasing hormone and cortisol in plasma, and on mood. Biol Psychol. 1995 Jun;40(3):251–65.

100 Willcock SM et al. Burnout and psychiatric morbidity in new medical graduates. Med J Aust. 2004;181(7):357–60.

101 Fahrenkopf AM, Sectish TC, Barger LK, et al. Rates of medication errors among depressed and burnt out residents: prospective cohort study. BMJ, doi:10.1136/bmj.39469.763218.BE (pub 7 February 2008).

102 Hallowell EM. Overloaded circuits: why smart people underperform. Harv Bus Rev. 2005 Jan;83(1):54–62, 116.

103 Schneider RH, Alexander CN, Staggers F, et al. Long-term effects of stress reduction on mortality in persons > or = 55 years of age with systemic hypertension. Am J Card. 2005;95(9):1060–4.

104 Sokejiana S, Kagamimori S. Working hours as a risk factor for acute myocardial infarction in Japan: case control study. BMJ 1998;317(7161)775–80.

105 Kusaka Y, Kondou H, Morimoto K. Healthy lifestyles are associated with higher natural killer cell activity. Prev Med. 1992 Sep;21(5):602–15.

106 Pelletier K. R. Mind-Body Health: Research, Clinical, and Policy Applications. Am J Health Promot 1992;6(5):345–358.

107 Glassman A, Helzer J, Covery L, et al. Smoking, smoking cessation, and major depression. JAMA 1990;264:1546–9.

108 Sutherland J. E. The link between stress and illness – Do our coping methods influence our health? Postgrad Med 1991;89 (1)159–164.

109 Magarey C. Meditation and Health. Pat Manag May 1989:89–101.

110 Kiecolt-Glasser J, et al. Psychoneuroimmunology: Can psychological interventions modulate immunity? J Consult Clinical Psych 1992;60(4):569–75.

111 Dillon K, et al. Positive emotional states and enhancement of the immune system. Int J Psych Med1986;15(1):13–18.

112 Lamontagne AD, Keegel T, Vallance D, et al. Job strain-attributable depression in a sample of working Australians: Assessing the contribution to health inequalities. BMC Pub Health. 2008;8(1):181.

113 Baldwin DC Jr, Daugherty SR. Sleep deprivation and fatigue in residency training: results of a national survey of first- and second-year residents. Sleep. 2004;27(2):217–23.

114 Landrigan CP, Rothschild JM, Cronin JW, et al. Effect of reducing interns' work hours on serious medical errors in intensive care units. N Engl J Med. 2004;351(18):1838–48.

115 Sexton JB, et al. Error, stress, and teamwork in medicine and aviation: cross sectional surveys. BMJ. 2000;320(7237):745–9.

116 Willich SN, Lowel H, Lewis M, et al. Weekly variation of acute myocardial infarction. Increased Monday risk in the working population. Circ. 1994;90(1):87–93.

117 Manfredini R, Casetta I, Paolino E, et al. Monday preference in onset of ischemic stroke. Am J Med 2001;111(5):401–3.

118 Vehvilainen AT, Kumpusalo EA, Takala JK. They call it stormy Monday; reasons for referral from primary to secondary care according to the days of the week. Brit J Gen Prac 1999;49(448):909–11.

119 Peters RW, Brooks MM, Zoble RG, et al. Chronobiology of acute myocardial infarction: cardiac arrhythmia suppression trial (CAST) experience. Am J Card 1996;78(11):1198–201.

120 Peters RW, McQuillan S, Resnick SK, et al. Increased Monday incidence of life-threatening ventricular arrhythmias. Experience with a third-generation implantable defibrillator. Circ 1996;94(6):1346–9.

121 Gump BB, Matthews KA. Are vacations good for your health? The 9-year mortality experience after the multiple risk factor intervention trial. Psychosom Med. 2000 Sep–Oct;62(5):608–12.

122 Bosma H, Peter R, Siegrist J, et al. Two alternative job stress models and the risk of coronary heart disease. Am J Public Health. 1998 Jan;88(1):68-74.

123 Theorell T, Tsutsumi A, Hallquist J, et al. Decision latitude, job strain, and myocardial infarction: a study of working men in Stockholm. The SHEEP Study Group. Stockholm Heart epidemiology Program. Am J Public Health. 1998 Mar;88(3):382-8.

124 Sokejiana S, Kagamimori S. Working hours as a risk factor for acute myocardial infarction in Japan: a case control study. BMJ 1998;317(7161):775-780.

125 Andel R, Crowe M, Pedersen NL, et al. Complexity of work and risk of Alzheimer's disease: a population-based study of Swedish twins. J Gerontol B Psychol Sci Soc Sci. 2005;60(5):P251–8.

126 Theorell T, Karasek RA. Current issues relating to psychosocial job strain and cardiovascular disease research. J Occup Health Psychol. 1996;1(1):9–26.

Erratum in: J Occup Health Psychol 1998;3(4):369.

127 Schneider RH, Alexander CN, Staggers F, et al. Long-term effects of stress reduction on mortality in persons > or = 55 years of age with systemic hypertension. Am J Card. 2005; 95(9):1060–4.

128 Orme-Johnson D. Medical care untilisation and the transcendental meditation program. Psychosom Med 1987;49:493–507.

129 Orme-Johnson D, Herron R. An innovative approach to reducing medical care utilisation and expenditures. Am J Man Care 1997;3:135–44.

130 Hassed C. *Know Thyself: the Stress Release Program.* Michelle Anderson Publishing, Melbourne, 2002.

131 Hassed C, de Lisle S, Sullivan G, Pier C. Enhancing the health of medical students: outcomes of an integrated mindfulness and lifestyle program. Adv Health Sci Educ Theory Pract. 2008 May 31. [Epub ahead of print]

132 Shapiro DH. Overview: clinical and physiological comparison of meditation with other self-control strategies. Am. J. Psych. 1982;139:267–273.

133 Michal M, Beutel ME, Jordan J, et al. Depersonalization, mindfulness, and childhood trauma. J Nerv Ment Dis. 2007;195(8):693–6.

134 Baer RA, Smith GT, Hopkins J, et al. Using self-report assessment methods to explore facets of mindfulness. Assessment. 2006;13(1):27–45.

135 Ivanovski B, Malhi G. The psychological and neurophysiological concomitants of mindfulness forms of meditation. Acta Neuropsychiatrica 2007;19:76–91.

136 Whitehouse WG, Dinges DF, Orne EC, et al. Psychological and immune effects of self-hypnosis training for stress management through the first semester of medical school. Psychosom Med 1996;58:249–63.

137 Kabat-Zinn et al. Effectiveness of meditation based stress reduction program in the treatment of anxiety disorders. Am J Psych 1992;149:936–943.

138 Teasdale J, Segal Z, Williams J, Mark G. How does cognitive therapy prevent depressive relapse and why should attention control (mindfulness) training help? Behav Res Ther 1995;33:25–39.

139 Teasdale J, Segal Z, Williams J, et al. Prevention of relapse/recurrence in major depression by mindfulness-based gognitive therapy. J Consul Clin Psychol 2000;68(4):615–23.

140 Ma SH, Teasdale JD. Mindfulness-based cognitive therapy for depression: replication and exploration of differential relapse prevention effects. J Consult Clin Psychol. 2004;72(1):31–40.

141 Shapiro S, Schwartz G, Bonner G. Effects of mind-fulness-based stress reduction on medical and pre-medical students. J Behav Med 1998;21(6): 581–99.

142 Soskis DA. Teaching meditation to medical students. J Religion and Health 1978;17:136–43.

143 Kelly JA, Bradlyn AS, Dubbert PM et al. Stress management training in medical school. J Med Ed 1982;57:91–9.

144 Dashef SS, Espey WM, Lazarus JA. Time-limited sensitivity groups for medical students. Am J Psych 1974;131:287–92.

145 Palan BM, Chandwani S. Coping with examination stress through hypnosis: an experimental study. Am J Clin Hypnos 1989;31:173–80.

146 Hilberman E, Konanc J, Perez-Reyes M et al. Support group for women in medical school: a first year program. J Med Ed 1975;50:867–75.

147 Speca M, Carlson L, Goodey E, Angen M. A randomised wait-list controlled trial: the effects of a mindfulness meditation based stress reduction program on mood and symptoms of stress in cancer patients. Psychosom Med 2000;62:613–22.

148 Carlson LE, Garland SN. Impact of mindfulness-based stress reduction (MBSR) on sleep, mood, stress and fatigue symptoms in cancer outpatients. Int J Behav Med. 2005;12(4):278–85.

149 Kaplan K, Goldenberg D, Galvin-Nadeau M. The impact of a meditation-based stress reduction program on fibromyalgia. Gen Hosp Psychiatry 1993;15:284–9.

150 Kabat-Zinn J, et al. Four-year follow-up of a meditation based program for the self-regulation of chronic pain: treatment outcomes and compliance. Clin J Pain 1987;2159–173.

151 Kristeller J, Hallett C. An exploratory study of a meditation-based intervention for binge eating disorder. J Health Psychol 1999;4:357–63.

152 Lazar SW, Kerr CE, Wasserman RH, et al. Meditation experience is associated with increased cortical thickness. Neuroreport. 2005;16(17):1893–7.

153 Duckworth AL, Seligman ME. Self-discipline outdoes IQ in predicting academic performance of adolescents. Psychol Sci. 2005 Dec;16(12):939-44.

154 Pagnoni G, Cekic M. Age effects on gray matter volume and attentional performance in Zen meditation. Neurobiol Aging. 2007;28(10):1623–7.

155 Weiss M, Nordlie JW, Siegel EP. Mindfulness-based stress reduction as an adjunct to outpatient psychotherapy. Psychother Psychosom. 2005;74(2):108–12.

156 Hassed, C. *Know Thyself.* Michelle Anderson Publishing, Melbourne 2002.

157 Mant A, Mattick RP, de Burgh S, et al. Benzodiazepine prescribing in general practice: dispelling some myths. Fam Pract. 1995 Mar;12(1): 37–43.

158 Mant A, de Burgh S, Mattick RP, Donnelly N, Hall W. Insomnia in general practice. Results from NSW General Practice Survey 1991–1992. Aust Fam Physic. 1996 Jan;Suppl 1:S15–8.

159 Janson C, Lindberg E, Gislason T, et al. Insomnia in men – a 10-year prospective population based study. Sleep 2001;24(4):425-30.

160 Kripke DF, Garfinkel L, Wingard DL, et al. Mortality associated with sleep duration and insomnia. Arch Gen Psych 2002;59(2):131–6.

161 Kojima M, Wakai K, Kawamura T, et al. Sleep patterns and total mortality: a 12-year follow-up study in Japan. J Epidemiol. 2000;10(2):87–93.

162 Cole SR, Kawachi I, Sesso HD, et al. Sense of exhaustion and coronary heart disease among college alumni. Am J Cardiol. 1999 Dec 15;84(12):1401–5.

163 Ayas NT, White DP, Manson JE, et al. A prospective study of sleep duration and coronary heart disease in women. Arch Intern Med 2003 Jan 27;163(2):205–9.

164 Bursztyn M, Stessman J. The siesta and mortality: twelve years of prospective observations in 70-year-olds. Sleep. 2005; 28(3):345–7.

165 Naska A, Oikonomou E, Trichopoulou A, et al. Siesta in healthy adults and coronary mortality in the general population. Arch Intern Med. 2007;167(3):296-301.

166 Burazeri G, Gofin J, Kark JD. Siesta and mortality in a Mediterranean population: a community study in Jerusalem. Sleep. 2003;26(5):578–84.

167 Stergiou GS, Vemmos KN, Pliarchopoulou KM, et al. Parallel morning and evening surge in stroke onset, blood pressure, and physical activity. Stroke. 2002;33(6):1480–6.

168 Irwin M, Clark C, Kennedy B et al. Nocturnal catecholamines and immune function in insomniacs, depressed patients, and control subjects. Brain, Behav Immun 2003;17(5):365–72.

169 Steiger A. Sleep and endocrinology. J Intern Med. 2003;254(1):13–22.

170 Holsboer-Trachsler E, Seifritz E. Sleep in depression and sleep deprivation: a brief conceptual review. World J Biol Psych. 2000;1(4):180-6.

171 Buysse DJ. Insomnia, depression and aging. Assessing sleep and mood interactions in older adults. Geriatrics 2004;59(2):47-51; quiz 52.

172 Riemann D, Voderholzer U. Primary insomnia: a risk factor for depression? J Affec Disord 2003; 76(1-3):255-9.

173 Cole MG. Dendukuri N. Risk factors for depression among elderly community subjects: a systematic review and metaanalysis. Am J Psych 2003;160(6):1147–56.

174 Mallon L, Broman J, Hetta J. Relationship between insomnia, depression, and mortality: a 12-year follow-up of older adults in the community. Int Psychogeriatr. 2000;12(3):295–306.

175 Morawetz, David. Insomnia and Depression: Which Comes First? Sleep Research Online 5(2): 77–81, 2003. http://

176 Germain A, Moul DE, Franzen PL, et al. Effects of a brief behavioural treatment for late-life insomnia: preliminary findings. J Clin Sleep Med. 2006;2(4):403–6.

177 Hohagen F, Rink K, Kappler C, et al. Prevalence and treatment of insomnia in general practice. A longitudinal study. Eur Arch Psychiatry Clin Neurosci 1993;242(6):329-36.

178 Leppamaki S, Partonen T, Vakkuri O et al. Effect of controlled-release melatonin on sleep quality, mood, and quality of life in subjects with seasonal or weather-associated changes in mood and behaviour. Eur Neuropsychopharmacol 2003;13(3):137–45.

179 Tooley GA, Armstrong SM, Norman TR, Sali A. Acute increases in night-time plasma melatonin levels following a period of meditation. Bio Psych 2000;53(1):69–78.

180 Massion AO, Teas J, Hebert JR, Wertheimer MD, Kabat-Zinn J. Meditation, melatonin and breast/ prostate cancer: hypothesis and preliminary data. Med Hypotheses 1995;44(1):39–46.

181 Merrill RM, Aldana SG, Greenlaw RL, et al. The effects of an intensive lifestyle modification program on sleep and stress disorders. J Nutr Health Aging. 2007 May-Jun; 11(3):242-8.

182 Youngstedt SD. Effects of exercise on sleep. Clin Sports Med. 2005 Apr;24(2):355-65, xi.

Chapter 3: Spirituality

1 Hassed C. Depression: dispirited or spiritually deprived? MJA 2000;173(10):545–7.

2 Matthews D, McCullough M, Larson D, et al. 'Religious commitment and health status: a review of the research and implications for family medicine.' Arch Fam Med 1998;7(2):118–24.

3 Reed P. Spirituality and wellbeing in terminally ill hospitalised patients. Res Nurs Health 1987;9:35–41.

4 Grosarth-Maticek R, Eysenck H. Prophylactic effects of psychoanalysis on cancer prone and coronary heart disease prone probands, as compared with control groups and behaviour therapy groups. Behav Ther Exp Psychiatry 1990;21(2):91–9.

5 Lukoff D, Fu F, Turner R. Cultural considerations in the assessment and treatment of religious and spiritual problems. Psychiatr Clin North Am 1995;18(3):467–84.

6 Matthews D, McCullough M, Larson D, et al. 'Religious commitment and health status: a review of the research and implications for family medicine.' Arch Fam Med 1998;7(2):118–24.

7 Resnick M, Bearman P, Blum R, et al. Protecting adolescents from harm; findings from the National Longitudinal Study on Adolescent Health. JAMA 1997;278(10):823–32.

8 Gartner J, Larson D, Allen G. Religious commitment and mental health: a review of the empirical literature. J Psych Theol 1991;19:6–25.

9 Koenig H, George L, Perterson B. Religiosity and remission of depression in medically ill older patients. Am J Psych1998; 155:536–42.

10 Gartner J, Larson D, Allen G. Religious commitment and mental health: a review of the empirical literature. J Psychol Theol 1991;19:6–25.

11 Comstock G, Partridge K. Church attendance and health. J Chronic Dis 1972;25:665–72.

12 Larson D., Wilson W. The religious life of alcoholics. South Med J 1980;73:723–7.

13 Moore R, Mead L, Pearson T. Youthful precursors of alcohol abuse in physicians. Am J Med 1990;88:332–6.

14 Fraser G, Sharlik D. Risk factors for all-cause and coronary heart disease mortality in the oldest old: the Adventist's Health Study. Arch Int Med 1997;157(19):2249–58.

15 Levin J, Vanderpool H. Is frequent religious

attendance really conducive to better health? Toward an epidemiology of religion. Soc Sci Med. 1987;24:589–600.

16 Kune G, Kune S, Watson L. Perceived religiousness is protective for colorectal cancer: data from the Melbourne Colorectal Cancer Study. J Royal Soc Med 1993;86:645–7.

17 Craigie F, Larson D, Liu I. References to religion in the Journal of Family Practice: dimensions and valency of spirituality. J Fam Pract 1990;30:477–80.

18 Hummer R, Rogers R, Nam C, et al. Religious involvement and U.S. adult mortality. Demog 1999;36(2):273–85.

19 Clark K, Friedman H, Martin L. A longitudinal study of religiosity and mortality risk. J Health Psych 1999;4(3):381–91.

20 Azari NP, Nickel J, Wunderlich G, et al. Neural correlates of religious experience. Eur J Neurosci. 2001;13(8):1649–52.

21 Persinger MA. Preadolescent religious experience enhances temporal lobe signs in normal young adults. Percep Motor Skills. 1991;72(2):453–4.

22 McCord G, Gilchrist VJ, Grossman SD et al. Discussing spirituality with patients: a rational and ethical approach. Ann Fam Med. 2004;2(4):356–61.

23 Hassed C. Western psychology meets Eastern philosophy. Aus Fam Phys 1999;28(10):1057–8.

24 Astin J. Why patients use alternative medicine: results of a national study. JAMA 1998;279(19):1548–53.

25 Koenig H, Cohen H, Blazer D, et al. Religious coping and depression in elderly, hospitalised medically-ill men. Am J Psych1992;149:1693–1700.

26 Williams D, Larson D, Buckler R, et al. Religion and psychological distress in a community sample. Soc Sci Med 1991;32:1257–62.

27 Oxman T, Freeman D, Manheimer E. Lack of social participation or religious strength and comfort as risk factors for death after cardiac surgery in the elderly. Psychosom Med 1995;57:5–15.

Chapter 4: Exercise

1 Bauman A. Trends in exercise prevalence in Australia. Comm Health Stud 1987;11:190–6.

2 Hauer K, et al. Intensive physical training in geriatric patients after severe falls and hip surgery. Age & Ageing. 2002;31:49–57.

3 Owen N, Bauman A. The descriptive epidemiology of physical inactivity in adult Australians. Int J Epidem., 1992;21:305–10.

4 Mastorakos G, Pavlatou M, Diamanti-Kandarakis E, et al. Exercise and the stress system. Hormones. 2005;4(2):73–89

5 Pedersen BK. Saltin B. Evidence for prescribing exercise as therapy in chronic disease. Scandi J Med Sci Sports. 2006;16 Suppl 1:3–63.

6 Brouwer BG, Visseren FL, van der Graaf Y; SMART Study Group. The effect of leisure-time physical activity on the presence of metabolic syndrome in patients with manifest arterial disease. The SMART study. Am Heart J. 2007 Dec;154(6):1146–52.

7 Lopez AD, Mathers CD, Ezzati M, et al. Global and regional burden of disease and risk factors, 2001: systematic analysis of population health data. Lancet 2006;367(9524):1747–57.

8 Kriska AM, Brach JS, Jarvis BJ, et al. Physical activity and gallbladder disease determined by ultrasonography. Med Sci Sports Exerci 2007;39(11):1927–32.

9 Ramakrishnan K, Scheid DC. Treatment options for insomnia. Am Fam Phys. 2007 Aug 15;76(4):517–26.

10 Australian Institute of Health and Welfare 2001. Heart, Stroke and Vascular Diseases – Australian Facts 2001. National Heart Foundation of Australia, National Stroke Foundation of Australia (Cardiovascular Disease Series No 14). AIWH Cat No CVD 13. AIWH, Canberra 2001

11 Allender S, Foster C, Scarborough P, Rayner M. The burden of physical activity-related ill health in the UK. J Epidemiol Comm Health. 2007 Apr;61(4):344–8.

12 Kampert J, Blair S, Barlow C, et al. Physical activity, fitness and all cause and cancer mortality. Annals Epidemiol. 1996;6:542–7.

13 Maiorana A, et al, Combined aerobic and resistance exercise training improves functional capacity and strength in CHF. J Appl Physiol. 2000;88:1565–70.

14 Linsted K, Tonstad S, Kuzma J. Self-reported of physical activity and patterns of mortality in Seventh Day Adventist men. J Clin Epidemiol 1991;44:355–364.

15 Lopez AD, Mathers CD, Ezzati M, et al. Global and regional burden of disease and risk factors, 2001: systematic analysis of population health data. Lancet 2006;367(9524):1747-57.

16 Kouris-Blazos A, Wahlqvist ML. Health economics of weight management: evidence and cost. Asia Pac J Clin Nut. 2007;16 Suppl 1:329–38.

17 Popkin BM, Kim S, Rusev ER, Du S, Zizza C. Measuring the full economic costs of diet, physical activity and obesity-related chronic diseases. Obes Rev. 2006 Aug;7(3):271–93.

18 Bensimhon DR, Kraus WE, Donahue MP. Obesity and physical activity: a review. Am Heart J. 2006;151(3):598–603.

19 Jones D, Hemphill W, Meyers E. Height, weight and other physical characteristics of NSW children. NSW Dept Health 1973.

20 Whitehead R, Paul A, Cole T. Trends in food energy intakes throughout childhood from one to eighteen years. Hum Nutr: Appl Nutr, 1982;36:57–6.

21 Janus ED, Laatikainen T, Dunbar JA, et al. Overweight, obesity and metabolic syndrome in rural southeastern Australia. Med J Aust. 2007 Aug 6;187(3):147-52.

22 Malm C, Celsing F, Friman G. Immune defense is both stimulated and inhibited by physical activity. Lakartidningen. 2005 Mar 14–20;102(11):867–8, 870, 873.

23 Resistance training improves muscle strength, functional level and self-reported health in patients with chronic obstructive pulmonary disease. Am Thorac Soc 99th Int Conf. 2003: CO42 Poster C33.

24 Adapted from Fiatarone-Singh M. (2007) Physical fitness and exercise. From Integrative Medicine Perspectives. AIMA, Melbourne.

Chapter 5: Nutrition

1 Barberger-Gateau P, Letenneur L, Deschamps V, et al. Fish, meat, and risk of dementia: cohort study. BMJ. 2002;325(7370):932–3.

2 Janatuinen EK, Kemppainen TA, Julkunen RJK, et al. No harm from five year ingestion of oats in coeliac disease. Gut 2002; 50:332-335.

3 American Gastroenterological Association Medical position statement: Gastroenterology, 2001;120: 1522–1525.

4 Nicholas L, Roberts D CK, Pond D. The role of the general practitioner and the dietician in patient nutrition management. Asia Pac J Clin Nutr. 2003;12(1):3–8.

5 Bourre JM. Dietary omega-3 fatty acids for women. Biomed Pharmacother. 2007;61 (2–3):105–12.

6 Griguol Chulich VI, León-Camacho M, Vicario Romero IM. Margarine's trans-fatty acid composition: modifications during the last decades and new trends. Arch Latinoam Nutr. 2005 Dec;55(4):367–73.

7 McCann D, Barrett A, Cooper A, et al. Food additives and hyperactive behaviour in 3-year-old and 8/9-year-old children in the community: a randomised, double-blinded, placebo-controlled trial. Lancet. 2007;370(9598):1560–7.

8 Lam F. and Brush B. Chlorophyll and wound healing; experimental and clinical study. Am J Surg 1950;80:204–10.

9 Yoshida A, et al. Therapeutic effect of chlorophyll-a in the treatment of patients with chronic pancreatitis. Gastroenterolog Japonica 1980;15(1) :49–61.

10 Adapted from Hark L, Deen D. Nutrition: the definitive Australian guide to eating for good health. Dorling Kindersley, Melbourne 2007.

11 Györéné KG, Varga A, Lugasi A. A comparison of chemical composition and nutritional value of organically and conventionally grown plant derived foods. Orv Hetil. 2006;147(43):2081–90.

12 Omenn GS, Goodman GE, Thornquist MD, et al. Effects of a combination of beta carotene and vitamin A on lung cancer and cardiovascular disease. N Engl J Med. 1996 May 2;334(18):1150–5.

13 Divisi D, Di Tommaso S, Salvemini S, et al. Diet and cancer. Acta Biomed. 2006 Aug;77(2):118–23.

14 Pryor WA, Stahl W, Rock CL. Beta carotene: From Biochemistry to Clinical Trials. Nut Rev. 2000;58:39–53.

15 Omenn GS. Chemoprevention of lung cancers: lessons from CARET, the beta-carotene and retinol efficacy trial, and prospects for the future. Eur J Cancer Prev. 2007 Jun;16(3):184–91.

16 Whitney EN and Rolfes SR. Understanding Nutrition. Wadsworth Thomson Learning. Belmont, 2002.

17 Jolly CA. Diet manipulation and prevention of aging, cancer and autoimmune disease. Curr Opin Clin Nutr Metab Care. 2005;8(4):382–7.

18 Gredilla R, Barja G. Minireview: the role of oxidative stress in relation to caloric restriction and longevity. Endocrinol 2005;146(9):3713–7.

19 Willcox DC, Willcox BJ, Todoriki H, et al. Caloric restriction and human longevity: what can we learn from the Okinawans? Biogerontol 2006 Jun 30; [Epub ahead of print]

20 Tsai AG, Wadden TA. Systematic review: an evaluation of major commercial weight loss programs in the United States. Ann Intern Med 2005;142(1):56–66.

21 Patton GC, Selzer R, Coffey C, et al. Onset of adolescent eating disorders: population based cohort study over 3 years. BMJ 1999;318(7186):765–8.

22 Gingras J, Fitzpatrick J, McCargar L. Body image of chronic dieters: lowered appearance evaluation and body satisfaction. J Am Diet Assoc 2004;104(10):1589–92.

23 Kausman R. Tips for long term weight management. Aus Fam Phys 2000;29(4):310–3.

24 Kausman R. If not dieting then what? Allen and Unwin. Melbourne, 2004.

Chapter 6: Connectedness

1 Miller M, Rahe R. Life changes scaling for the 1990's J Psychosom Res. 1997;43(3): 279–92.

2 House JS, Landis KR, Umberson D. Social relationships and health. Science 1988;241:540–5.

3 Lantz PM, House JS, Lepkowski JM, et al. Socioeconomic factors, health behaviours, and mortality: results from a nationally representative prospective study of US adults. JAMA 1998;279(21):1703–8.

4 Cohen S, Doyle WJ, Turner R, et al. Sociability and susceptibility to the common cold. Psychol Sci. 2003 Sep;14(5):389–95.

5 Glass TA, de Leon CM, Marottoli RA, Berkman LF. Population based study of social and productive activities as predictors of survival among elderly Americans. BMJ 1999;319:478–83.

6 Hemingway H, Marmot M. Evidence based cardiology: psychosocial factors in the aetiology and prognosis of coronary heart disease. Systematic review of prospective cohort studies. BMJ 1999;318(7196):1460–7.

7 Mookadam F, Arthur HM. Social support and its relationship to morbidity and mortality after acute myocardial infarction: systematic overview. Arch Intern Med. 2004 Jul 26;164(14):1514–8.

8 Berkman L, Leo-Summers L, Horwitz R. Emotional support and survival after AMI: a prospective population-based study of the elderly. Ann Int Med 1992;117:1003–9.

9 Ruberman W, et al. Psychosocial influences on mortality after AMI. N Engl J Med 1984;311:552–9.

10 Resnick MD, Bearman P, Blum R, et al. Protecting adolescents from harm; findings from the National Longitudinal Study on Adolescent Health. JAMA 1997;278(10):823–32.

11 McKelvey R, Davies L, Pfaff J, et al. Psychological

distress and suicidal ideation among 15–24 year olds presenting to a general practice: a pilot study. ANZ J Psychiat 1998;32(3):344–8.

12 Lantz PM, House JS, Lepkowski JM, et al. Socioeconomic factors, health behaviours, and mortality: results from a nationally representative prospective study of US adults. JAMA 1998;279(21):1703–8.

13 Davey CG, Yücel M, Allen NB. The emergence of depression in adolescence: Development of the prefrontal cortex and the representation of reward. Neurosci Biobehav Rev. 2007 May 16; [Epub ahead of print]

14 Whittle S, Yücel M, Fornito A, et al. Neuroanatomical correlates of temperament in early adolescents. J Am Acad Child Adolesc Psychiatry. 2008;47(6):682–93.

15 Bushman BJ, Baumeister RF, Stack AD. Catharsis, aggression, and persuasive influence: self-fulfilling or self-defeating prophecies? J Pers Soc Psychol. 1999 Mar;76(3):367–76.

16 Iribarren C, Sidney S, Bild DE, et al. Association of hostility with coronary artery calcification in young adults: the CARDIA study. Coronary Artery Risk Development in Young Adults. JAMA 2000;283(19):2546–51.

17 Forero R, McLellan L, Rissel C, Bauman A. Bullying behaviour and psychosocial health among school students in New South Wales, Australia: cross sectional survey. BMJ 1999;319:344–8, 348–51.

18 Hallfors DD, Waller MW, Bauer D et al. Which comes first in adolescence – sex and drugs or depression? Am J Prev Med. 2005;29(3):163–70.

19 Davey CG, Yücel M, Allen NB. The emergence of depression in adolescence: Development of the prefrontal cortex and the representation of reward. Neurosci Biobehav Rev. 2007 May 16; [Epub ahead of print]

20 Marazziti D, Akiskal HS, Rossi A, Cassano GB. Alteration of the platelet serotonin transporter in romantic love. Psychol Med. 1999 May;29(3):741–5.

21 Cramer D, Donachie M. Psychological health and change in closeness in platonic and romantic relationships. J Soc Psychol. 1999 Dec;139(6): 762–7.

22 Jaffe DH, Manor O, Eisenbach Z, Neumark YD. The protective effect of marriage on mortality in a dynamic society. Ann Epidemiol. 2007;17(7):540–7.

23 Kiecolt-Glaser J, Newton T. Marriage and health: his and hers. Psych Bull. 2001;127(4):472–503.

24 Litwak, E, Messeri, P. Organisational theory, social supports, and mortality rates: A theoretical convergence. Am Soc Rev 1989;54:49–66.

25 Ross C, Mirowsky J, Goldsteen, K. The impact of the family on health: The decade in review. J Marriage Fam 1990;52:1059–1078.

26 Hibbard JH, Pope CR. The quality of social roles as predictors of morbidity and mortality. Soc Sci Med 1993;36:217–225.

27 Appelberg K, Romanov, K, Heikkila K, et al.

Interpersonal conflict as a predictor of work disability: A follow-up study of 15,348 Finnish employees. J Psychosom Res1996;40:157–167.

28 Beach SRH, Fincham FD, Katz J. Marital therapy in the treatment of depression: Toward a third generation of therapy and research. Clin Psych Rev 1998;18:635–661.

29 Lee C, Gramotnev H. Life transitions and mental health in a national cohort of young Australian women. Develop Psychol. 2007;43(4):877–88.

30 Glenn ND, Weaver CN. The contribution of marital happiness to global happiness. J Marr Fam1981;43:161–168.

31 Hooley J M, Teasdale JD. Predictors of relapse in unipolar depressives: Expressed emotion, marital distress, and perceived criticism. J Abnorm Psych 1989;98:229–235.

32 Whitton SW, Olmos-Gallo PA, Stanley SM, et al. Depressive symptoms in early marriage: predictions from relationship confidence and negative marital interaction. J Fam Psych. 2007;21(2):297–306.

33 Carels RA, Sherwood A, Blumenthal JA. Psychosocial influences on blood pressure during daily life. Int J Psychophysiol 1998;28:117–129.

34 Orth-Gomér K, Wamala SP, Horsten M, et al. Marital stress worsens prognosis in women with coronary heart disease: the Stockholm Female Coronary Risk Study. JAMA. 2000;284:3008–3014.

35 Hart CL, Hole DJ, Lawlor DA, et al. Effect of conjugal bereavement on mortality of the bereaved spouse in participants of the Renfrew/Paisley Study. J Epidemiol Comm Health. 2007;61(5):455–60.

36 Phillips AC, Carroll D, Burns VE, et al. Bereavement and marriage are associated with antibody response to influenza vaccination in the elderly. Brain Behav Immun. 2006;20(3):279–89.

37 Verbrugge L. Sex differentials in health. Pub Health Rep 1982;97:417–37.

38 Kiecolt-Glaser JK, Fisher LD, Ogrocki P, et al. Marital quality, marital disruption, and immune function. Psychosom Med. 1987 Jan-Feb; 49(1):13-34.

39 Kiecolt-Glaser JK, Kennedy S, Malkoff S, et al. Marital discord and immunity in males. Psychosom Med. 1988 May-Jun;50(3):213-29.

40 Goodwin S. The marital relationship and health in women with chronic fatigue and immune dysfunction syndrome: Views of wives and husbands. Nurs Res1997;46:138–146.

41 Flor H, Breitenstein C, Birbaumer N, et al. A psychophysiological analysis of spouse solicitousness towards pain behaviours, spouse interaction, and pain perception. Behav Ther 1995;26:255–272.

42 Spiegel D, Sephton SE, Terr AI, et al. Effects of psychosocial treatment in prolonging cancer survival may be mediated by neuroimmune pathways. Ann NY Acad Sci 1998. 840:674–83.

43 Tuschen-Caffier B, Florin I, Krause W, et al. Cognitive–behavioural therapy for idiopathic infertile couples. Psychother Psychosom1999;68:15–21.

44 Baker B, Helmers K, O'Kelly B, et al. Marital

cohesion and ambulatory blood pressure in early hypertension. Am J Hypertens 1999;12:227–230.

45 Pecchioni LL, Sparks L. Health information sources of individuals with cancer and their family members. Health Comm. 2007;21(2):143–51.

46 Heinicke BE, Paxton SJ, McLean SA, et al. Internet-delivered targeted group intervention for body dissatisfaction and disordered eating in adolescent girls: a randomized controlled trial. J Abnorm Child Psych. 2007;35(3):379–91.

Chapter 7: Environment

1 Yencken D, Porter L. A Just and Sustainable Australia. September 2001. Published on behalf of the Australian Collaboration by the Australian Council of Social Service, Melbourne.

2 ABC Radio National Health Report transcript 19 Jan 2004: 'Dirty Diesel'.

3 Valent F, Little D, Bertollini R, et al. Burden of disease attributable to selected environmental factors and injury among children and adolescents in Europe. Lancet. 2004;363(9426):2032–9.

4 Jerrett M, Buzzelli M, Burnett RT, DeLuca PF. Particulate air pollution, social confounders, and mortality in small areas of an industrial city. Soc Sci Med. 2005;60(12):2845–63.

5 Pope CA, Burnett RT, Thun MJ, et al. Lung cancer, cardiopulmonary mortality, and long-term exposure to fine particulate air pollution. JAMA. 2002;287(9):1132–41.

6 Brauer C, Kolstad H, Orbaek P, et al. The sick building syndrome: a chicken and egg situation? Int Arc Occupat Enviro Health. 2006; 79(6):465-71.

7 Wyon DP. The effects of indoor air quality on performance and productivity. Indoor Air. 2004;14 Suppl 7:92–101.

8 Hackshaw AK, Law MR, Wald NJ. The accumulated evidence on lung cancer and environmental tobacco smoke. BMJ. 1997;315(7114):980–8.

9 Fichtenberg CM, Glantz SA. Effect of smoke-free workplaces on smoking behaviour: systematic review. BMJ. 2002;325(7357):188.

10 Solomon G, Schettler T. (2002) Ch 9, pp147–62, Environmental Endocrine Disruption, in Life Support: the environment and human health. MIT Press, Massachusetts.

11 Christensen M. Noise levels in a general surgical ward: a descriptive study. J Clin Nurs. 2005;14(2):156–64.

12 Willich SN, Wegscheider K, Stallmann M, Keil T. Noise burden and the risk of myocardial infarction. Eur Heart J. 2005 Nov 24; [Epub ahead of print]

13 Ristovska G, Gjorgjev D, Pop Jordanova N. Psychosocial effects of community noise: cross sectional study of school children in urban center of Skopje, Macedonia. Croat Med J. 2004;45(4):473–6.

14 Good M. Effects of relaxation and music on postoperative pain: a review. J Advanc Nurs 1996;24(5):905–14.

15 O'Callaghan C. Pain, music creativity and music

therapy in palliative care. Am J Hospice Pallia Care 1996;13(2):43–9.

16 Standley J, Hanser S. Music therapy research and applications in pediatric oncology treatment. J Pediat Oncol Nurs 1995;12(1):3–8.

17 Allen K, Blascovich J. Effects of music on cardiovascular reactivity among surgeons. JAMA 1994;272(11):882–4.

18 Augustin P, Hains A. Effect of music on ambulatory surgery patient's preoperative anxiety. AORN J 1996;63(4):750–8.

19 Krumhansl C. An exploratory study of musical emotions and psychophysiology. Can J Exper Psych 1997;51(4):336–53.

20 Kneafsey R. The therapeutic use of music in a care of the elderly setting: a literature review. J Clin Nurs 1997;6(5):341–6.

21 Rauscher F, Shaw G, Ky K. Listening to Mozart enhances spatial-temporal reasoning: towards a neurophysiologic basis. Neuroscience Letters 1995;185(1):44–7.

22 Gardiner M, Fox A, Knowles F, et al. Learning improved by arts training. Nature 1996;381(6580):284.

23 Rauscher F, Shaw G, Lenine L, et al. Music training causes long-term enhancement of preschool children's spatial-temporal reasoning. Neurolog Res 1997;19(1):2–8.

24 McCraty R, Barrios-Choplin B, Atkinson M, et al. The effect of different types of music on mood, tension, and mental clarity. Alt Ther Health Med 1998;4(1):75–84.

25 Hanser S, Thompson L. Effects of a music therapy strategy on depressed older adults. J Gerontol 1994;49(6):265–9.

26 Chlan L. Psychophysiologic responses of mechanically ventilated patients of music: a pilot study. Am J Crit Care 1995;4(3):233–8.

27 Guzzetta C. Effects of relaxation and music therapy on patients in a coronary care unit with presumptive acute myocardial infarction. Heart and Lung 1989;18(6):609–16.

28 Field T, Martinez A, Nawrocki T, et al. Music shifts frontal EEG in depressed adolescents. Adolesc 1998; 33(129):109–16.

29 Kabuto M, Nageyama T, Nitta H. EEG power spectrum changes due to listening to pleasant music and their relation to relaxation effects. Jap J Hyg 1993;48(4):807–18.

30 Kalliopuska M, Ruokonen I. A study with a follow-up of the effect of music education on holistic development of empathy. Percep Motor Skills 1993;76(1):131–7.

31 Charnetski C, Brennan F, Harrison J. Effect of music and auditory stimuli on secreatory immunoglobulin A. Percep Motor Skills 1998;87(3):1163–70.

32 Kumar AM, Tims F, Cruess DG, et al. Music therapy increases serum melatonin levels in patients with Alzheimer's disease. Alt Ther Health Med.

1999;5(6):49–57.

33 Mills B. Effects of music on assertive behaviour during exercise by middle-schoolage students. Percep Motor Skills 1996;83(2):423–6.

34 Robinson T, Weaver J, Zillman D. Exploring the relation between personality and the appreciation of rock music. Psycholog Rep 1996;78(1):259–69.

35 McCraty R, Barrios-Choplin B. Atkinson M, et al. The effect of different types of music on mood, tension, and mental clarity. Alt Ther Health Med 1998;4(1):75–84.

36 Martin G, Clarke M, Pearce C. Adolescent suicide: music preference as an indicator of vulnerability. J Am Acad Child & Adol Psychiatry 1993;32(3):530–5.

37 Young R, Sweeting H, West P. Prevalence of deliberate self harm and attempted suicide within contemporary Goth youth subculture: longitudinal cohort study. BMJ. 2006;332(7549):1058–61.

38 Martino SC, Collins RL, Elliott MN, et al. Exposure to degrading versus nondegrading music lyrics and sexual behaviour among youth. Pediatrics 2006;118(2):e430–41.

39 Godfrey R, Julien M. Urbanisation and health. Clin Med. 2005;5(2):137–41. 343

40 Stephens C. Urbanisation: the implications for health. Afr Health. 1996;18(2):14–5.

41 Sim M. Bushfires: are we doing enough to reduce the human impact? Occ Env Med 2002;59(4):215–216.

42 Communications, Environment, Information Technology and the Arts Committee, 'The heat is on: Australia's greenhouse future', Canberra: Commonwealth of Australia, 2000.

43 Lucas RM, Repacholi MH, McMichael AJ. Is the current public health message on UV exposure correct? Bull World Health Organ. 2006 Jun;84(6):485–91.

44 Janda M, Kimlin MG, Whiteman DC, et al. Sun protection messages, vitamin D and skin cancer: out of the frying pan and into the fire? Med J Aust. 2007 Jan 15;186(2):52–4.

45 Robinson PD, Högler W, Craig ME, et al. The re-emerging burden of rickets: a decade of experience from Sydney. Arch Dis Child. 2006;91(7):564–8.

46 Matsuoka LY, Ide L, Wortsman J, et al. Sunscreens suppress cutaneous vitamin D3 synthesis. J Clin Endocrinol Metab 1987;64:1165–8.

47 Holick MF. Sunlight and vitamin D for bone health and prevention of autoimmune diseases, cancers, and cardiovascular disease. Am J Clin Nutr. 2004 Dec;80(6 Suppl):1678S–88S.

48 Khaw KT. Temperature and cardiovascular mortality. Lancet 1995;345:337–8.

49 Grimes DS, Hindle E, Dyer T. Sunlight, cholesterol and coronary heart disease. Q J Med 1996;89:579–89.

50 Scragg R, Jackson R, Holdaway IM, et al. Myocardial infarction is inversely associated with plasma 25-hydroxyvitamin D3 levels: a community-based study. Int J Epidemiol 1990;19:559–63.

51 MacPherson A. Bacso J. Relationship of hair calcium concentration to incidence of coronary heart disease.

Sci Total Environ 2000;255(1–3):11–9.

52 Krause R, Buhring M, Hopfenmuller W, Holick MF, Sharma AM. Ultraviolet B and blood pressure. Lancet 1998;352:709–10.

53 Grant WB, Garland CF, Holick MF. Comparisons of estimated economic burdens due to insufficient solar ultraviolet irradiance and vitamin D and excess solar UV irradiance for the United States. Photochem Photobiol. 2005;81(6):1276–86.

54 Grant WB. An estimate of premature cancer mortality in the U.S. due to inadequate doses of solar ultraviolet-B radiation. Cancer 2002;94(6):1867–75.

55 Tuohimaa P, Pukkala E, Scelo G, et al. Does solar exposure, as indicated by the non-melanoma skin cancers, protect from solid cancers: vitamin D as a possible explanation. Eur J Cancer. 2007 Jul;43(11):1701–12.

56 John EM, Koo J, Schwartz GG. Sun exposure and prostate cancer risk: evidence for a protective effect of early-life exposure. Cancer Epidemiol Biomarkers Prev. 2007 Jun;16(6):1283–6.

57 Arthey S, Clarke VA. Suntanning and sun protection: a review of the psychological literature. Soc Sci Med 1995;40:265–74.

58 Molin J, Mellerup E, Bolwig T. et al. The influence of climate on development of winter depression. J Affec Disord 1996;37(2–3):151–5.

59 Chew KSY, McCleary R. The spring peak in suicides: a cross-national analysis. Soc Sci Med 1995;40:223–30.

60 Marusic A. Suicide mortality in Slovenia: regional variation. Crisis: J Crisis Interven Suici 1998;19(4):159–66.

61 Avery DH, Eder DN, Bolte MA, et al. Dawn simulation and bright light in the treatment of SAD: a controlled study. Biolog Psychi 2001;50(3):205–16.

62 McGrath J, Selten JP, Chant D. Long-term trends in sunshine duration and its association with schizophrenia birth rates and age at first registration – data from Australia and the Netherlands. Schizophren Res 2002;54 (3):199–212.

63 Dealberto MJ. Why are immigrants at increased risk for psychosis? Vitamin D insufficiency, epigenetic mechanisms, or both? Med Hypotheses. 2007;68(2):259–67.

64 Utiger RD. The need for more vitamin D. N Engl J Med 1998;338:828–9.

65 Lamberg-Allardt CJ, Outila TA, Karkkainen MU, et al. Vitamin D deficiency and bone health in healthy adults in Finland: could this be a concern in other parts of Europe? J Bone Min Res 2001;16(11): 2066–73.

66 Falkenbach A. Physical exercise, nutrition and sunshine exposure for the prevention of osteoporosis. Forschende Komplementarmedizin und Klassische Naturheilkunde 2001;8(4):196–204.

67 McMichael AJ, Hall AJ. Does immuno suppressive ultraviolet radiation explain the latitude gradient for multiple sclerosis? Epidemiol 1997;8:642-5.

68 O'Reilly MA, O'Reilly PM. Temporal influences

on relapses of multiple sclerosis. Europ Neurology 1991;31(6):391-5.

69 Esparza ML, Sasaki S, Kesteloot H. Nutrition, latitude, and multiple sclerosis mortality: an ecologic study. Am J Epidem 1995;142:733–7.

70 Freedman DM, Dosemeci M, Alavanja MC. Mortality from multiple sclerosis and exposure to residential and occupational solar radiation: a case-control study based on death certificates. Occupat Environ Med 2000;57(6):418–21.

71 van der Mei IA, Ponsonby AL, Blizzard L, Dwyer T. Regional variation in multiple sclerosis prevalence in Australia and its association with ambient ultraviolet radiation. Neuroepidemiol 2001; 20:168–74.

72 van der Mei IA, Ponsonby AL, Dwyer T, et al. Past exposure to sun, skin phenotype, and risk of multiple sclerosis: case-control study. BMJ. 2003 Aug 9; 327(7410): 316.

73 Dahlquist G, Mustonen L. Childhood onset diabetes – time trends and climatological factors. Int J Epidemiol 1994;23(6):1234–41.

74 Y, Amital H, Shoenfeld Y. Vitamin D and autoimmunity: new aetiological and therapeutic considerations. Ann Rheum Dis. 2007;66(9): 1137–42.

75 Arnson Cantorna MT. Vitamin D and its role in immunology: multiple sclerosis, and inflammatory bowel disease. Prog Biophys Mol Biol. 2006;92(1): 60–4.

76 Surkan PJ, Zhang A, Trachtenberg F, Daniel DB, et al. Neuropsychological function in children with blood lead levels <10mug/dL. Neurotoxicol 2007 Jul 25; [Epub ahead of print].

77 Nigg JT, Knottnerus GM, Martel MM, et al. Low Blood Lead Levels Associated with Clinically Diagnosed Attention-Deficit/ Hyperactivity Disorder and Mediated by Weak Cognitive Control. Biol Psychi. 2007 Sep 12; [Epub ahead of print]

78 Ahlbom A, Day N, Feychting M, et al. A pooled analysis of magnetic fields and childhood leukemia. Br J Cancer. 2000;83:692–698.

79 Hardell L, Carlberg M, Soderqvist F, et al. Long-term use of cellular phones and brain tumours: increased risk associated with use for > or =10 years. Occup Environ Med. 2007;64(9):626–32.

80 Mild KH, Hardell L, Carlberg M. Pooled analysis of two Swedish case-control studies on the use of mobile and cordless telephones and the risk of brain tumours diagnosed during 1997–2003. Int J Occup Saf Ergon. 2007;13(1):63–71.

81 Klaeboe L, Blaasaas KG, Tynes T. Use of mobile phones in Norway and risk of intracranial tumours. Eur J Cancer Prev. 2007;16(2):158–64.

82 Lahkola A, Auvinen A, Raitanen J, et al. Mobile phone use and risk of glioma in 5 North European countries. Int J Cancer. 2007;120(8):1769–75.

83 Feizi AA, Arabi MA. Acute childhood leukemias and exposure to magnetic fields generated by high voltage overhead power lines – a risk factor in Iran. Asian Pac J Cancer Prev. 2007 Jan–Mar;8(1):69–72.

84 Henshaw DL, Reiter RJ. Do magnetic fields cause increased risk of childhood leukemia via melatonin disruption? Bioelectromag. 2005;Suppl 7:S86–97.

85 Adapted from Hoptman N & K. *Help Yourself to Health*. Millennium Books, Melbourne, 1996.

PART 2 – PUTTING THE PILLARS INTO PRACTICE

Chapter 8: Changing behaviour

1 Kivimaki M, Leino-Arjas P, Luukkonen R, et al. Work stress and risk of cardiovascular mortality: prospective cohort study of industrial employees. BMJ. 2002;325(7369):857.

2 Plato's *Republic*, book 4.

3 'Health Promotion is powerful, effective, and cheap!' Dr Rob Moodie.

4 Kiecolt-Glaser J, Glaser R. Stress and the immune system: human studies. In Tasman A. and Riba M. (eds.) Annl Rev Psychiat 1991;11:169–80.

PART 3 – PREVENTION AND MANAGEMENT

Chapter 10: Heart disease and stroke

1 Rozanski A, Blumenthal J, Kaplan J. Impact of psychosocial factors on the pathogenesis of cardiovascular disease and implications for therapy. Circulat 1999;99(16):2192–217

2 McCraty R, Atkinson M, Tiller W, et al. The effects of emotions on short-term power spectrum analysis of heart-rate variability. Am J Cardiol 1995;76(14): 1089–93.

3 Strike PC, Perkins-Porras L, Whitehead DL, et al. Triggering of acute coronary syndromes by physical exertion and anger: clinical and sociodemographic characteristics. Heart. Published online first: 6 January 2006. doi:10.1136/hrt.2005.077362

4 Everson S, Kaplan G, Goldberg D, et al. Anger expression and incident stroke: prospective evidence from the Kuipio ischaemic heart disease study. Stroke 1999;30(3):523–8

5 Weissman M, Markowitz J, Ouellette R. et al. Panic disorder and cardiovascular/ cerebrovascular problems: results from a community survey. Am J Psych 1990;147(11):1504–8.

6 Simonsick E, Wallace R, Blazer D, Berkman L. Depressive symptomatology and hypertension-associated morbidity and mortality in older adults. Psychosom Med 1995;57(5):427–35.

7 Appels A, Otten F. Exhaustion as precursor of cardiac death. Br J Clin Psych 1992;31(3):351–6.

8 Appels A, Kop W, Bar F. Vital exhaustion, extent of atherosclerosis, and the clinical course after successful percutaneous transluminal coronary angioplasty. Eur Heart J 1995;16(12):1880–5.

9 Hemingway H, Marmot M. Evidence-based cardiology: psychosocial factors in the aetiology

and prognosis of coronary heart disease. BMJ 1999;318(7196):1460–7.

10 Rugulies R. Depression as a predictor for coronary heart disease. a review and metaanalysis. Am J Prev Med. 2002;23(1):51–61.

11 Rozanski A, Blumenthal J, Kaplan J. Impact of psychosocial factors on the pathogenesis of cardiovascular disease and implications for therapy. Circulat. 1999;99(16):2192–2217

12 Ogawa K, Tsuji I, Shiono K, Hisamichi S. Increased acute myocardial infarction mortality following the 1995 Great Hanshin-Awaji earthquake in Japan. Int J Epidemiol 2000;29(3):449–55.

13 Dobson AJ, Alexander HM, Malcolm JA, Et al. Heart attacks and the Newcastle earthquake. Med J Aust1991;155(11–12):757–61.

14 Willich SN, Lowel H, Lewis M, et al. Weekly variation of acute myocardial infarction. Increased Monday risk in the working population. Circulat. 1994;90(1):87–93.

15 Manfredini R, Casetta I, Paolino E, et al. Monday preference in onset of ischemic stroke. Am J Med 2001;111(5):401–3.

16 Peters RW, Brooks MM, Zoble RG, et al. Chronobiology of acute myocardial infarction: cardiac arrhythmia suppression trial (CAST) experience. Am J Card 1996;78(11):1198–201.

17 Peters RW, McQuillan S, Resnick SK, et al. Increased Monday incidence of life-threatening ventricular arrhythmias. Experience with a third-generation implantable defibrillator. Circulat. 1996;94(6):1346–9.

18 Vehvilainen AT, Kumpusalo EA, Takala JK. They call it stormy Monday; reasons for referral from primary to secondary care according to the days of the week. Brit J Gen Prac 1999;49(448):909–11.

19 Strike PC, Perkins-Porras L, Whitehead DL, et al. Triggering of acute coronary syndromes by physical exertion and anger: clinical and sociodemographic characteristics Heart. Published online first: 6 January 2006. doi:10.1136/hrt.2005.077362

20 Gump BB, Matthews KA. Are vacations good for your health? The 9-year mortality experience after the multiple risk factor intervention trial. Psychosom Med. 2000;62(5):608–12.

21 Kop WJ, Vingerhoets A, Kruithof GJ, Gottdiener JS. Risk factors for myocardial infarction during vacation travel. Psychosom Med. 2003;65(3):396–401.

22 Kirkup W, Merrick DW. A matter of life and death: population mortality and football results. J Epidemiol Comm Health. 2003;57(6):429–32.

23 Carroll D, Ebrahim S, Tilling K, et al. Admissions for myocardial infarction and World Cup football: database survey. BMJ. 2002;325(7378):1439–42.

24 Wilbert-Lampen U, Leistner D, Greven S, et al. Cardiovascular Events during World Cup Soccer. NEJM 2008; 358 (5):475–483.

25 Sokejiana S, Kagamimori S. Working hours as a risk factor for acute myocardial infarction in Japan: a case control study. BMJ 1998;317(7161):775–780.

26 Steptoe A, Kunz-Ebrecht S, Owen N, et al. Socioeconomic status and stress-related biological responses over the working day. Psychosom Med 2003;65(3):461–70.

27 Steptoe A, Kunz-Ebrecht S, Owen N, et al. Influence of socioeconomic status and job control on plasma fibrinogen responses to acute mental stress. Psychosom Med 2003;65(1):137–44.

28 Ishizaki M, Martikainen P, Nakagawa H. Marmot M. The relationship between employment grade and plasma fibrinogen level among Japanese male employees. YKKJ Research Group. Atherosclerosis 2000;151(2):415–21.

29 Kurl S, Laukkanen JA, Rauramaa R, et al. Systolic blood pressure response to exercise stress test and risk of stroke. Stroke. 2001;32(9):2036–41.

30 Linden W, Stossel C, Maurice J. Psychosocial interventions for patients with coronary artery disease: a meta-analysis. Arch Int Med 1996;156(7):745–52.

31 Blumenthal J et al. Stress management and exercise training in cardiac patients with myocardial ischaemia. Arch Int Med 1997;157:2213–23.

32 Wenneberg SR, Schneider RH, Walton KG, et al. A controlled study of the effects of the Transcendental Meditation program on cardiovascular reactivity and ambulatory blood pressure. Int J Neurosci 1997;89:15–28.

33 Alexander CN, Schneider R, Claybourne M, Sheppard W, Staggers F, Rainforth M, et al. A trial of stress reduction for hypertension in older African Americans, II: sex and risk factor subgroup analysis. Hypertension 1996;28:228–37.

34 Castillo-Richmond A, Schneider R, Alexander C, et al. Effects of stress reduction on carotid atherosclerosis in hypertensive African Americans. Stroke 2000;31:568–73.

35 Schneider RH, Alexander CN, Staggers F, et al. Long-term effects of stress reduction on mortality in persons > or = 55 years of age with systemic hypertension. Am J Card. 2005;95(9):1060–4.

36 Maselko J, Kubzansky L, Kawachi I, et al. Religious service attendance and allostatic load among high-functioning elderly. Psychosom Med. 2007;69(5): 464–72.

37 King DE, Mainous AG III, Steyer TE, et al. The relationship between attendance at religious services and cardiovascular infl ammatory markers. In J Psychi Med. 2001;31(4):415–25.

38 Powell LH, Shahabi L, Thoresen CE. Religion and spirituality. Linkages to physical health. Am Psychol. 2003;58(1):36–52.

39 Obisesan T, Livingston I, Trulear HD, Gillum F. Frequency of attendance at religious services, cardiovascular disease, metabolic risk factors and dietary intake in Americans: an age-stratified exploratory analysis. Int J Psychi Med. 2006;36(4):435–48.

40 Berlin J, Colditz G. A meta analysis of physical activity in the prevention of coronary heart disease.

Am J Epidemiol 1990;132:612–28.

41 Hamer M. Exercise and psychobiological processes: implications for the primary prevention of coronary heart disease. Sports Med. 2006;36(10):829–38.

42 Strike PC, Perkins-Porras L, Whitehead DL, et al. Triggering of acute coronary syndromes by physical exertion and anger: clinical and sociodemographic characteristics Heart. Published Online First: 6 January 2006. doi:10.1136/hrt.2005.077362

43 American College of Sports Medicine. American Heart Association. Exercise and acute cardiovascular events: placing the risks into perspective. Med Sci Sports Exercise. 2007;39(5):886–97.

44 Thompson PD, Franklin BA, Balady GJ, et al. American Heart Association Council on Nutrition, Physical Activity and Metabolism. American Heart Association Council on Clinical Cardiology. American College of Sports Medicine. Exercise and acute cardiovascular events placing the risks into perspective: a scientific statement from the American Heart Association Council on Nutrition, Physical Activity, and Metabolism and the Council on Clinical Cardiology. Circulat. 2007;115(17):2358–68.

45 Braith RW, Stewart KJ. Resistance exercise training: its role in the prevention of cardiovascular disease. Circulat. 2006;113 (22):2642–50.

46 Manson JE, et al. Walking compared with vigorous exercise for the prevention of cardiovascular events in women. N Eng J Med 2002 Sep 5;347:716–25.

47 Fleg JL. Exercise therapy for elderly heart failure patients. Clin Geriat Med. 2007;23(1):221–34.

48 Maiorana A, et al. Combined aerobic and resistance exercise training improves functional capacity and strength in CHF. J Appl Physiol. 2000;88:1565–70.

49 Maiorana A, O'Driscoll G, Dembo L, et al. Effect of aerobic and resistance exercise training on vascular function in heart failure. Am J Physiol Heart Circ Physiol. 2000;279(4):H1999–2005.

50 Shinton R, Sagar G. Lifelong exercise and stroke. BMJ. 1993; 307: 231–34.

51 Eliasson M, Asplund K, Evrin P. Regular leisure time physical activity predicts high levels of tissue plasminogen activator. Intern J Epidemiol. 1996; 25: 1182–1188.

52 Fagard R, Tipton C. Physical activity, fitness and hypertension in Bouchard C (Ed), Physical activity and health, Human Kinetics Press. 1994; pp 633–655.

53 Edwards KM, Ziegler MG, Mills PJ. The potential anti-inflammatory benefits of improving physical fitness in hypertension. J Hypertens. 2007;25(8): 1533–42.

54 Kelley G, Mc Clellan P. Antihypertensive effects of aerobic exercise – a brief meta analytic review. Am J Hypertens.1994;7:115–19.

55 Moore S. Physical activity, fitness and atherosclerosis. In Bouchard C, Shepherd R, Stephens J, (Eds). Physical activity, fitness and health. Human Kinetics Publishers, Illinois, pp 570–77.

56 Sdringola S, Nakagawa K, Nakagawa Y, et al. Combined intense lifestyle and pharmacologic lipid treatment further reduce coronary events and myocardial perfusion abnormalities compared with usual-care cholesterol-lowering drugs in coronary artery disease. J Am Coll Cardiol. 2003 Jan 15;41(2):263-72

57 Tsatsoulis A, Fountoulakis S. The protective role of exercise on stress system dysregulation and comorbidities. Ann NY Acad Sci. 2006;1083:196–213.

58 Miriam C, De Souza AF, Walker PA, et al. National Heart Foundation of Australia. A review of the relationship between dietary fat and cardiovascular disease. Aust J Nutr Diet 1999;56(4 Suppl):S5–S22

59 Meneely, G and Batterbee, H. High sodium-low potassium environment and hypertension. Am J Cardiology, 1976;38:.768–81

60 Appel LJ, Moore TJ, Obarzanek E, Wollmer WM, et al. A clinical trial of the effects of dietary patterns on blood pressure. N Engl J Med 1997; 1117–24

61 Balk EM, Lichtenstein AH, Chung M, et al. Effects of omega-3 fatty acids on serum markers of cardiovascular disease risk: A systematic review. J Atherosclerosis.2006.02.012

62 Albert CM, Hennekens CH, O'Donnell CJ, et al. Fish consumption and risk of sudden cardiac death. JAMA 1998;279:23–8.

63 Studer M, Briel M, Leimenstoll B, et al. Effect of different antilipidemic agents and diets on mortality: a systematic review. Arch Intern Med. 2005;165(7): 725–30.

64 Keogh A, Fenton S, Leslie C, et al. Randomised double-blind, placebo-controlled trial of coenzyme Q10 therapy in class II and III systolic heart failure. Heart Lung Circulat 2003; 12: 135–141

65 Soja A, Mortensen S. Treatment of congestive heart failure with Coenzyme Q10 illuminated by meta-analysis of clinical trials, Mol. Aspects Med. 1997; 18 (Suppl.): 159–68.

66 Rosenfeldt FL, Pepe S, Linnane A, et al. Coenzyme Q10 protects the aging heart against stress. Ann. NY Acad. Sci. 2002; 959:355–59.

67 He FJ, Nowson CA, MacGregor GA. Fruit and vegetable consumption and stroke: meta-analysis of cohort studies. Lancet. 2006;367(9507):320–6.

68 Sumner MD, Elliott-Eller M, Weidner G et al. Effects of pomegranate juice consumption on myocardial perfusion in patients with coronary heart disease. Am J Cardiol. 2005;96(6):810–4.

69 Trichopoulou A, et al. Mediterranean diet and survival among patients with coronary heart disease in Greece. Arch Intern Med. 2005;165(8):929–35.

70 Trichopoulou A, et al. Modified Mediterranean diet and survival: EPIC-elderly prospective cohort study. BMJ. 2005;330(7498):991.

71 Bartley M, Fitzpatrick R, Firth D, Marmot M. Social distribution of cardiovascular disease risk factors: change among men in England 1984–1993. J Epidemiol Comm Health 2000;54(11):806–14.

72 Bosma H, Marmot MG, Hemingway H et al. Low job control and risk of coronary heart disease in the Whitehall II (prospective cohort) study. BMJ 1997;

314: 558–65

73 *Work in America: Report of a special task-force to the Secretary of Health, Education and Welfare.* Cambridge, MA:MIT Press, 1973.

74 Berkman L., Syme S. Social networks, host resistance and mortality: a nine year follow-up study of Alameda County residents. Am J Epidemiol 1979;109:186–204.

75 Boden-Albala B, Litwak E, Elkind MS, et al. Social isolation and outcomes post stroke. Neurolog. 2005;64(11):1888–92.

76 Luecken LJ. Childhood attachment and loss experiences affect adult cardiovascular and cortisol function. Psychosom Med 1998 Nov-Dec;60(6):765–72.

77 Cancado JE, Braga A, Pereira LA, et al. Clinical repercussions of exposure to atmospheric pollution. Jornal Brasileiro De Pneumologia: Publicacao Oficial Da Sociedade Brasileira De Pneumologia E Tisilogia. 32 Suppl 2:S5–11, 2006.

78 Willich SN, Wegscheider K, Stallmann M, Keil T. Noise burden and the risk of myocardial infarction. Eur Heart J. 2005 Nov 24; [Epub ahead of print]

79 Wang CH, Hsiao CK, Chen CL, et al. A review of the epidemiologic literature on the role of environmental arsenic exposure and cardiovascular diseases. Toxicol App Pharmacol. 2007;222(3):315–26.

80 Newbold RR, Padilla-Banks E, Snyder RJ, et al. Developmental exposure to endocrine disruptors and the obesity epidemic. Repro Toxicol. 2007;23(3):290–6.

81 Navas-Acien A, Guallar E, Silbergeld EK, Rothenberg SJ. Lead exposure and cardiovascular disease – a systematic review. Enviro Health Persp. 2007;115(3):472–82.

82 Virtanen JK, Rissanen TH, Voutilainen S, et al. Mercury as a risk factor for cardiovascular diseases. J Nut Biochem. 2007;18(2):75–85.

83 Kivimaki M, Ferrie JE, Brunner E, et al. Justice at work and reduced risk of coronary heart disease among employees: the Whitehall II Study. Arch Intern Med. 2005;165(19):2245–51.

84 Holick MF. Vitamin D: importance in the prevention of cancers, Type-1 diabetes, heart disease, and osteoporosis. Am J Clin Nut. 2004;79(3):362–71.

85 Ornish, D. Dr. *Dean Ornish's Program for Reversing Heart Disease: the only system scientifically proven to reverse heart disease without drugs or surgery.* Random House, 1990.

86 Ornish D, et al. Can lifestyle changes reverse coronary heart disease? Lancet 1990;336:129–133.

87 News. US insurance company covers lifestyle therapy. BMJ. 1993;307:465.

88 Penninx BW, Beekman AT, Honig A, et al. Depression and cardiac mortality: results from a community-based longitudinal study. Arch Gene Psych. 2001;58(3):221–7.

89 Ornish D., Scherwitz L., Billings J., et al. Intensive lifestyle changes for reversal of coronary heart disease. JAMA 1998;280:2001–7.

Chapter 11: Cancer

1 http://www.wcrf-uk.org/research_science/recommendations.lasso

2 Brown KW, Levy AR, Rosberger Z, Edgar L. Psychological distress and cancer survival: a follow-up 10 years after diagnosis. Psychosom Med. 2003;65(4):636–43.

3 Spiegel D, Giese-Davis J. Depression and cancer: mechanisms and disease progression. Biol Psychiat. 2003;54(3):269–82.

4 Falagas ME, Zarkadoulia EA, Ioannidou EN et al. The effect of psychosocial factors on breast cancer outcome: a systematic review. Breast Cancer Res. 2007;9(4):R44.

5 Oerlemans M, van den Akker M, Schuurman AG, et al. A meta-analysis on depression and subsequent cancer risk. Clin Pract Epidemiol Ment Health. 2007;3:29.

6 Brown KW, Levy AR, Rosberger Z, Edgar L. Psychological distress and cancer survival: a follow-up 10 years after diagnosis. Psychosom Med. 2003;65(4):636–43.

7 Penninx BW, Guralnik JM, Pahor M, et al. Chronically depressed mood and cancer risk in older persons. J Natl Cancer Inst. 1998;90(24):1888–93.

8 Serraino D, Pezzotti P, Fratino L, et al. Chronically depressed mood and cancer risk in older persons. J Natl Cancer Inst. 1999 Jun 16;91(12):1080–1.

9 Steel JL, Geller DA, Gamblin TC, Olek MC, Carr BI. Depression, immunity, and survival in patients with hepatobiliary carcinoma. J Clin Oncol. 2007;25(17):2397–405.

10 Faller H, Bulzebruck H, Drings P, Lang H. Coping, distress, and survival among patients with lung cancer. Archives of General Psychiatry. 1999;56(8):756–62.

11 Greer S, Morris T, Pettingale KW, Haybittle JL. Psychological response to breast cancer and 15 year outcome. Lancet. 1990;1:49–50.

12 Rogentine GN, Van Kammen DP, Fox BH, et al. Psychological factors in the prognosis of malignant melanoma: a prospective study. Psychosom Med. 1979;41:647–655.

13 Richardson J, Zarnegar Z, Bisno B, Levine A. Psychosocial status at initiation of cancer treatment and survival. J Psychosomatic Essence of Health TEXT.indd 388 Research 1990;34(2):189–201.

14 Montazeri A, Gillis CR, McEwen J. Quality of life in patients with lung cancer: a review of literature from 1970 to 1995. Chest. 1998;113:467–481.

15 Coates A, Gebski V, Signorini D, et al. for the Australian New Zealand Breast Cancer Trials Group. Prognostic value of quality-of-life scores during chemotherapy for advanced breast cancer. J Clin Oncol. 1992;10:1833–1838.

16 Dancey J, Zee B, Osoba D, et al. Quality of life scores: an independent prognostic variable in a general population of cancer patients receiving chemotherapy. Qual Life Res. 1997;6:151–158.

17 Coates AS, Hurny C, Peterson HF, et al. Quality-of-life scores predict outcome in metastatic but not early breast cancer. International Breast Cancer Study

Group. J Clin Oncol. 2000;18(22):3768–74.

18 Butow P, Coates A, Dunn S. Psychosocial predictors of survival in metastatic melanoma. J Clinical Oncology 1999;17(12):3856–63.

19 Falagas ME, Zarkadoulia EA, Ioannidou EN et al. The effect of psychosocial factors on breast cancer outcome: a systematic review. Breast Cancer Res. 2007;9(4):R44.

20 Falagas ME, Zarkadoulia EA, Ioannidou EN, et al. The effect of psychosocial factors on breast cancer outcome: a systematic review. Breast Cancer Res. 2007;9(4):R44.

21 Gottlieb BH, Wachala ED. Cancer support groups: a critical review of empirical studies. Psychooncol. 2007;16(5):379–400.

22 Spiegel D, et al. Effect of psychosocial treatment on survival of patients with metastatic breast cancer. Lancet 1989;2:888–891.

23 Fawzy F, et al. Malignant melanoma; Effects of an early structured psychiatric intervention, coping and affective state on recurrence and survival six years later. Arch Gen Psych 1993;50:681–89.

24 Fawzy FI, Canada AL, Fawzy NW. Malignant melanoma: effects of a brief, structured psychiatric intervention on survival and recurrence at 10-year follow-up. Arch Gen Psychi 2003;60(1):100–3.

25 Richardson JL, Shelton DR, Krailo M, Levine AM. The effect of compliance with treatment on survival among patients with hematologic malignancies. J Clin Oncol 1990;8:356–64.

26 Kuchler T, Henne-Bruns D, Rappat S, et al. Impact of psychotherapeutic support on gastrointestinal cancer patients undergoing surgery: survival results of a trial. Hepato-Gastroenterol. 1999;46(25):322–35.

27 Ratcliffe MA, Dawson AA, Walker LG. Personality Inventory L-scores in patients with Hodgkin's disease and non Hodgkin's lymphoma. Psychooncol 1995;4:39–45.

28 Kuchler T, Bestmann B, Rappat S, et al. Impact of psychotherapeutic support for patients with gastrointestinal cancer undergoing surgery: 10-year survival results of a randomized trial. J Clin Oncol. 2007;25(19):2702–8.

29 Cunningham AJ, Edmonds CV, Phillips C, et al. A prospective, longitudinal study of the relationship of psychological work to duration of survival in patients with metastatic cancer. Psycho-Oncol. 2000;9(4):323–39.

30 Edelman S, Lemon J, Bell DR, et al. Effects of group CBT on the survival time of patients with metastatic breast cancer. Psycho-Oncology. 1999;8(6):474–81.

31 Ilnyckyj A, Farber J, Cheang MC, Weinerman BH. A randomized controlled trial of psychotherapeutic intervention in cancer patients. Ann R Coll Phys Surg Can 1994;27:93–6.

32 Linn MW, Linn BS, Harris R. Effects of counseling for late stage cancer patients. Cancer 1982;49:1048–55.

33 Goodwin PJ, Leszcz M, Ennis M, et al. The effect of group psychosocial support on survival in metastatic breast cancer. N Engl J Med 2001;345:1719–26.

34 Kissane DW, Grabsch B, Clarke DM, et al. Supportive-expressive group therapy for women with metastatic breast cancer: survival and psychosocial outcome from a randomized controlled trial. Psychooncol. 2007;16(4):277–86.

35 Fawzy FI. Psychosocial interventions for patients with cancer: what works and what doesn't. Eur J Cancer 1999;35(11):1559–64.

36 Cunningham A, Phillips C, Lockwood G, et al. Association of involvement in psychological self-regulation with longer survival in patients with metastatic cancer: an exploratory study. Advan Mind-Body Med 2000;16(4):276–87.

37 Rehse B, Pukrop R. Effects of psychosocial interventions on quality of life in adult cancer patients: meta analysis of 37 published controlled outcome studies. Patient Educ Couns. 2003;50(2):179–86.

38 Visintainer MA, Volpicelli JR, Seligman ME. Tumor rejection in rats after inescapable or escapable shock. Science. 1982;216(4544):437–9.

39 Watson M, Homewood J, Haviland J, Bliss JM. Influence of psychological response on breast cancer survival: 10-year follow-up of a population-based cohort. Europ J Cancer. 2005;41(12):1710–4.

40 Schulman P, Keith D, Seligman ME. Is optimism heritable? A study of twins. Behav Res Ther.1993;31(6):569–74.

41 Petticrew M, Bell R, Hunter D. Influence of psychological coping on survival and recurrence in people with cancer: systematic review. BMJ. 2002;325(7372):1066.

42 Spiegel D, Giese-Davis J. Depression and cancer: mechanisms and disease progression. Biol Psychiatry. 2003;54(3):269–82.

43 Rabbitts J. Chromosomal translocations in human cancer. Nature 1994;372:143.

44 Abercrombie HC, Giese-Davis J, Sephton S, et al. Flattened cortisol rhythms in metastatic breast cancer patients. Psychoneuroendocrinol. 2004;29(8):1082–92.

45 Sephton SE. Sapolsky RM. Kraemer HC. Spiegel D. Diurnal cortisol rhythm as a predictor of breast cancer survival. J Nat Cancer Instit. 2000;92(12):994–1000.

46 Turner-Cobb JM, Sephton SE, Koopman C, et al. Social support and salivary cortisol in women with metastatic breast cancer. Psychosom Med. 2000;62(3):337–45.

47 Oliver R. Does surgery disseminate or accelerate cancer? Lancet 1995;346:1506.

48 Chrousos G. The HPA axis and immune mediated inflammation. N Engl J Med 1995;332:1351.

49 Kearney R. From theory to practice – The implications of the latest psychoneuroimmunology research and how to apply them. MIH Conference Proceedings 1998;171–88.

50 Bushell WC. From molecular biology to anti-aging cognitive-behavioral practices: the pioneering research

of Walter Pierpaoli on the pineal and bone marrow foreshadows the contemporary revolution in stem cell and regenerative biology. Ann N Y Acad Sci. 2005;1057:28–49.

51 Chrousos G. The HPA axis and immune mediated inflammation. N Engl J Med 1995;332:1351.

52 Kearney R. From theory to practice – The implications of the latest psychoneuroimmunology research and how to apply them. MIH Conference Proceedings 1998;171–88.

53 Holmgren L, et al. Dormancy of micrometastases; Balanced proliferation and apoptosis in the presence of angiogenesis suppression. Nature Med 1995;1:149.

54 Kune S, et al. Recent life change and large bowel cancer. J Clin Epidemiol 1991;44:57–68.

55 Kiecolt-Glaser J, Stephens R, Lipetz P, et al. Distress and DNA repair in human lymphocytes. J Behav Med 1985;8(4):311–20.

56 Irie M, Asami S, Nagata S, et al. Relationships between perceived workload, stress and oxidative DNA damage. Int Arch Occup Environ Health 2001;74(2):153–7.

57 Irie M, Asami S, Nagata S et al. Psychological factors as a potential trigger of oxidative DNA damage in human leukocytes. Jpn J Cancer Res 2001;92(3):367–76.

58 Irie M, Asami S, Nagata S, et al. Psychological mediation of a type of oxidative DNA damage, 8-hydroxydeoxyguanosine, in peripheral blood leukocytes of non-smoking and non-drinking workers. Psychother Psychosom 2002;71(2):90–6.

59 Tomei LD, Kiecolt-Glaser JK, Kennedy S, Glaser R. Psychological stress and phorbol ester inhibition of radiation-induced apoptosis in human peripheral blood leukocytes. Psychi Res.1990;33(1):59–71.

60 Pero RW, Roush GC, Markowitz MM, Miller DG. Oxidative stress, DNA repair, and cancer susceptibility. Cancer Detect Prev 1990;14(5):555–61.

61 Kiecolt-Glaser JK, Robles TF, Heffner KL, et al. Psycho-oncology and cancer: psychoneuroimmunology and cancer. Ann Oncol. 2002;13 Suppl 4:165–9.

62 Miller SC, Pandi-Perumal SR, Esquifino AI, et al. The role of melatonin in immuno-enhancement: potential application in cancer. Int J Experi Path. 2006;87(2):81–7.

63 Lissoni P. Biochemotherapy with standard chemotherapies plus the pineal hormone melatonin in the treatment of advanced solid neoplasms. Pathologie Biologie. 2007;55(3–4):201–4.

64 Mills E, Wu P, Seely D, Guyatt G. Melatonin in the treatment of cancer: a systematic review of randomized controlled trials and meta-analysis. J Pineal Res. 2005;39(4):360–6.

65 Maestroni GJ, Conti A, Pierpaoli W. Role of the pineal gland in immunity. J. Neuroimmunol. 1986;13:19–30.

66 Pierpaoli W. Neuroimmunomodulation of aging. a program in the pineal gland. Ann. NY Acad. Sci. 1998;840:491–497.

67 Reiter R and Robinson J. In *Melatonin* Bantam

Books: New York, London 1995.

68 Panzer A, Viljoen M. The validity of melatonin as an oncostatic agent. J Pineal Res. 1997;22(4):184–202.

69 Sephton S, Spiegel D. Circadian disruption in cancer: a neuroendocrine-immune pathway from stress to disease?. Brain Behav Immun. 2003;17(5):321–8.

70 Franzese E, Nigri G. Night work as a possible risk factor for breast cancer in nurses. Correlation between the onset of tumors and alterations in blood melatonin levels. Prof Inferm. 2007;60(2):89–93.

71 Massion AO, Teas J, Hebert JR, Wertheimer MD, Kabat-Zinn J. Meditation, melatonin and breast/ prostate cancer: hypothesis and preliminary data. Med Hypoth. 1995;44(1):39–46.

72 Tooley GA, Armstrong SM, Norman TR, Sali A. Acute increases in night-time plasma melatonin levels following a period of meditation. Biolog Psych 2000;53(1):69–78.

73 Kearney R. From theory to practice – The implications of the latest psychoneuroimmunology research and how to apply them. MIH Conference Proceedings 1998;171–88.

74 Brzezinski A. Melatonin in humans. N Engl J Med 1997;336:186.

75 Weindruch R, Sohal RS. Seminars in medicine of the Beth Israel Deaconess Medical Center. Caloric intake and aging. N Engl J Med. 1997 Oct 2;337(14):986-94

76 Heuther G. Melatonin synthesis in the GI tract and the impact on nutritional factors on circulating melatonin. Annals NY Acad Sci 1994;719:146.

77 Cronin AJ, Keifer JC, Davies MF, et al. Melatonin secretion after surgery. Lancet. 2000 Oct 7;356(9237):1244-5.

78 Lutgendorf SK, Johnsen EL, Cooper B et al. Vascular endothelial growth factor and social support in patients with ovarian carcinoma. Cancer 2002;95(4):808–15.

79 Onogawa S, Tanaka S, Oka S, et al. Clinical significance of angiogenesis in rectal carcinoid tumors. Oncol Rep 2002;9(3):489–94.

80 Thaker PH, Han LY, Kamat AA, et al. Chronic stress promotes tumor growth and angiogenesis in a mouse model of ovarian carcinoma. Nat Med. 2006 Jul 23; [Epub ahead of print]

81 Carlson LE, Speca M, Faris P, Patel KD. One year pre-post intervention follow-up of psychological, immune, endocrine and blood pressure outcomes of mindfulness-based stress reduction (MBSR) in breast and prostate cancer outpatients. Brain Behav Immun. 2007;21(8):1038–49.

82 Kune G, Kune S, Watson L. Perceived religiousness is protective for colorectal cancer: data from the Melbourne Colorectal Cancer Study. J Royal Soc Med.1993;86:645–7.

83 Jim HS, Andersen BL. Meaning in life mediates the relationship between social and physical functioning and distress in cancer survivors. Br J Health Psychol. 2007;12(Pt 3):363–81.

84 Astin J, Harkness E, Ernst E. The efficacy of

'Distant Healing': A systematic review of randomised trials. Ann Int Med 2000;132(11):903–10.

85 http://www.wcrf-uk.org/cancer_ prevention/index.lasso

86 Slattery M, Potter J, Caan B, et al. Energy balance and colon cancer – beyond physical activity. Cancer Res. 1997;57:75–80.

87 Colditz G, Cannuscio C, Grazier A. Physical activity and reduced risk of colon cancer. Cancer Caus Cont. 1997;8:649–667.

88 Thune I, Lund E. The influence of physical activity on lung cancer risk. Int J Cancer. 1997;70:57–62.

89 Rockhill B, Willett WC, Hunter DJ, et al. A prospective study of recreational physical activity and breast cancer risk. Arch Intern Med. 1999 Oct 25;159(19):2290-6.

90 McTiernan, et al. Recreational physical activity and the risk of breast cancer in post menopausal women: The Women's Health Initiative Cohort Study. JAMA 2003;290:1331–1336.

91 Thune I, Lund E. The influence of physical activity on lung cancer risk. Int J Cancer 1997;70:57–62.

92 Holmes MD, Chen WY, Feskanich D, et al. Physical activity and survival after breast cancer diagnosis. JAMA. 2005;293(20):2479–86.

93 Pierce JP, Stefanick ML, Flatt SW, et al. Greater survival after breast cancer in physically active women with high vegetable-fruit intake regardless of obesity. J Clin Oncol. 2007;25(17):2345–51.

94 Giovannucci EL, Liu Y, Leitzmann MF, et al. A prospective study of physical activity and incident and fatal prostate cancer. Arch Intern Med. 2005;165(9):1005–10.

95 Haydon AM, Macinnis RJ, English DR, Giles GG. Effect of physical activity and body size on survival after diagnosis with colorectal cancer. Gut. 2006 Jan;55(1):62-7.

96 Morgan G, Ward R, Barton M. The contribution of cytotoxic chemotherapy to 5-year survival in adult malignancies. Clin Oncol (R Coll Radiol). 2004 Dec;16(8):549-60.

97 Galvao DA, Newton RU. Review of exercise intervention studies in cancer patients. J Clin Oncol. 2005;23(4):899–909.

98 Borjesson M, Karlsson J, Mannheimer C. Relief of pain by exercise. Increased physical activity can be a part of the therapeutic program in both acute and chronic pain. Lakartidningen. 2001;98(15):1786–91.

99 Doll R, Peto R. The causes of cancer: quantitative estimates of avoidable risks of cancer in the United States today. J. Natl. Cancer Inst. 1981;66 1196–1265.

100 Key TJ, Allen NE, Spencer EA, et al. The effect of diet on risk of cancer. Lancet 2002;360:861–868.

101 Ahn J, Gammon MD, Santella RM, et al. Associations between breast cancer risk and the catalase genotype, fruit and vegetable consumption, and supplement use. Am J Epidemiol. 2005 Nov 15;162(10):943-52. Epub 2005 Sep.

102 Moss RW. Do antioxidants interfere with radiation therapy for cancer? Integr Cancer Ther. 2007 Sep;6(3):281–92.

103 Kritchevsky D. Caloric restriction and experimental carcinogenesis. Toxicol Sci. 1999 Dec;52(2 Suppl):13–6.

104 Miller M. Can reducing caloric intake also help reduce cancer? J Natl Cancer Inst. 1998 Dec 2;90(23):1766–7.

105 Miller M. Can reducing caloric intake also help reduce cancer? J Natl Cancer Inst. 1998 Dec 2;90(23):1766–7.

106 Chlebowski RT, Blackburn GL, Thomson CA, et al. Dietary fat reduction and breast cancer outcome: interim efficacy results from the Women's Intervention Nutrition Study. J Natl Cancer Inst. 2006 Dec 20;98(24):1767-76.

107 Bandera EV, Kushi LH, Moore DF, et al. Consumption of animal foods and endometrial cancer risk: a systematic literature review and meta-analysis. Cancer Caus Cont. 2007;18(9):967–88. Epub 2007 Jul 19.

108 Pierce JP, Stefanick ML, Flatt SW, et al. Greater survival after breast cancer in physically active women with high vegetable-fruit intake regardless of obesity. J Clin Oncol. 2007;25(17):2345–51.

109 Rock CL, Flatt SW, Natarajan L, et al. Plasma carotenoids and recurrence-free survival in women with a history of breast cancer. J Clin Oncol. 2005 Sep 20;23(27):6631-8.

110 Divisi D, Di Tommaso S, Salvemini S, et al. Diet and cancer. Acta Biomed. 2006 Aug;77(2):118–23.

111 D.T.H. Verhoeven, R.A. Goldbohm, G. van Poppel, H. Verhagen, P.A. van den Brandt. Epidemiological studies on Brassica vegetables and cancer risk. Cancer Epidemiol. Biomarkers Prev. 1996;5: 733–748

112 Brennan P, Hsu CC, Moullan N, et al. Effect of cruciferous vegetables on lung cancer in patients stratified by genetic status: a mendelian randomisation approach. Lancet. 2005;366(9496):1558–60.

113 Traka M, Gasper AV, Melchini A, et al. Broccoli consumption interacts with GSTM1 to perturb oncogenic signalling pathways in the prostate. PLoS ONE. 2008 Jul 2;3(7):e2568.

114 Conway C, et al. Disposition of glucosinolates and sulforaphane in humans after ingestion of steamed and fresh broccoli. Nut Cancrt 2000;38(2):168–78.

115 Fleischauer AT, Arab L. Garlic and cancer: a critical review of the epidemioiological literature. J. Nutr. 2001;131: 1032S–1040S.

116 Madgee PJ, Rowland IR. Phytooestrogens, their mechanism of action: current evidence for a role in breast and prostate cancer. Br. J. Nut 2004; 91:513–531.

117 Cotterchio M; Boucher BA, Manno M, et al. Dietary phytoestrogen intake is associated with reduced colorectal cancer risk. J. Nutri; Dec 2006;136,12;Health Module,3046

118 Verheus M, van Gils CH, Keinan-Boker L, et al. Plasma phytoestrogens and subsequent breast cancer risk. J Clin Oncol. 2007 Feb 20;25(6):648-55.

119 Larsson SC, Kumlin M, Ingelman-Sundberg M et al. Dietary long chain n-3 fatty acids for

the prevention of cancer: a review of potential mechanisms. Am. J. Clin. Nutr. 2004; 79: 935–945

120 Pelletier K. Mind-body health: research, clinical and policy applications. Am J Health Promot 1992; 6(5):345–58.

121 House J, Landis K, Umberson D. Social relationships and health. Science 1988;241:540–5.

122 Falagas ME, Zarkadoulia EA, Ioannidou EN, et al. The effect of psychosocial factors on breast cancer outcome: a systematic review. Breast Cancer Res. 2007 Jul 17;9(4):R44 [Epub ahead of print]

123 Kune G. *Reducing the Odds: a manual for the prevention of cancer.* Allen and Unwin. Sydney, 1999.

124 Taylor R, Najafi F, Dobson A. Meta-analysis of studies of passive smoking and lung cancer: effects of study type and continent. Int J Epidemiol. 2007 Oct;36(5):1048–59.

125 Davis S, Mirick DK. Residential magnetic fields, medication use, and the risk of breast cancer. Epidemiol. 2007 Mar;18(2):266–9.

126 Henshaw DL, Reiter RJ. Do magnetic fields cause increased risk of childhood leukemia via melatonin disruption? Bioelectromagnet. 2005;Suppl 7:S86–97.

127 Andrieu N, Easton DF, Chang-Claude J, et al. Effect of chest X-rays on the risk of breast cancer among BRCA1/2 mutation carriers in the international BRCA1/2 carrier cohort study: a report from the EMBRACE, GENEPSO, GEO-HEBON, and IBCCS Collaborators' Group. J Clin Oncol. 2006 Jul 20;24(21):3361–6.

128 Ornish D, Weidner G, Fair WR, et al. Intensive lifestyle changes may affect the progression of prostate cancer. J Urol. 2005;174(3):1065–9.

Chapter 12: Diabetes

1 Crespo PS, Prieto Perera JA, Lodeiro FA, Azuara LA. Metabolic syndrome in childhood. Public Health Nutr. 2007 Oct;10(10A):1121–5.

2 Steyn NP, Mann J, Bennett PH, et al. Diet, nutrition and the prevention of Type-2 diabetes. Public Health Nutr. 2004;7(1A):147–65.

3 Sepa A, Ludvigsson J. Psychological stress and the risk of diabetes-related autoimmunity: a review article. Neuroimmunomodulat. 2006;13(5–6):301–8.

4 Surwit RS, van Tilburg MA, Zucker N, et al. Stress management improves long-term glycemic control in Type-2 diabetes. Diabetes Care 2002;25(1):30–4.

5 Fitchett G, Murphy PE, Kim J, et al. Religious struggle: prevalence, correlates and mental health risks in diabetic, congestive heart failure, and oncology patients. Int J Psychiatry Med. 2004;34(2):179–96.

6 Polzer RL, Miles MS. Spirituality in African Americans with diabetes: self-management through a relationship with God. Qual Health Res. 2007 Feb;17(2):176–88.

7 Giles BG, Findlay CS, Haas G, et al. Integrating conventional science and aboriginal perspectives on diabetes using fuzzy cognitive maps. Soc Sci Med. 2007 Feb;64(3):562–76.

8 Helmrich S, Ragland D, Paffenbarger R. Prevention of non-insulin dependent diabetes mellitus with physical activity. Med Sci Sports Exerc. 1994;26: 649–660.

9 Williams PT, Franklin B. Vigorous Exercise and Diabetic, Hypertensive, and Hypercholesterolemia Medication Use. Med Sci Sports Exerc. 2007 Nov;39(11):1933–1941.

10 Norris JM, Yin X, Lamb MM, et al. Omega-3 polyunsaturated fatty acid intake and islet autoimmunity in children at increased risk for Type-1 diabetes. JAMA. 2007 Sep 26;298(12): 1420–8.

11 Tuomilehto J, Linström J, Eriksson JG, et al. Prevention of Type-2 Diabetes Mellitus by changes in lifestyle among subjects with impaired glucose tolerance. N Engl J Med, 2001;334:1343–1350.

12 Choudhary P. Review of dietary recommendations for diabetes mellitus. Diabetes Res Clinical Prac. 2004;65:S9–15.

13 Barclay AW, Flood VM, Rochtchina E, et al. Glycemic index, dietary fiber, and risk of Type-2 diabetes in a cohort of older Australians. Diabetes Care. 2007 Nov;30(11):2811–3.

14 Brand-Miller J, Hayne S, Petocz P, Colagiuri S. Low-glycemic index diets in the management of diabetes: a meta-analysis of randomized controlled trials. Diabetes Care. 2003 Aug;26(8):2261–7.

15 Dietitians Association of Australia review paper Glycaemic index in diabetes management. Aust J Nutr and Dietetics 1997; 54:57–63

16 Sydney University Glycemic Index Research Service (SUGiRS)

17 White AM, Johnston CS. Vinegar ingestion at bedtime moderates waking glucose concentrations in adults with well-controlled Type-2 diabetes. Diabetes Care. 2007 Nov;30(11):2814–5.

18 Sipetic S, Vlajinac H, Marinkovi J, et al. Stressful life events and psychological dysfunctions before the onset of type 1 diabetes mellitus. J Pediatr Endocrinol Metab. 2007 Apr;20(4):527-34.

19 Biros E, Jordan MA, Baxter AG. Genes mediating environment interactions in Type-1 diabetes. Rev Diabet Stud. 2005 Winter;2(4):192–207.

20 Dahlquist G, Mustonen L. Childhood onset diabetes – time trends and climatological factors. Int J Epidemiol 1994;23(6):1234–41.

Chapter 13: Multiple sclerosis

1 Ackerman KD, Stover A, Heyman R, et al. Relationship of cardiovascular reactivity, stressful life events, and multiple sclerosis disease activity. Brain Behav Immun. 2003;17(3):141–51.

2 Marsland AL, Bachen EA, Cohen S, et al. Stress, immune reactivity and susceptibility to infectious disease. Physiol Behav. 2002;77(4–5):711–6.

3 Mohr DC, Hart SL, Julian L, Cox D, Pelletier D. Association between stressful life events and exacerbation in multiple sclerosis: a meta-analysis. BMJ. 2004 Mar 27;328(7442):731.

4 Mohr DC, Goodkin DE, Nelson S, et al. Moderating

effects of coping on the relationship between stress and the development of new brain lesions in multiple sclerosis. Psychosom Med. 2002;64(5):803–9.

5 Mohr DC, Goodkin DE, Bacchetti P, et al. Psychological stress and the subsequent appearance of new brain MRI lesions in MS. Neurology. 2000;55(1):55–61.

6 Mohr DC, Cox D. Multiple sclerosis: empirical literature for the clinical health psychologist. J Clin Psychol. 2001;57(4):479–99.

7 Lalive PH, Burkhard PR, Choffl on M. TNF-alpha and psychologically stressful events in healthy subjects: potential relevance for multiple sclerosis relapse. Behav Neurosci. 2002 Dec;116(6):1093–7.

8 Wood GJ, Bughi S, Morrison J, et al. Hypnosis, differential expression of cytokines by T-cell subsets, and the hypothalamopituitary-adrenal axis. Am J Clin Hypn 2003 Jan;45(3):179–96

9 Carlson LE, Speca M, Patel KD, Goodey E. Mindfulness-based stress reduction in relation to quality of life, mood, symptoms of stress, and immune parameters in breast and prostate cancer outpatients. Psychosom Med. 2003;65(4):571–81.

10 Davidson RJ, Kabat-Zinn J, Schumacher J, Rosenkranz M, Muller D, Santorelli SF, Urbanowski F, Harrington A, Bonus K, Sheridan JF. Alterations in brain and immune function produced by mindfulness meditation. Psychosom Med. 2003 Jul–Aug;65(4):564–70.

11 Büssing A, Ostermann T, Matthiessen PF. Role of religion and spirituality in medical patients: confirmatory results with the SpREUK questionnaire. Health Qual Life Outcomes. 2005 Feb 10;3:10.

12 Tesar N, Baumhackl U, Kopp M, Gunther V. Effects of psychological group therapy in patients with multiple sclerosis. Acta Neurologica Scandinavica. 107(6):394–9, 2003 Jun.

13 Sutherland G, Andersen MB. Exercise and multiple sclerosis: physiological, psychological, and quality of life issues. J Sports Med Phys Fitness 2001; 41:421–32.

14 Sadovnick AD, Remick RA, Allen J, et al. Depression and multiple sclerosis. Neurology 1996; 46:628–32.

15 Stuifbergen AK, Blozis SA, Harrison TC, et al. Exercise, functional limitations, and quality of life: A longitudinal study of persons with multiple sclerosis. Arch Phys Med Rehabil 2006; 87:935–943.

16 Ornish D, Brown SE, Scherwitz LW, et al. Can lifestyle changes reverse coronary heart disease? The Lifestyle Heart Trial. Lancet. 1990;336(8708):129–33.

17 Swank RL. Dugan BB. Effect of low saturated fat diet in early and late cases of multiple sclerosis. Lancet. 1990;336(8706):37–9.

18 Swank RL, Multiple sclerosis: fat-oil relationship. Nutrition. 1991;7(5):368–76.

19 Fitzgerald G, Harbige LS, Forti A, Crawford MA. The effect of nutritional counselling on diet and plasma EFA status in multiple sclerosis patients over 3 years. Hum Nutr Appl Nutr 1987; 41:297–310.

20 Dworkin RH, Bates D, Millar JH, Paty DW. Linoleic acid and multiple sclerosis: a reanalysis of three double-blind trials. Neurology 1984; 34:1441–5.

21 Nordvik I, Myhr KM, Nyland H, Bjerve KS. Effect of dietary advice and n-3 supplementation in newly diagnosed MS patients. Acta Neurol Scand. 2000;102(3):143–9.

22 Weinstock-Guttman B, Baier M, Park Y, et al. Low fat dietary intervention with omega-3 fatty acid supplementation in multiple sclerosis patients. Prostagland Leukot Essent Fatty Acids. 2005;73(5):397–404.

23 National Institute for Clinical Excellence, UK. http://www.nice.org.uk/guidance/CG8

24 Gallai V, Sarchielli P, Trequattrini A, et al. Cytokine secretion and eicosanoid production in the peripheral blood mononuclear cells of MS patients undergoing dietary supplementation with n-3 polyunsaturated fatty acids. J Neuroimmunol 1995; 56:143–53.

25 Lauer K. The risk of multiple sclerosis in the U.S.A. in relation to sociogeographic features: a factor-analytic study. J Clin Epidemiol 1994; 47:43–8.

26 Ghadirian P, Jain M, Ducic S et al. Nutritional factors in the aetiology of Multiple Sclerosis: a case control study in Montreal, Canada. Int J Epidemiol. 1998;27:845–52.

27 Sepcic J, Mesaros E, Materljan E, Sepic-Grahovac D. Nutritional factors and multiple sclerosis in Gorski Kotar, Croatia. Neuroepidemiol. 1993; 12:234–40.

28 Gusev E, Boiko A, Lauer K, Riise T, Deomina T. Environmental risk factors in MS: a case-control study in Moscow. Acta Neurol Scand 1996; 94:386–94.

29 Malosse D, Perron H, Sasco A, Seigneurin JM. Correlation between milk and dairy product consumption and multiple sclerosis prevalence: a worldwide study. Neuroepidemiol. 1992; 11:304–12.

30 Das UN. Is there a role for saturated and long-chain fatty acids in multiple sclerosis? Nutrition. 2003;19(2):163–6.

31 Embry AF, Snowdon LR, Veith R. Vitamin D and seasonal fl uctuations of gadolinium-enhancing magnetic resonance imaging lesions in multiple sclerosis. Ann Neurol. 2000;48:271–2.

32 Hayes CE. Vitamin D: a natural inhibitor of multiple sclerosis. Proceedings of the Nutrition Society. 2000;59(4):531–5.

33 Goldberg P. Multiple sclerosis: decreased relapse rate through dietary supplementation with calcium, magnesium and vitamin D. Med Hypoth. 1986;21:193–200.

34 Munger KL, Levin LI, Hollis BW, Howard NS, Ascherio A. Serum 25-hydroxyvitamin D levels and risk of multiple sclerosis. JAMA. 2006;296(23):2832–8.

35 Embry AF, Snowdon LR, Vieth R. Vitamin D and seasonal fl uctuations of gadolinium-enhancing magnetic resonance imaging lesions in multiple sclerosis. Ann Neurol 2000; 48:271–2.

36 Munger KL, Zhang SM, O'Reilly E, et al. Vitamin D intake and incidence of multiple sclerosis. Neurology. 2004;62(1):60–5.

37 Strenge H. The relationship between psychological

stress and the clinical course of multiple sclerosis. An update. Psychother Psychosom Med Psychol. 2001;51(3–4):166–75.

38 Homo-Delarche F, Fitzpatrick F, Christeff N, et al. Sex steroids, glucocorticoids, stress and autoimmunity. J Ster Biochem Molec Biol. 1991;40(4–6):619–37.

39 O'Reilly MA, O'Reilly PM. Temporal influences on relapses of multiple sclerosis. Euro Neurol. 1991;31(6):391–5.

40 McMichael AJ, Hall AJ. Does immunosuppressive ultraviolet radiation explain the latitude gradient for multiple sclerosis? Epidemiol. 1997;8:642–5.

41 Esparza ML, Sasaki S, Kesteloot H. Nutrition, latitude, and multiple sclerosis mortality: an ecologic study. Am J Epidemiol. 1995;142:733–7.

42 Hutter CD, Laing P. Multiple sclerosis: sunlight, diet, immunology and aetiology. Med Hypoth. 1996;46(2):67–74.

43 Freedman DM, Dosemeci M, Alavanja MC. Mortality from multiple sclerosis and exposure to residential and occupational solar radiation: a case-control study based on death certificates. Occupat Enviro Med. 2000;57(6):418–21.

44 van der Mei IA, Ponsonby AL, Blizzard L, Dwyer T. Regional variation in multiple sclerosis prevalence in Australia and its association with ambient ultraviolet radiation. Neuroepidemiol. 2001; 20:168–74.

45 Freedman DM, Dosemeci M, Alavanja MC. Mortality from multiple sclerosis and exposure to residential and occupational solar radiation: a case-control study based on death certificates. Occupat Enviro Med. 2000;57(6):418–21.

46 van der Mei IA, Ponsonby AL, Blizzard L, Dwyer T. Regional variation in multiple sclerosis prevalence in Australia and its association with ambient ultraviolet radiation. Neuroepidemiol. 2001; 20:168–74.

47 van der Mei IA, Ponsonby AL, Dwyer T, et al. Past exposure to sun, skin phenotype, and risk of multiple sclerosis: case-control study. BMJ. 2003 Aug 9; 327(7410): 316.

48 Green MH, Petit-Frere C, Clingen PH, et al. Possible effects of sunlight on human lymphocytes. J Epidemiol. 1999;9(6 Suppl): S48–57.

Chapter 14: Asthma

1 Isenberg SA, Lehrer PM, Hochron S. The effects of suggestion and emotional arousal on pulmonary function in asthma: a review and a hypothesis regarding vagal mediation. Psychosom Med. 1992 Mar-Apr;54(2):192-216.

2 Lehrer PM. Emotionally triggered asthma: a review of research literature and some hypotheses for self-regulation therapies. Appl Psychophysiol Biofeedback. 1998 Mar;23(1):13–41

3 Lehrer PM, Isenberg S, Hochron SM. Asthma and emotion: a review. J Asthma. 1993;30(1):5–21

4 Mrazek D. 'Psychiatric complications of paediatric asthma.' Ann All.1992;69:285–90.

5 Mrazek D, et al. 'Early asthma onset: Consideration of parenting issues.' J Am Acad Child Adolesc Psychi.

1991;30:277–82.

6 Lehrer PM. Emotionally triggered asthma: a review of research literature and some hypotheses for self-regulation therapies. App Psychophysiol Biofeedback. 1998;23(1):13–41.

7 Strunk RC, Mrazek DA, Fuhrmann GS, LaBrecque JF. Physiologic and psychological characteristics associated with deaths due to asthma in childhood. A case-controlled study. JAMA. 1985 Sep 6;254(9):1193–8.

8 Klinnert MD, Mrazek PJ, Mrazek DA. Early asthma onset: the interaction between family stressors and adaptive parenting. Psychiatry. 1994 Feb;57(1):51–61.

9 Godfrey S, et al. Demonstration by placebo response in asthma by means of exercise testing. J Psychosom Res 1973;17:291–97.

10 Huntley A, White AR, Ernst E. Relaxation therapies for asthma: a systematic review. Thorax. 2002 Feb;57(2):127-31.

11 Peper E, Tibbetts V. Fifteen-month follow-up with asthmatics utilizing EMG/incentive inspirometer feedback. Biofeedback Self Regul. 1992 Jun;17(2): 143-51.

12 Devine EC. Meta-analysis of the effects of psychoeducational care in adults with asthma. Res Nurs Health. 1996 Oct;19(5):367-76.

13 Lehrer PM, Sargunaraj D, Hochron S. Psychological approaches to the treatment of asthma. J Consult Clin Psychol. 1992 Aug; 60(4):639-43

14 Lehrer PM. Emotionally triggered asthma: a review of research literature and some hypotheses for self-regulation therapies. App Psychophysiol Biofeedback. 1998;23(1):13–41.

15 Lehrer PM. Emotionally triggered asthma: a review of research literature and some hypotheses for self-regulation therapies. App Psychophysiol Biofeedback. 1998;23(1):13–41.

16 Murphy AI, Lehrer PM, Karlin R, et al. Hypnotic susceptibility and its relationship to outcome in the behavioral treatment of asthma: some preliminary data. Psychol Rep. 1989 Oct; 65(2):691–8.

17 Morrison JB. Chronic asthma and improve-ment with relaxation induced by hypnotherapy. J R Soc Med. 1988 Dec;81(12):701–4.

18 Smyth JM, Stone AA, Hurewitz A, Kaell A. Effects of writing about stressful experiences on symptom reduction in patients with asthma or rheumatoid arthritis: a randomized trial. JAMA. 1999 Apr 14;281(14):1304–9.

19 Brown D. Evidence-based hypnotherapy for asthma: a critical review. Int J Clin Exp Hypn. 2007;55(2):220–49.

20 Nagarathna R, et al. Yoga for bronchial asthma: a controlled study. BMJ 1985;291:1077–1079

21 Nagendra H, Nagarathna R. An integrated approach of yoga therapy for bronchial asthma: a 3–54 month prospective study. J Asthm. 1986;23(3):123–137.

22 Singh V, Wisniewski A, Britton J, et al. Effects of Yoga breathing exercises (pranayama) on airway reactivity in subjects with asthma. Lancet

1990;335:1381–3.

23 Weiner P, et al. Inspiratory muscle training in patients with bronchial asthma. Chest 1992;102: 1357–61.

24 Slader CA, Reddel HK, Spencer LM, et al. A double-blind randomised controlled trial of two different breathing techniques in the management of asthma. Thorax. 2006 Jun 5; [Epub ahead of print]

25 Bowler S, Green A, Mitchell C. Buteyko breathing techniques in asthma: a blinded randomised controlled trial. MJA 1998;169:573–4.

26 van Olphen J, Schulz A, Israel B, et al. Religious involvement, social support, and health among African-American women on the east side of Detroit. J Gen Intern Med. 2003 Jul;18(7):549–57.

27 Fulton RA, Moore CM. Spiritual care of the school-age child with a chronic condition. J Pediatr Nurs. 1995 Aug;10(4):224–31.

28 Lucas SR, Platts-Mills TA. Paediatric asthma and obesity. Paediatr Respir Rev. 2006 Dec;7(4):233–8.

29 Parameswaran K, Todd DC, Soth M. Altered respiratory physiology in obesity. Can Respir J. 2006 May–Jun;13(4):203–10.

30 Ram FS, Robinson SM, Black PN, Picot J. Physical training for asthma. Cochrane Database Syst Rev. 2005 Oct 19;(4):CD001116.

31 Hallal PC, Victora CG, Azevedo MR, Wells JC. Adolescent physical activity and health: a systematic review. Sports Med. 2006;36(12):1019–30.

32 Bock SA, Food-related asthma and basic nutrition. J Asth, 1983;20:377–81.

33 Oehling, A. Importance of food allergy in childhood asthma. Allergol. Immunopathol. Suppl., 1981;IX:71–3.

34 Tarlo SM, Sussman GL. Asthma and anaphylactoid reactions to food additives. Can Fam Phys. 1993 May;39:1119-23.

35 Mickleborough TD, Gotshall RW, Cordain L, et al. Dietary salt alters pulmonary function during exercise in exercise-induced asthmatics. J Sports Sci. 2001 Nov;19(11):865-73.

36 L Chatzi, G, Apostolaki, I, Bibakis, I, et al. Protective effect of fruits, vegetables and the Mediterranean diet on asthma and allergies among children in Crete. Thorax 2007;62(8):677–683.

37 Hodge L, Peat JK, Salome C. Increased consumption of polyunsaturated oils may be a cause of increased prevalence of childhood asthma. ANZ J Med 1994;24:727.

38 Haby MM, Peat JK, Marks GB, et al. Asthma in preschool children: prevalence and risk factors. Thorax. 2001 Aug;56(8):589–95.

39 B D Patel, A A Welch, S A Bingham, et al. Dietary antioxidants and asthma in adults. Thorax 2006;61:388–393

40 L Chatzi, G, Apostolaki, I, Bibakis, I, et al. Protective effect of fruits, vegetables and the Mediterranean diet on asthma and allergies among children in Crete. Thorax 2007;62(8):677–683.

41 Woods RK, Walters EH, Raven JM, et al. Food and nutrient intakes and asthma risk in young adults. Am J Clin Nutr 2003;78:414–21.

42 Nishimura T, Wang LY, Kusano K, Kitanaka S. Flavonoids that mimic human ligands from the whole plants of Euphorbia lunulata. Chem Pharm Bull (Tokyo). 2005 Mar;53(3):305-8

43 Lundberg JM, Saria A. Capsaicin-induced desensitization of airway mucosa to cigarette smoke, mechanical and chemical irritants. Nature 1983;302:251–3.

44 Hodge L, Salome CM, Peat JK, et al. Consumption of oily fish and childhood asthma risk. Med J Aust. 1996 Feb 5;164(3):137-40.

45 Reisman J, Schachter HM, Dales RE, et al. Treating asthma with omega-3 fatty acids: where is the evidence? A systematic review. BMC Complement Altern Med. 2006 Jul 19;6:26.

46 Troisi RJ, Willett WC, Weiss ST, et al. A prospective study of diet and adult-onset asthma. Am J Respir Crit Care Med. 1995 May;151(5):1401-8.

47 Thien FC, Woods RK, Walters EH. Oily fish and asthma – a fishy story? Further studies are required before claims can be made of a beneficial effect of oily fish consumption on asthma. Med J Aust. 1996 Feb 5;164(3):135-6.

48 Patel BD, Welch AA, Bingham SA, et al. Dietary antioxidants and asthma in adults. Thorax. 2006;61(5):388–93.

49 Hatch GE. Asthma, inhaled oxidants, and dietary antioxidants. Am J Clin Nutr. 1995 Mar;61(3 Suppl): 625S-630S.

50 Ram FS, Rowe BH, Kaur B. Vitamin C supplementation for asthma. Cochrane Database Syst Rev. 2004;(3):CD000993.

51 Kaslow JE. Double-blind trial of pyridoxine (vitamin B6) in the treatment of steroid-dependent asthma. Ann All. 1993;71(5):492.

52 Reynolds RD, Natta CL. Depressed plasma pyridoxal phosphate concentrations in adult asthmatics. Am J Clin Nutr. 1985;41(4):684–8.

53 Skobeloff EM, Spivey WH, McNamara RM, Greenspon L. Intravenous magnesium sulfate for the treatment of acute asthma in the emergency department. JAMA. 1989 Sep 1; 262(9):1210–3.

54 Strunk RC, Mrazek DA, Fuhrmann GS, et al. Physiologic and psychological characteristics associated with deaths due to asthma in childhood. A case-controlled study. JAMA. 1985;254(9): 1193–8.

Chapter 15: Healthy ageing

1 Lenaz G, Bovina C, D'Aurelio M, et al. Role of mitochondria in oxidative stress and aging. Ann NY Acad Sci 2002;959:199–213.

2 Barrett-Connor E, Grady D, Stefanick ML. The rise and fall of menopausal hormone therapy. Annu Rev Pub Health 2005;26:115–40.

3 Michaud C, Murray C, Bloom B. Burden of disease: implications for future research. JAMA 2001;285(5):535–9.

4 Health United States cited in Breslow L, Breslow N. Health Practices and Disability: some evidence from Alameda County. Prev Med. 1993;22:86–95.

5 Vaupel J. Quotation from The Washington Quarterly, cited in http://www. abc.net.au/health/regions/features/death/ default.htm

6 Olshansky SJ. In search of Methuselah: estimating the upper limits to human longevity. Science 1990;250:634.

7 Fries J. Aging, natural death, and the compression of morbidity. NE J Med. 1980;303:130–5.

8 nceph.anu.edu.au

9 Inglehart R. Globalisation and Postmodern Values. Washington Quarterly 2000;23(1):215–28.

10 Mathers CD, Vos ET, Stevenson CE, Begg SJ. The Australian Burden of Disease Study: measuring the loss of health from diseases, injuries and risk factors. Med J Aust. 2000;172(12):592–6.

11 Rozanski A, Blumenthal J, Kaplan J. Impact of psychosocial factors on the pathogenesis of cardiovascular disease and implications for therapy. Circulat. 1999;99(16):2192–217.

12 Ten S, Maclaren N. Insulin resistance syndrome in children. J Clin Endocrinol Metab. 2004 Jun;89(6):2526–39.

13 Millar J. System performance is the real problem. Healthc Pap. 2001;2(1):79–84, discussion 86–9.

14 Yates LB, Djoussé L, Kurth T, et al. Exceptional Longevity in Men: Modifiable Factors Associated With Survival and Function to Age 90 Years. Arch Intern Med. 2008;168(3):284–290.

15 Human Population Laboratory, California Department of Public Health. Alameda County Population, 1965. Series A, No. 7, 1966.

16 Wiley J, Camacho T. Lifestyle and future health: evidence from the Alameda County Study. Prev Med. 1980;9:1–21.

17 Bushell WC. From molecular biology to anti-aging cognitive-behavioral practices: the pioneering research of Walter Pierpaoli on the pineal and bone marrow foreshadows the contemporary revolution in stem cell and regenerative biology. Ann NY Acad Sci. 2005;1057:28–49.

18 Valliant G, Mukamal K. Successful aging. Am J Psychi. 2001;158(6):839–47.

19 Levy BR, Slade MD, Kunkel SR, Kasl SV. Longevity increased by positive self-perceptions of aging. J Personal Soci Psych. 2002;83(2):261–70.

20 Hummer R, Rogers R, Nam C, et al. Religious involvement and US adult mortality. Demography 1999;36(2):273–85.

21 Everitt AV, Le Couteur DG. Life extension by calorie restriction in humans. Ann NY Acad Sci 2007;1114:428–33.

22 Sohal RS, Weindruch R. Oxidative stress, caloric restriction, and aging. Science 1996; 273: 59–63.

23 Roth GS, Lane MA, Ingram DK, et al. Biomarkers of caloric restriction may predict longevity in humans. Science. 2002 Aug 2;297 (5582):811.

24 Lin SJ, Ford E, Haigis M, Liszt G, Guarente L.

Calorie restriction extends yeast life span by lowering the level of NADH. Genes Dev. 2004;18(1):12–6.

25 Weinert BT, Timiras PS. Invited review: Theories of ageing. J Appl Physiol. 2003;95(4):1706–16.

26 Anisimov VN. Insulin/IGF-1 signaling pathway driving aging and cancer as a target for pharmacological intervention. Exp Gerontol. 2003;38(10):1041–9.

27 Franco OH, Bonneux L, de Laet C, et al. The Polymeal: a more natural, safer, and probably tastier (than the Polypill) strategy to reduce cardiovascular disease by more than 75%. BMJ 2004;329:1447–1450.

28 Ramassamy C. Emerging role of polyphenolic compounds in the treatment of neurodegenerative diseases: a review of their intracellular targets. Eur J Pharmacol. 2006 Sep 1;545(1):51–64.

29 Khan N, Mukhtar H. Tea polyphenols for health promotion. Life Sci. 2007 Jul 26;81(7):519–33.

30 Visioli F, Hagen TM. Nutritional strategies for healthy cardiovascular aging: focus on micronutrients. Pharmacol Res. 2007 Mar;55(3):199–206.

31 Bengmark S. Impact of nutrition on ageing and disease. Curr Opin Clin Nutr Metab Care. 2006 Jan;9(1):2–7.

32 Visioli F, Hagen TM. Nutritional strategies for healthy cardiovascular aging: focus on micronutrients. Pharmacol Res. 2007 Mar;55(3):199–206.

33 Bengmark S. Impact of nutrition on ageing and disease. Curr Opin Clin Nutr Metab Care. 2006 Jan;9(1):2–7.

34 Tapsell LC, Hemphill I, Cobiac L, et al. Health benefits of herbs and spices: the past, the present, the future. Med J Aust. 2006 Aug 21;185(4 Suppl):S4–24.

35 Galeone C, Pelucchi C, Talamini R, et al. Onion and garlic intake and the odds of benign prostatic hyperplasia. Urology. 2007 Oct;70(4):672–6.

36 Jefremov V, Zilmer M, Zilmer K, et al. Antioxidative effects of plant polyphenols: from protection of G protein signaling to prevention of age-related pathologies. Ann NY Acad Sci. 2007 Jan;1095:449–57.

37 Wallace DC. A mitochondrial paradigm of metabolic and degenerative diseases, aging, and cancer: a dawn for evolutionary medicine. Annu Rev Genet 2005;39:359–407.

38 Melov S, Ravenscroft J, Malik S, et al. Extension of life-span with superoxide dismutase/catalase mimetics. Science 2000;289:1567–1569.

39 Kagan T, Davis C, Lin L, Zakeri Z. Coenzyme Q10 can in some circumstances block apoptosis, and this effect is mediated through mitochondria. Ann NY Acad Sci 1999;887:31–47.

40 Perls TT, Reisman NR, Olshansky SJ. Provision or distribution of growth hormone for "antiaging": clinical and legal issues. JAMA 2005;294(16): 2086–90.

41 Yen SS, Morales AJ, Khorram O. Replacement of DHEA in aging men and women. Potential remedial effects. Ann NY Acad Sci 1995;774:128–42.

42 Seeman T, Kaplan G, Knudsen L et al. Social

network ties and mortality among the elderly in the Alameda County Study. Am J Epidemiol. 1987;126:714–23.

Chapter 16: Arthritis

1 Clegg DO, Reda DJ, Harris CL, et al. Glucosamine, chondroitin sulfate, and the two in combination for painful knee osteoarthritis. N Engl J Med. 2006;354(8):795–808.

2 Najm WI, Reinsch S, Hoehler F, et al. S-adenosyl methionine (SAMe) versus celecoxib for the treatment of osteoarthritis symptoms: a double-blind cross-over trial. [ISRCTN36233495]. BMC Musculoskelet Disord. 2004 Feb 26;5:6.

3 Homo-Delarche F, Fitzpatrick F, Christeff N et al. Sex steroids, glucocorticoids, stress and autoimmunity. Steroid Biochem Molec Biol 1991;40:619–37.

4 De Vellis R, De Vellis B, McEvoy H et al. Predictors of pain and functioning in arthritis. Health Educ Res: Theory Pract. 1986;1:61–7.

5 Zautra A, Hoffman J, Potter P, et al. Examination of changes in interpersonal stress as a factor in disease exacerbations among women with rheumatoid arthritis. Ann Behav Med. 1997;19(3):279–86.

6 Papageorgiou C, Panagiotakos DB, Pitsavos C, et al. Association between plasma inflammatory markers and irrational beliefs; the ATTICA epidemiological study. Prog Neuropsychopharmacol Biol Psychiatry. 2006 Jul 14; [Epub ahead of print]

7 Pace TW, Mletzko TC, Alagbe O, et al. Increased stress-induced infl ammatory responses in male patients with major depression and increased early life stress. Am J Psychiatry. 2006;163(9):1630–3.

8 Ottonello M. Cognitive-behavioral interventions in rheumatic diseases. G Ital Med Lav Ergon. 2007 Jan–Mar;29(1 Suppl A):A19–23.

9 Smyth J, et al. Effects of writing about stressful experiences on symptom reduction in patients with asthma or rheumatoid arthritis. A randomised trial. JAMA 1999;281:1304–9.

10 Young LD. Psychological factors in rheumatoid arthritis. J Consult Clin Psych. 1992;60(4):619–27.

11 Mitton DL, Treharne GJ, Hale ED, et al. The health and life experiences of mothers with rheumatoid arthritis: A phenomenological study. Musculoskelet Care. 2007 Sep 24; [Epub ahead of print]

12 Frohnauer A, Neff A, Knechtle B. Does running increase the risk of osteoarthritis? Schweiz Rundsch Med Prax. 2006 Aug 30;95(35):1305–16.

13 Eckstein F, Hudelmaier M, Putz R. The effects of exercise on human articular cartilage. J Anat. 2006 Apr;208(4):491–512.

14 Wilk KE, Briem K, Reinold MM, et al. Rehabilitation of articular lesions in the athlete's knee. J Orthop Sports Phys Ther. 2006 Oct;36(10):815–27.

15 Sowers MF, Yosef M, Jamadar D, et al. BMI vs body composition and radiographically defined osteoarthritis of the knee in women: a 4-year follow-up study. Osteoarth Cart. 2007 Sep 19; [Epub ahead of print]

16 Stenholm S, Sainio P, Rantanen T, et al. Effect of co-morbidity on the association of high body mass index with walking limitation among men and women aged 55 years and older. Aging Clin Exp Res. 2007 Aug;19(4):277–83.

17 Minor M. Physical activity and the management of arthritis. Ann Behav Med. 1991;13:117–24.

18 Simonsick E. Risk due to inactivity in physically capable older adults. American Journal of Public Health. 1993;83:1443–1450.

19 Mayoux Benhamou MA. Reconditioning in patients with rheumatoid arthritis. Ann Readapt Med Phys. 2007 Jul;50(6):382–5, 377–81.

20 Neuberger GB, Aaronson LS, Gajewski B, et al. Predictors of exercise and effects of exercise on symptoms, function, aerobic fitness, and disease outcomes of rheumatoid arthritis. Arthritis Rheum. 2007 Aug 15;57(6):943–52.

21 Lee MS, Pittler MH, Ernst E. Tai chi for rheumatoid arthritis: systematic review. Rheumatol (Oxford). 2007 Nov;46(11):1648–51.

22 Clark KL. Nutritional considerations in joint health. Clin Sports Med. 2007 Jan;26(1):101–18.

23 McAlindon TE, Biggee BA. Nutritional factors and osteoarthritis: recent developments. Curr Opin Rheumatol. 2005 Sep;17(5):647–52.

24 Berkow SE, Barnard N. Vegetarian diets and weight status. Nutr Rev. 2006 Apr;64(4):175–88.

25 Kjeldsen-Kragh J, Haugen M, Borchgrevink CF, et al. Controlled trial of fasting and one-year vegetarian diet in rheumatoid arthritis. Lancet 1991;338(8772):899–902.

26 Kjeldsen-Kragh J. Rheumatoid arthritis treated with vegetarian diets. Am J Clin Nutr 1999;70(suppl):594S–600S.

27 Ameye LG, Chee WS. Osteoarthritis and nutrition. From nutraceuticals to functional foods: a systematic review of the scientific evidence. Arth Res Ther. 2006;8(4):R127.

28 Lee S, Gura KM, Kim S, et al. Current clinical applications of omega-6 and omega-3 fatty acids. Nutr Clin Pract. 2006 Aug;21(4):323–41.

29 Goldberg RJ, Katz J. A meta-analysis of the analgesic effects of omega-3 polyunsaturated fatty acid supplementation for inflammatory joint pain. Pain. 2007 May;129(1–2):210–23.

30 Matsuzaki T, Takagi A, Ikemura H, et al. Intestinal microflora: probiotics and autoimmunity. J Nutr. 2007 Mar;137(3 Suppl 2):798S–802S.

31 McAlindon TE. Nutraceuticals: do they work and when should we use them? Best Pract Res Clin Rheumatol. 2006 Feb;20(1):99–115.

32 Machtey I, and Ouaknine L, "tocopherol in osteoarthristis: a controlled pilot study", J Am Geriat Soc, 1978, 26, pp328–30

33 Walker AF, Bundy R, Hicks SM, Middleton RW. Bromelain reduces mild acute knee pain and improves well-being in a dose-dependent fashion in an open study of otherwise healthy adults. Phytomed. 2002 Dec;9(8):681–6.

34 Kovalenko VN, Shuba NM, Golovatskiy IV, Bortkevich OP, Yasinskaya VA. Estimation of efficacy of basic therapy of rheumatoid arthritis on the basis of systemic enzyme therapy: results of five-year monitoring. Int J Immunother 2001;XVII (2/3/4):129–33.

35 Dunn JM, Wilkinson JM. Naturopathic management of rheumatoid arthritis. Mod Rheumatol 2005;15:87–90.

36 Zautra AJ, Hoffman JM, Matt KS, et al. An examination of individual differences in the relationship between interpersonal stress and disease activity among women with rheumatoid arthritis. Arth Care Res 1998;11:271–279.

37 Weigl M, Cieza A, Cantista P, et al. Determinants of disability in chronic musculoskeletal health conditions: a literature review. Eura Medicophys. 2007 Nov 9; [Epub ahead of print]

38 Klareskog L, Padyukov L, Rönnelid J, Alfredsson L. Genes, environment and immunity in the development of rheumatoid arthritis. Curr Opin Immunol. 2006 Dec;18(6):650–5.

Chapter 17: Mental health

1 Kirsch I, Moore TJ, Scoboria A, Nicholls SS (2002) The emperor's new drugs: An analysis of antidepressant medication data submitted to the U.S. Food and Drug Administration. Prev Treat 5 article 23. Available: http://journals.apa.org/prevention/volume5/pre0050023a.html.

2 Kirsch I, Deacon BJ, Huedo-Medina TB, Scoboria A, Moore TJ, et al. Initial Severity and Antidepressant Benefits: A Meta-Analysis of Data Submitted to the Food and Drug Administration PLoS Medicine 2008 Feb;5(2):e45 doi:10.1371/journal. pmed.0050045

3 Wilkinson G. Anxiety: recognition and treatment in general practice. Oxford: Radcliffe Medical Press, 1992.

4 Dantzer R. Somatization: a psychoneuroimmune perspective. Psychoneuroendocrinol. 2005;30(10):947–52.

5 Southwick SM, Vythilingam M, Charney DS. The psychobiology of depression and resilience to stress: implications for prevention and treatment. Annu Rev Clin Psychol. 2005;1:255–91.

6 Oei TP, Dingle G. The effectiveness of group cognitive behaviour therapy for unipolar depressive disorders. J Affect Disord. 2007 Aug 21; [Epub ahead of print]

7 Chu BC, Harrison TL. Disorder-specific Effects of CBT for Anxious and Depressed Youth: A Meta-analysis of Candidate Mediators of Change. Clin Child Fam Psychol Rev. 2007 Dec;10(4):352–372.

8 James A, Soler A, Weatherall R. Cognitive behavioural therapy for anxiety disorders in children and adolescents. Cochrane Database Syst Rev. 2005 Oct 19;(4):CD004690.

9 Kraus CA, Kunik ME, Stanley MA. Use of cognitive behavioral therapy in late-life psychiatric disorders. Geriatrics. 2007 Jun;62(6):21–6.

10 Waddell C, Hua JM, Garland OM, et al. Preventing mental disorders in children: a systematic review to inform policy-making. Can J Pub Health. 2007 May–Jun;98(3):166–73.

11 Doering LV, Cross R, Vredevoe D, et al. Infection, depression, and immunity in women after coronary artery bypass: a pilot study of cognitive behavioral therapy. Altern Ther Health Med. 2007 May–Jun;13(3):18–21.

12 Sjösten N, Kivelä SL. The effects of physical exercise on depressive symptoms among the aged: a systematic review. Int J Geriatr Psychiatry. 2006 May;21(5):410–8.

13 Byrne A, Byrne DG: The effect of exercise on depression, anxiety and other mood states: a review. J Psychosom Res 1993;13(3): 160–170.

14 Warburton DE, Nicol CW, Bredin SS. Health benefits of physical activity: the evidence. CMAJ. 2006 Mar 14;174(6):801–9.

15 Chaouloff F: Effects of acute physical exercise on central serotonergic systems. Med Sci Sports Exerc 1997; 29(1):58–62.

16 King AC, Oman RF, et al. Moderate-intensity exercise and self-rated quality of sleep in older adults. JAMA 1997;277(1):32–37.

17 Lombard CB. What is the role of food in preventing depression and improving mood, performance and cognitive function? Med J Aust. 2000 Nov 6;173 Suppl:S104-5.

18 Peet M. International variations in the outcome of schizophrenia and the prevalence of depression in relation to national dietary practices: an ecological analysis. Br J Psychiatry. 2004 May;184:404–8.

19 Ross BM, Seguin J, Sieswerda LE. Omega-3 fatty acids as treatments for mental illness: which disorder and which fatty acid? Lipids Health Dis. 2007 Sep 18;6(1):21.

20 Sanchez-Villegas A, Henriquez P, Figueiras A, et al. Long chain omega-3 fatty acids intake, fish consumption and mental disorders in the SUN cohort study. Eur J Nutr. 2007 Sep;46(6):337–46.

21 Parker G, Crawford J. Chocolate craving when depressed: a personality marker. Br J Psychiatry. 2007 Oct;191:351–2.

22 Hintikka J, Tolmunen T, Tanskanen A, Viinamäki H. High vitamin B12 level and good treatment outcome may be associated in major depressive disorder. BMC Psychi 2003,3:17.

23 Coppen, Alec, and Christina Bolander-Gouaille. Treatment of depression: time to consider folic acid and vitamin B12. J Psychopharmacol. 2005;19(1):59.

24 Taylor MJ, Carney SM, Goodwin GM, Geddes JR. Folate for depressive disorders: systematic review and meta-analysis of randomized controlled trials. J Psychopharm acol. 2004; 18: 251–256.

25 Bressa GM. S-adenosyl-1-methionine (SAMe) as antidepressant: meta-analysis of clinical studies. Acta Neurologica Scandinavica 1994; Suppl. 154: 7–14.

26 Hintikka J, Tolmunen T, Tanskanen A, Viinamäki H.
High vitamin B12 level and good treatment outcome

may be associated in major depressive disorder. BMC Psychi 2003,3:17.

27 Coppen, Alec, and Christina Bolander-Gouaille. Treatment of depression: time to consider folic acid and vitamin B12. J Psychopharmacol. 2005;19(1):59.

28 Birdsall T. 5-Hydroxytryptophan: A Clinically-Effective Serotonin Precursor. Alt Med Rev. Volume 3, Number 4 1998.

29 Beard JL, et al. Maternal Iron Deficiency Anaemia Affects Postpartum Emotions and Cognition. J Nutr. 135: 267–272, 2005.

30 Whalen DJ, Silk JS, Semel M, et al. Caffeine Consumption, Sleep, and Affect in the Natural Environments of Depressed Youth and Healthy Controls. J Pediatr Psychol. 2007 Oct 25; [Epub ahead of print]

31 Haraguchi H, Yoshida N, Ishikawa H, et al. Protection of mitochondrial functions against oxidative stresses by isofl avans from Glycyrrhiza glabra. J Pharm Pharmacol. 2000 Feb;52(2):219–23.

32 Ross BM, Seguin J, Sieswerda LE. Omega-3 fatty acids as treatments for mental illness: which disorder and which fatty acid? Lipids Health Dis. 2007 Sep 18;6(1):21.

33 Palatnik A, Frolov K, Fux M, Benjamin J. Double-blind, controlled, crossover trial of inositol versus fluvoxamine for the treatment of panic disorder. J Clin Psychopharmacol, 2001;21:335–9.

34 Saeed SA, Bloch RM, Antonacci DJ. Herbal and Dietary Supplements for Treatment of Anxiety Disorders. Am Fam Physician 2007;76:549–56.

35 McKay DL, Blumberg JB. A review of the bioactivity and potential health benefits of chamomile tea (Matricaria recutita L.). Phytother Res. 2006 Jul;20(7):519–30.

36 Liebert MA. A synergistic effect of a daily supplement for 1 month of 200 mg magnesium plus 50 mg Vitamin B6 for the relief of anxiety-related premenstrual symptoms: a randomized, double-blind, crossover study. J Wom Health Gender-Based Med. Volume 9, Number 2, 2000.

37 Carroll C, Ring M, Suter G, et al. The effects of an oral multivitamin combination with calcium, magnesium, and zinc on psychological well-being in healthy young male volunteers: a double-blind placebo-controlled trial, Psychopharmacol. (2000) 150:220–225.

38 Carroll C, Ring M, Suter G, et al. The effects of an oral multivitamin combination with calcium, magnesium, and zinc on psychological well-being in healthy young male volunteers: a double-blind placebo-controlled trial, Psychopharmacol. (2000) 150:220–225.

39 Cornelius MD, Goldschmidt L, DeGenna N, Day NL. Smoking during teenage pregnancies: effects on behavioral problems in offspring. Nicotine Tob Res. 2007 Jul;9(7):739–50.

40 Szyszkowicz M. Air pollution and emergency department visits for depression in edmonton, Canada. Int J Occup Med Environ Health.

2007;20(3):241–5.

41 Levitan RD. The chronobiology and neurobiology of winter seasonal affective disorder. Dialogues Clin Neurosci. 2007;9(3):315–24.

42 McGrath J, Selten JP, Chant D. Long-term trends in sunshine duration and its association with schizophrenia birth rates and age at first registration – data from Australia and the Netherlands. Schizophr Res. 2002 Apr 1;54(3):199–212.

Chapters 18: Brain health and dementia

1 Plassman BL, Langa KM, Fisher GG, et al. Prevalence of dementia in the United States: the aging, demographics, and memory study. Neuroepidemiol. 2007;29(1–2):125–32.

2 Hall CB, Derby C, LeValley A, et al. Education delays accelerated decline on a memory test in persons who develop dementia. Neurol. 2007 Oct 23;69(17):1657–64.

3 Ngandu T, von Strauss E, Helkala EL, et al. Education and dementia: what lies behind the association? Neurol. 2007 Oct 2;69(14):1442–50.

4 Kaduszkiewicz H. Zimmermann T. Beck-Bornholdt HP. et al. Cholinesterase inhibitors for patients with Alzheimer's disease: systematic review of randomised clinical trials. BMJ. 2005;331(7512):321–7.

5 Peters R. Ageing and the brain. Postgrad Med J. 2006;82(964):84–8.

6 Mattson MP, Duan W, Chan SL, et al. Neuroprotective and neurorestorative signal transduction mechanisms in brain aging: modification by genes, diet and behaviour. Neurobiol Aging 2002;23(5):695–705.

7 Morocz M, Kalman J, Juhasz A, et al. Elevated levels of oxidative DNA damage in lymphocytes from patients with Alzheimer's disease. Neurobiol Aging 2002;23(1):47–53.

8 Wilson RS, Evans DA, Bienias JL, Mendes de Leon CF, Schneider JA, Bennett DA. Proneness to psychological distress is associated with risk of Alzheimer's disease. Neurol. 2003;61(11):1479–85.

9 Draper B, MacCuspie-Moore C, Brodaty H. Suicidal ideation and the 'wish to die' in dementia patients: the role of depression. Age Ageing. 1998 Jul;27(4):503–7.

10 Paterniti S, Verdier-Taillefer MH, Dufouil C, Alperovitch A. Depressive symptoms and cognitive decline in elderly people. Longitudinal study. Br J Psychiatry. 2002 Nov;181:406–10.

11 Pomara N, Doraiswamy PM, Willoughby LM, et al. Elevation in plasma Abeta42 in geriatric depression: a pilot study. Neurochem Res. 2006 Mar;31(3):341–9. Epub 2006 Apr 1.

12 Pedersen WA, Wan R, Mattson MP. Impact of aging on stress-responsive neuroendocrine systems. Mech Ageing Dev. 2001;122(9):963–83.

13 Lindstrom HA, Fritsch T, Petot G, et al. The relationships between television viewing in midlife and the development of Alzheimer's disease in a case-control study. Brain Cogn. 2005 Jul;58(2):

157–65.

14 Friedland RP, Fritsch T, Smyth K, et al. Patients with Alzheimer's disease have reduced activities in midlife compared with healthy control-group members. Proceedings of the National Academy of Science USA, 10.1073/pnas.061002998

15 Scarmeas N, Levy G, Tang MX, et al. Influence of leisure activity on the incidence of Alzheimer's disease. Neurol. 2001;57(12):2236–42.

16 Simons LA, Simons J, McCallum J, et al. Lifestyle factors and risk of dementia: Dubbo Study of the elderly. Med J Aust. 2006 Jan 16;184(2):68–70.

17 Bernhardt T, Seidler A, Frolich L. The effect of psychosocial factors on risk of dementia. [Review] Fortschritte der Neurologie-Psychiatrie 2002;70(6):283–8.

18 Bernhardt TM, Seidler A, Frolich L. The effect of psychosocial factors on risk of dementia. [Review] Fortschritte der Neurologie-Psychiatrie 2002;70(6):283–8.

19 Fratiglioni L, Wang HX. Brain reserve hypothesis in dementia. J Alzheimers Dis. 2007 Aug;12(1):11–22.

20 Lindberg DA. Integrative review of research related to meditation, spirituality, and the elderly. Geriatr Nurs. 2005 Nov–Dec;26(6):372–7.

21 Spurlock WR. Spiritual well-being and caregiver burden in Alzheimer's caregivers. Geriatr Nurs. 2005 May–Jun;26(3):154–61.

22 Kaufman Y, Anaki D, Binns M, Freedman M. Cognitive decline in Alzheimer disease: Impact of spirituality, religiosity, and QOL. Neurology. 2007 May 1;68(18):1509–14.

23 MacKinlay EB, Trevitt C. Spiritual care and ageing in a secular society. Med J Aust. 2007 May 21;186 (10 Suppl):S74–6.

24 Kramer AF, Erickson KI, Colcombe SJ. Exercise, cognition, and the aging brain. J Appl Physiol. 2006 Oct;101(4):1237–42.

25 Wang L, Larson FB, Bowen JD, van Belle G. Performance-based physical function and future dementia in older people. Arch Int Med. 2006 May 22;166(10):1115-20.

26 Lautenschlager NT, Almeida OP. Physical activity and cognition in old age. Curr Opin Psychiatry. 2006 Mar;19(2):190–3.

27 Laurin D, Verreault R, Lindsay J, et al. Physical activity and risk of cognitive impairment and dementia in elderly persons. Arch Neurol. 2001;58(3):498–504.

28 Van de Winckel A, Feys H, De Weerdt W, Dom R. Cognitive and behavioural effects of music-based exercises in patients with dementia. Clin Rehabil. 2004;18(3):253–60.

29 Lautenschlager NT, Almeida OP. Physical activity and cognition in old age. Curr Opin Psychiatry. 2006 Mar;19(2):190–3.

30 Singh-Manoux A, Hillsdon M, Brunner E, Marmot M. Effects of Physical Activity on Cognitive Functioning in Middle Age: Evidence From the Whitehall II Prospective Cohort Study. Am J Public Health. 2005;95(12):2252–2258.

31 Mattson MP, Chan SL, Duan W. Modification of brain aging and neurodegenerative disorders by genes, diet and behaviour. Physiol Rev 2002;82(3):637–72.

32 Lau FC, Shukitt-Hale B, Joseph JA. Nutritional intervention in brain aging: reducing the effects of infl ammation and oxidative stress. Subcell Biochem. 2007;42:299–318.

33 Kalmijn S, van Boxtel MPJ, Ocké M. Dietary intake of fatty acids and fish in relation to cognitive performance at middle age. Neurol. 2004;62:275–280.

34 Lim WS, Gammack JK, Van Niekerk J, Dangour AD. Omega 3 fatty acid for the prevention of dementia. Cochrane Database Syst Rev. 2006;(1):CD005379.

35 Wolters M, Strohle A, Hahn A. Cobalamin: a critical vitamin in the elderly. Preventive Medicine 2004;39:1256–1266.

36 Kropiunigg U, Sebek K, Leonhardsberger A, et al. Psychosocial risk factors for Alzheimer's disease. Psychotherapie, Psychosomatik, Medizinische Psychologie 1999;49(5):153–9.

37 Helmer C, Damon D, Letenneur L, et al. Marital status and risk of Alzheimer's disease: a French population-based cohort study. Neurol. 1999;53(9):1953–8.

38 Brooker DJ, Woolley RJ. Enriching opportunities for people living with dementia: the development of a blueprint for a sustainable activity-based model. Aging Ment Health. 2007 Jul;11(4):371–83.

39 Tyas SL, Manfreda J, Strain LA, Montgomery PR. Risk factors for Alzheimer's disease: a population-based, longitudinal study in Manitoba, Canada. Int J Epidemiol. 2001 Jun;30(3):590–7.

40 Dosunmu R, Wu J, Basha MR, Zawia NH. Environ-mental and dietary risk factors in Alzheimer's disease. Expert Rev Neurother. 2007 Jul;7(7):887–900.

41 Monnet-Tschudi F, Zurich MG, Boschat C, et al. Involvement of environmental mercury and lead in the etiology of neurodegenerative diseases. Rev Environ Health. 2006 Apr–Jun;21(2):105–17.

Chapter 19: Healthy Immunity

1 Goriely S, Goldman M. From tolerance to autoimmunity: is there a risk in early life vaccination? J Comp Pathol. 2007 Jul;137 Suppl 1:S57–61.

2 Messina G, Lissoni P, Bartolacelli E, et al. A psychoncological study of lymphocyte subpopulations in relation to pleasure-related neurobiochemistry and sexual and spiritual profile to Rorschach's test in early or advanced cancer patients. J Biol Regul Homeost Agents. 2003 Oct–Dec;17(4):322–6.

3 Sephton SE, Koopman C, Schaal M, et al. Spiritual expression and immune status in women with metastatic breast cancer: an exploratory study. Breast J. 2001 Sep–Oct;7(5):345–53.

4 Folkman S, Chesney MA, Cooke M, et al. Caregiver burden in HIV-positive and HIV-negative partners of men with AIDS. J Consult Clin Psychol. 1994 Aug;62(4):746–56.

5 Timmons BW. Paediatric exercise immunology:

health and clinical applications. Exerc Immunol Rev. 2005;11:108–44.

6 Phillips AC, Burns VE, Lord JM. Stress and exercise: Getting the balance right for aging immunity. Exerc Sport Sci Rev. 2007 Jan;35(1):35–9.

7 Chin A Paw MJ, de Jong N, et al. Immunity in frail elderly: a randomized controlled trial of exercise and enriched foods. Med Sci Sports Exerc. 2000 Dec;32(12):2005–11.

8 Woods JA, Vieira VJ, Keylock KT. Exercise, inflammation, and innate immunity. Neurol Clin. 2006 Aug;24(3):585–99.

9 Nixon S, O'Brien K, Glazier RH, Tynan AM. Aerobic exercise interventions for adults living with HIV/AIDS. Cochrane Database Syst Rev. 2005 Apr 18;(2):CD001796.

10 Gleeson M. Immune system adaptation in elite athletes. Curr Opin Clin Nutr Metab Care. 2006 Nov;9(6):659–65.

11 Chandra RK. Nutrition and the immune system: an introduction, Am J Nut. 1997:66:460S–3S.

12 Walker WA. Role of nutrients and bacterial colonization in the development of intestinal host defense. J Ped Gastroent Nut. 2000;30(2):S2–S7.

13 Sanchez A, et al. Role of sugars in human neutrophillic phagocytosis, Am J Clin Nutr, 1973;26(1):180–4.

14 Ishikawa H, Saeki T, Otani T, et al. Aged garlic extract prevents a decline of NK cell number and activity in patients with advanced cancer. J Nutr. 2006 Mar;136(3 Suppl):816S– 820S.

15 Webb AL, Villamor E. Update: effects of antioxidant and non-antioxidant vitamin supplementation on immune function. Nutr Rev. 2007 May;65(5):181–217.

16 Wintergerst ES, Maggini S, Hornig DH. Contribution of selected vitamins and trace elements to immune function. Ann Nutr Metab. 2007;51(4):301–23.

17 Borchers AT, Stern JS, Hackman RM, et al. Mushrooms, tumors and immunity. Proc Soc Exp Biol Med 1999;221:281–293.

18 Chandra RK. Nutrition and the immune system: an introduction, Am J Clinical Nutrition 1997:66:460S–3S.

19 Scrimshaw NS, SanGiovanni JP. Synergism of nutrition, infection, and immunity: an overview. Am J Clin Nutr. 1997 Aug;66(2):464S–477S.

20 Chandra RK, et al. Iron status: immunocompetence and susceptibility to infection. In Jacob A (ed) Ciba Foundation symplasium on iron metabolism. Amsterdam: Elsevier, I 977:249-68.

21 Bourlioux P, Pochart P. Nutritional and health properties of yogurt, World Rev Nutr Diet 1988;56:217–58.

22 Roller M, Clune Y, Collins K, et al. Consumption of prebiotic inulin enriched with oligofructose in combination with the probiotics Lactobacillus rhamnosus and Bifidobacterium lactis has minor effects on selected immune parameters in polypectomised and colon cancer patients. Br J Nutr.

2007 Apr;97(4):676–84.

23 Guandalini S. The influence of gluten: weaning recommendations for healthy children and children at risk for celiac disease. Nestle Nutr Workshop Ser Pediatr Program. 2007;60:139–51; discussion 151–5.

24 Knip M, Akerblom HK. Early nutrition and later diabetes risk. Adv Exp Med Biol. 2005;569:142–50.

25 Subramanian S, Campbell BJ, Rhodes JM. Bacteria in the pathogenesis of inflammatory bowel disease. Curr Opin Infect Dis. 2006 Oct;19(5):475–84.

26 Matsuzaki T, Takagi A, Ikemura H, et al. Intestinal microflora: probiotics and autoimmunity. J Nutr. 2007 Mar;137(3 Suppl 2):798S–802S.

27 Shanahan F. Probiotics in inflammatory bowel disease – therapeutic rationale and role. Adv Drug Del Rev 56 (2004) 809–818*.

28 Ferguson LR, Shelling AN, Browning BL, et al. Genes, diet and inflammatory bowel disease. Mutat Res. 2007 Sep 1;622(1–2):70–83.

29 Trebble TM, Arden NK, Wootton SA, et al. Fish oil and antioxidants alter the composition and function of circulating mononuclear cells in Crohn disease, Am J Clin Nutr 2004;80:1137–44.

30 Mahmud N, Weir DG. The urban diet and Crohn's disease: is there a relationship? Eur J Gastroenterol Hepatol 2001;13(2):93–95.

31 Shoda R, Matsueda K, Yamato S, et al. Epidemiologic analysis of Crohns disease in Japan: increased dietary intake of nK6 polyunsaturated fatty acids and animal protein relates to the increased incidence of Crohns disease in Japan. Am J Clin Nutr 1996;63(5):741–745.

32 Russel M, Engels L, Muris J, et al. Modern life in the epidemiology of infl ammatory bowel disease: a case control study with special emphasis on nutritional factors. Eur J Gastroenterol Hepatol 1998;10(3): 235–237.

33 Persson P, Ahlbom A & Hellers G. Diet and inflammatory bowel disease: a case-control study, Epidemiology 1992;3(1):47–52.

34 Sonnenberg A. Geographic and temporal variations of sugar and margarine consumption in relation to Crohn's disease. Digestion 1988;41(3):161–171.

35 Mishkin B, Mishkin S. Dietary fads and gut mysteries versus nutrition with a grain of common sense. Can J Gastroenterol 1997;11(4):371–375.

36 Fukuda M, Kanauchi O, Araki Y, et al. Prebiotic treatment of experimental colitis with germinated barley foodstuff: a comparison with probiotic or antibiotic treatment. International Journal of Molecular Medicine 2002;9:65–70.

37 Bengmark S. Bioecological control of inflammatory bowel disease, Clinical Nutrition 2007;26:169–181.

38 Margherita T, Cantorna, Vitamin D and its role in immunology: Multiple sclerosis,and inflammatory bowel disease, Progress in Biophysics and Molecular Biology 92 (2006) 60–64

39 Gasche C, Lomer MC, Cavill I, Weiss G. Iron, anaemia, and inflammatory bowel diseases. Gut 2004;53:1190–7.

40 Razack R, Seidner DL. Nutrition in inflammatory bowel disease. Curr Opin Gastroenterol. 2007 Jul;23(4):400–5.

41 Noverr MC, Huffnagle GB. The 'microflora hypothesis' of allergic diseases. Clin Exp Allergy. 2005 Dec;35(12):1511–20.

42 Schoetzau A, Filipiak-Pittroff B, Franke K, et al. Effect of exclusive breast-feeding and early solid food avoidance on the incidence of atopic dermatitis in high-risk infants at 1 year of age. Pediatr Allergy Immunol 2002;13:234–42.

43 Halken S. Prevention of allergic disease in childhood: clinical and epidemiological aspects of primary and secondary allergy prevention, Pediatr Allergy Immunol 2004:15(Suppl. 16):9–32.

44 Hodge L, Salome CM, Woolcock AJ. Factors associated with bronchial hyper-responsiveness in Australian adults and children. Eur Respir J 1992:5:921–9.

45 Pistelli R, Forastiere F, Corbo GM, et al. Respiratory symptoms and bronchial responsiveness are related to dietary salt intake and urinary potassium excretion in male children. Eur Respir J 1993:6: 517–22.

46 Soutar A, Seaton A, Brown K. Bronchial reactivity and dietary antioxidants. Thorax 1997:52:166–70.

47 Marko Kalliomaki; Seppo Salminen; Tuija Poussa; Heikki Arvilommi; Erika Isolauri, Probiotics and prevention of atopic disease: 4-year follow-up of a randomised.The Lancet; May 31, 2003; 361, 9372; Health Module, pg. 1869

48 Wassenberg J, Ciuffreda D, Bart PA, et al. Modern nutrition and development of new allergies. Rev Med Suisse. 2007 Apr 25;3(108):1032–4, 1036–7.

49 Cohen S, Doyle WJ, Turner R, et al. Sociability and susceptibility to the common cold. Psychol Sci. 2003 Sep;14(5):389–95.

50 Schleifer SJ, Keller SE, Camerino M, et al. Suppression of lymphocyte stimulation following bereavement. JAMA. 1983 Jul 15;250(3):374–7.

51 Kiecolt-Glaser JK, Fisher LD, Ogrocki P, et al. Marital quality, marital disruption, and immune function. Psychosom Med. 1987 Jan–Feb;49(1): 13–34.

52 Gao L, Tsai YJ, Grigoryev DN, Barnes KC. Host defense genes in asthma and sepsis and the role of the environment. Curr Opin Allergy Clin Immunol. 2007 Dec;7(6):459–67.

Chapter 20: Chronic fatigue

1 Crawley E, Smith GD. Is chronic fatigue syndrome (CFS/ME) heritable in children, and if so, why does it matter? Archives of Disease in Childhood 2007;92:1058–1061.

2 Working Group of the Royal Australasian College of Physicians. Chronic fatigue syndrome. Clinical practice guidelines–2002. Med J Aust. 2002 May 6; 176 Suppl:S23–56.

3 Ibid.

4 Wyller VB. The chronic fatigue syndrome–an update. Acta Neurol Scand Suppl. 2007;187:7–14.

5 Kato K, Sullivan PF, Evengård B, Pedersen NL. Premorbid predictors of chronic fatigue. Arch Gen Psychiatry. 2006 Nov;63(11):1267–72.

6 Sharpe M, Hawton K, Simkin S, et al. Cognitive behaviour therapy for the chronic fatigue syndrome: a randomised controlled trial. BMJ 1996; 312:22–26.

7 Sharpe M. Cognitive behaviour therapy for chronic fatigue syndrome: efficacy and implications. Am J Med 1998; 105: 104S–109S.

8 Cho HJ, Hotopf M, Wessely S. The placebo response in the treatment of chronic fatigue syndrome: a systematic review and meta-analysis. Psychosom Med. 2005 Mar–Apr;67(2):301–13.

9 Wallman KE, Morton AR, Goodman C, et al. Randomised controlled trial of graded exercise in chronic fatigue syndrome. Med J Aust. 2004 May 3;180(9):444–8.

10 Logan AC, Wong C. Chronic Fatigue Syndrome: Oxidative stress and dietary Modifications. Alt Med Rev. 2001;6(5):450–9.

11 Jenkins M, Rayman M. Nutrient intake is unrelated to nutrient status in patients with chronic fatigue syndrome. J Nut Enviro Med 2005;15(4):177–189.

12 Lundell K, Qazi S, Eddy L, Uckun FM. Clinical activity of folinic acid in patients with chronic fatigue syndrome, Arzneimittelforschung 2006:56:399–404

13 Puri BK, Holmes J, Hamilton G. Eicosapentaenoic acid-rich essential fatty acid supplementation in chronic fatigue syndrome associated with symptom remission and structural brain changes. Int J Clin Pract 2004;58(3):297–299.

14 Teitelbaum JE, Johnson C, St Cyr J. The use of D-ribose in chronic fatigue syndrome and fibromyalgia: a pilot study. J Altern Complement Med. 2006 Nov;12(9):857–62.

Chapter 21: Genetics

1 Levine A. The tumour suppressor genes. Ann Rev Biochem. 1993;62:623–51.

2 Interview, cited in Micho Kaku, Visions: How Science Will Revolutionise the 21st Century, 1997.

3 Gidron Y, Russ K, Tissarchondou H, Warner J. The relation between psychological factors and DNA-damage: a critical review. Biol Psychol. 2006 Jun;72(3):291–304.

4 Adachi S, Kawamura K, Takemoto K. Oxidative damage of nuclear DNA in liver of rats exposed to psychological stress. Cancer Res. 1993;53(18):4153–5.

5 Fischman H, Pero R, Kelly D. Psychogenic stress induces chromosomal and DNA damage. Int J Neurosci. 1996;84 (1–4):219–27.

6 Cohen L, Marshall G, Cheng L, et al. DNA repair capacity in healthy medical students during and after exam stress. J Beh Med 2000;23(6):531–45.

7 Ramos JM, Ruiz A, Colen R, et al. DNA repair and breast carcinoma susceptibility in women. Cancer. 2004;100(7):1352-7.

8 Kiecolt-Glaser J, Glaser R. Psychoneuroimmunology and immunotoxicology: implications for

carcinogenesis. Psychosom Med. 1999;61(3):271–2.

9 McEwen BS. Protective and damaging effects of stress mediators: central role of the brain. Dialogues Clin Neurosci. 2006;8(4):367–81.

10 Banerjee B, Vadiraj HS, Ram A, et al. Effects of an integrated yoga program in modulating psychological stress and radiation-induced genotoxic stress in breast cancer patients undergoing radiotherapy. Integr Cancer Ther. 2007 Sep;6(3):242–50.

11 Self D, Nestler E. Relapse to drug seeking: neural and molecular mechanisms. Drug Alc Dep. 998;51 (1–2):49–60.

12 Cui Y, Gutstein W, Jabr S, et al. Control of human vascular smooth muscle cell proliferation by sera derived from 'experimentally stressed' individuals. Oncol Rep. 1998;5(6):1471–4.

13 Lopez J, Chalmers D, Little K, et al. Regulation of serotonin 1A, glucocorticoid, and mineralocorticoid receptor in rat and human hippocampus: implications for the neurobiology of depression. Biolog Psychi. 1998;43(8):547–73.

14 Benes F. The role of stress and dopamine-GABA interactions in the vulnerability for schizophrenia. J Psychi Res. 1997;31(2):257–75.

15 Mrazek DA, Klinnert M, Mrazek PJ, Brower A, McCormick D, Rubin B, Ikle D, Kastner W, Larsen G, Harbeck R, Jones J. Prediction of early-onset asthma in genetically at-risk children. Pediatr Pulmonol. 1999;27(2):85–94.

16 Szyf M, Weaver I, Meaney M. Maternal care, the epigenome and phenotypic differences in behavior. Reprod Toxicol. 2007 Jul;24(1):9–19.

17 Duric V, McCarson KE. Persistent pain produces stress-like alterations in hippocampal neurogenesis and gene expression. J Pain. 2006;7(8):544–55.

18 Epel ES, Blackburn EH, Lin J, et al. Accelerated telomere shortening in response to life stress. Proc Natl Acad Sci U S A. 2004 Dec 7;101(49):17312–5.

19 Simon NM, Smoller JW, McNamara KL, et al. Telomere shortening and mood disorders: preliminary support for a chronic stress model of accelerated aging. Biol Psychi. 2006 Sep 1;60(5):432–5.

20 Epel ES, Lin J, Wilhelm FH, et al. Cell aging in relation to stress arousal and cardiovascular disease risk factors. Psychoneuroendocrinol. 2006;31(3):277–87.

21 Li QZ, Li P, Garcia GE, et al. Genomic profiling of neutrophil transcripts in Asian Qigong practitioners: a pilot study in gene regulation by mind-body interaction. J Altern Complement Med. 2005 Feb;11(1):29–39.

22 Kendler KS, Liu XQ, Gardner CO, et al. Dimensions of religiosity and their relationship to lifetime psychiatric and substance use disorders. Am J Psychiatry. 2003 Mar;160(3):496–503.

23 Timberlake DS, Rhee SH, Haberstick BC, et al. The moderating effects of religiosity on the genetic and environmental determinants of smoking initiation. Nicotine Tob Res. 2006 Feb;8(1):123–33.

24 Radak Z, Chung HY, Goto S. Exercise and hormesis: oxidative stress-related adaptation for successful aging. Biogerontol. 2005;6(1):71–5.

25 Kritchevsky D. Caloric restriction and experimental carcinogenesis. Hybrid Hybridomics. 2002 Apr;21(2):147–51.

26 Pittaluga M, Parisi P, Sabatini S, et al. Cellular and biochemical parameters of exercise-induced oxidative stress: relationship with training levels. Free Radic Res. 2006 Jun;40(6):607–14.

27 Radák Z, Apor P, Pucsok J, et al. Marathon running alters the DNA base excision repair in human skeletal muscle. Life Sci. 2003 Feb 21;72(14):1627–33.

28 Tsai K, Hsu TG, Hsu KM, et al. Oxidative DNA damage in human peripheral leukocytes induced by massive aerobic exercise. Free Radic Biol Med. 2001 Dec 1;31(11):1465–72.

29 Mathers JC, Coxhead JM, Tyson J. Nutrition and DNA repair–potential molecular mechanisms of action. Curr Cancer Drug Targets. 2007 Aug;7(5):425–31.

30 Mathers JC. Nutritional modulation of ageing: genomic and epigenetic approaches. Mech Ageing Dev. 2006 Jun;127(6):584–9.

31 Kritchevsky D. Caloric restriction and cancer. J Nutr Sci Vitaminol (Tokyo). 2001 Feb;47(1):13–9.

32 Kritchevsky D. Caloric restriction and cancer. J Nutr Sci Vitaminol (Tokyo). 2001 Feb;47(1):13–9.

33 Kritchevsky D. Caloric restriction and experimental carcinogenesis. Toxicol Sci. 1999 Dec;52(2 Suppl):13-6.

34 Miller M. Can reducing caloric intake also help reduce cancer? J Natl Cancer Inst. 1998 Dec 2;90(23):1766-7.

35 Gonzalez, C, Najera, O, Cortes, E, et al. Hydrogen peroxide-induced DNA damage and DNA repair in lymphocytes from malnourished children. Enviro Molec Mutagen. 2002;39:33–42.

36 Wei Q, Shen H, Wang LE, et al. Association between low dietary folate intake and suboptimal cellular DNA repair capacity. Cancer Epidemiol Biomarkers Prev. 2003 Oct;12(10):963–9.

37 Sheng Y, Pero RW, Olsson AR, et al. DNA repair enhancement by a combined supplement of carotenoids, nicotinamide, and zinc. Cancer Detec Prev. 1998;22:284–292.

38 Tomasetti M, Alleva R, Borghi B, Collins AR. In vivo supplementation with coenzyme Q10 enhances the recovery of human lymphocytes from oxidative DNA damage. FASEB J. 2001;15:1425–1427.

39 Astley SB, Elliott RM, Archer DB, et al. Evidence that dietary supplementation with carotenoids and carotenoid-rich foods modulates the DNA damage: repair balance in human lymphocytes. B J Nurt. 2004;91:63–72.

40 Machowetz A, Poulsen HE, Gruendel S, et al. Effect of olive oils on biomarkers of oxidative DNA stress in Northern and Southern Europeans. FASEB J. 2007 Jan;21(1):45–52.

41 Yonezawa Y, Hada T, Uryu K, et al. Mechanism of cell cycle arrest and apoptosis induction by conjugated eicosapentaenoic acid, which is a mammalian DNA polymerase and topoisomerase inhibitor. Int J Oncol.

2007 May;30(5):1197–204

42 Self D, Nestler E. Relapse to drug seeking: neural and molecular mechanisms. Drug Alc Dep. 1998;51(1–2):49–60.

43 Howes OD, McDonald C, Cannon M, et al. Pathways to schizophrenia: the impact of environmental factors. Int J Neuropsychopharmacol. 2004;7 Suppl 1:S7–S13.

44 Moskvina V, Farmer A, Swainson V, et al. Interrelationship of childhood trauma, neuroticism, and depressive phenotype. Depress Anxiety. 2006 Aug 9; [Epub ahead of print]

45 Meaney MJ, Szyf M. Maternal care as a model for experience-dependent chromatin plasticity? Trends Neurosci. 2005;28(9):456–63.

46 van Dellen A, Blakemore C, Deacon R, et al. Delaying the onset of Huntington's in mice. Nature. 2000;404(6779):721–2.

Appendix 1

1. Wilson DMC, Ciliska D. Lifestyle assessment: part 1: development and use of the FANTASTIC checklist. Can Fam Physician 1984;30:1527–32. Wilson DMC, Nielsen E, Ciliska D. Lifestyle assessment: testing the FANTASTIC instrument. Can Fam Physician 1984;30:1863-6.

Index

cancer, 152–3, 229
diabetes, 154, 241
health promotion, 165
heart disease, 152, 202
immunity, 317
melatonin, 79, 229, 247
mental health, 153, 298
multiple sclerosis, 154, 246–8
psoriasis, 153
schizophrenia, 153, 298
Seasonal Affective Disorder, 79, 153, 298
UV radiation, 151, 229
vitamin D, 115, 151–4, 246–8, 282
super foods, 223–6, 323
sympathetic nervous system (SNS), 21, 23, 45, 191, 244, 252
syphilis, 300

tai chi, 101, 279, 289
T-cells, 308
tea, 222, 240, 257, 294
chamomile, 296
decaffeinated, 294
green tea, 225, 271, 331
telomerase, 329
telomeres, 329
testosterone, 24, 260, 266
thermal effect of food (TEF), 96
thyroid problems
chronic fatigue syndrome cause, 319
dementia, 301
relaxation reducing, 48
tiredness, 191
tiredness, 191
insulin and, 232
sleep problems see sleep
vital exhaustion, 191
TNF-alpha, 215
tomatoes, 224, 271
Transcendental Meditation, 50, 52, 194
transient ischaemic attack (TIA), 188
tryptophan, 255–6
turmeric, 226, 272

ulcerative colitis, 315
unemployment, 43, 192, 296
urinary tract infection, 38, 301

vaccinations, 310
vascular dementia, 300
vascular endothelial growth factor (VEGF), 217, 218
vegetables see fruit and vegetables
vegetarian diet, 126

VicHealth, 3, 165, 352
vital exhaustion, 191
vitamins
B group, 114, 126, 258, 293, 296, 305, 313, 315
recommended daily intake (RDI), 113–15
supplements, 257–8
vitamin A, 113, 114, 313
vitamin C, 112, 115, 257, 272, 281, 294, 313
vitamin D, 113, 115, 151–4, 202, 229, 241, 246–8, 281, 282, 313, 315
vitamin E, 112, 115, 200, 257, 272, 305, 313
vitamin K, 115

water
environment, 145–6
intake, 111–12
pollution, 146
weight, 95–7
basal metabolic rate (BMR), 95, 96
body mass index (BMI), 94–5
cancer prevention, 209
immunity and, 313
management see weight management
overweight see obesity and overweight
thermal effect of food (TEF), 96
weight management, 125–8
achievable goals, 127
body image, 128
calorie restriction, 125
diabetes, 237
exercise, 128
non-hungry eating, 127
positive attitude towards food, 127
6 steps, 126–8
slowing down, 128
special diets, 126
white blood cells, 34, 35, 308–9
B-cells, 308
immuno-suppression, 36, 309
lifestyle affecting, 43
low count, 34
lymphocytes, 308
NK cells, 35, 43, 212, 308, 311
self/non-self discrimination, 36, 309
spirituality, 311
T-cells, 308
whole foods, 121
workplace stress, 44–7
associated problems, 44
burnout, 40, 42, 45
cardiovascular disease risk, 45, 189,